Medical Terminology

A Text/Workbook

Fourth Edition

Alice V. Prendergast, RN, BSN, MA

Frances L. Fulton, RN, BS, MS, CAS, CASE

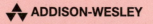 **ADDISON-WESLEY**

An Imprint of Addison Wesley Longman, Inc.

Menlo Park, California • Reading, Massachusetts • New York • Harlow, England
Don Mills, Ontario • Sydney • Mexico City • Madrid • Amsterdam

Medical Terminology
A Text/Workbook

Fourth Edition

Alice V. Prendergast, RN, BSN, MA

Frances L. Fulton, RN, BA, MF, CAS, CASE

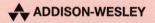
ADDISON-WESLEY

An Imprint of Addison Wesley Longman, Inc.

Menlo Park, California • Reading, Massachusetts • New York • Harlow, England
Don Mills, Ontario • Sydney • Mexico City • Madrid • Amsterdam

Senior Editor	Erin M. Mulligan
Editorial Assistant	Kim Crowder
Managing Editor	Wendy Earl
Production Editor	Michele Mangelli
Text Designer	Vargas/Williams/Design
Cover Designer	Yvo Riezebos Design
Manufacturing Supervisor	Merry Free Osborn

Care has been taken to confirm the accuracy of information presented in this book. The authors, editors, and publisher, however, cannot accept any responsibility for errors or omissions or for the consequences from application of the information in this book and make no warranty, express or implied, with respect to its contents.

The authors and publisher have exerted every effort to ensure that drug selections and dosages set forth in this text are in accord with current recommendation and practice at time of publication. However, in view of ongoing research, changes in government regulations, and the constant flow of information relating to drug therapy and drug reactions, the reader is urged to check the package inserts of all drugs for any changes in indications of dosage and for added warnings and precautions. This is particularly important when the recommended agent is a new and/or infrequently employed drug.

Cover image: © Copyright 1996. CIBA-GEIGY Corporation. Reprinted with permission from the Clinical Symposia, illustrated by Frank Netter, M.D. All rights reserved.

Library of Congress Cataloging-in-Publication Data

Prendergast, Alice, 1914–
    Medical terminology: a text/workbook/Alice V. Prendergast,
Frances L. Fulton.--4th ed.
        p. cm.
    Includes bibliographical references and index.
    ISBN 0-8053-9368-4
    1. Medicine--Terminology--Examinations, questions, etc.
I. Fulton, Frances L.   II. Title.
R123.P72   1996
610'.14--DC20   96-35083
                                                          CIP

ISBN 0-8053-9368-4

    3 4 5 6 7 8 9 10-CRK-00 99 98

Addison Wesley Longman, Inc.
2725 Sand Hill Road
Menlo Park, California 94025

Preface

Audience

Medical Terminology: A Text/Workbook was originally written to accompany a one-semester allied health course for students in medical reception, medical secretarial, medical records, medical transcription, medical assisting, emergency medical technology, and unit clerking. Nursing programs at all levels have found this book to be a valuable supplement to the basic curriculum for their students, and other allied health professions discovered that their students also benefited from a directed, focused approach to learning medical terminology. This fourth edition is suitable for students of occupational therapy, physical therapy, radiology technology, laboratory technology, chiropractic studies, veterinary science, and similar professions.

As health-related issues become increasingly important in all areas of our lives, many industries have also realized that their personnel need a solid grounding in medical terminology. This text can meet the needs of insurance adjusters, court reporters, paralegals, attorneys, legal secretaries, pharmaceutical company employees, and insurance secretaries. And finally, individuals who are interested in knowing more about their own conditions and prescriptions will find this book of great value.

Goals of the Text

When the first edition of *Medical Terminology* was published in 1977, the original author, Alice Prendergast, had been teaching the subject for six years and had used all of the popular texts then available. Although some were excellent books, none proved satisfactory because they simply offered too much material to cover in a one-semester course. They included more than most students in the allied health fields needed or could reasonably assimilate in a short course; the result was discouragement. As we began to revise the current edition, we found that few books address students' needs in a succinct manner. *Medical Terminology* continues to be the exception.

Instead of presenting an exhaustive list of every known medical word and forcing the students to try to memorize what is in essence a dictionary, this text was designed to help the student learn the basic construction of medical words. Our workbook format makes it easy to learn the basics of terminology by providing immediate learning reinforcement. Through constant practice, repetition, and simplified explanations, the student can acquire a solid foundation that not only aids retention of the vocabulary learned in this text, but also facilitates understanding new vocabulary encountered in subsequent course work, as well as a myriad of professional employment environments.

The text accomplishes these goals by assuming no extensive knowledge of anatomy and physiology or any other previous learning that does not occur naturally in the course of daily living. Therefore, it is an ideal foundation reference text for all allied health majors, especially students from foreign countries and students returning to school after a prolonged period away. The book offers concrete learning activities in the form of worksheets and self-tests, with answers provided to allow immediate feedback and progress evaluation.

In the fourth edition, the new coauthor, Frances Fulton, focused on maintaining the integrity of the original text and incorporating the useful suggestions of the many reviewers who have used the text for a number of years. She also expanded and updated the text to reflect current medical information. Drawing on her background in nursing, teaching, and graduate studies in education, she addressed the learning needs of a varied student population. Pronunciations were added for auditory learners. A new color and new figures were added for visual learners. Health Promotion Tips in Part 2 address each body system in terms of the reader's own health.

New to the Fourth Edition

Medical Terminology includes updated information, features, and format, while maintaining the hallmark features that students and instructors consistently praise. New features include:

■ **Updated content**

All chapters have been reviewed and updated to ensure students are exposed to the latest in terminology.

■ **Pronunciations**

Pronunciations have been added throughout the workbook to all medical terms that may be difficult to pronounce.

■ **Two-color design**

A second color has been incorporated in order to highlight certain features and help visual learners and others navigate through the text.

■ **More student review exercises**

Five Check Your Progress sections that correspond with review tests have been added throughout the text.

■ **Streamlined organization**

In Part 1, covering basic terminology and word structure, Chapters 6, 7, and 8 have been reorganized in a more logical, easier to use manner. Part 2, focusing on body systems, has been fine-tuned so that each chapter is consistent and well organized. The Reproductive System chapter of the third edition is now separated into two chapters, Chapters 22 and 23, that address the male and female reproductive systems as well as specific new information on genetics, obstetrics, neonatology, and sexually transmitted diseases. The information on the endocrine system and psychiatric terms has been expanded as well.

■ **Health Promotion Tips**

The chapters in Part 2 of the text contain the new feature Health Promotion Tips, which gives important advice to readers on how to stay healthy.

■ **Veterinary terms**

Finally, a useful listing of veterinary terms has been included inside the back cover.

Hallmark Features

■ **Tests**

A feature unique to our book is the inclusion of actual tests in the text. Instructors, of course, may wish to use their own or combine theirs with the ones given, to suit individual needs. More tests are provided than are needed; some may be used as additional exercises. By studying actual tests, students can better learn all the information and succeed in the course. For Part 2 chapters on body systems, an alternate test is also provided. Many tests include dictation for spelling.

■ **Pronunciation**

In the fourth edition, new terms are shown either with their pronunciation or with the stressed syllable in boldface type. Thus students can learn how to say terms at the same time they learn to recognize and spell them. A key to pronunciation is inside the front cover. It should be remembered that pronunciation may vary somewhat in different settings and in different parts of the country, and many words can be pronounced in more than one way.

■ **Case Histories**

There are sample case histories in each body system chapter. As in actual medical practice, these are not consistent in form. Some use abbreviations for headings, laboratory data, and other information, and others spell them out. These inconsistencies have been retained purposely so that the student can see how actual reports vary in form, completeness, and clarity.

■ **Illustrations**

As in the previous editions, the illustrations are ones that are not readily found in every text. They are generally simple and straightforward in order to give students the clearest possible example of what is being discussed. Illustration plates of excellent quality can be found in most medical dictionaries and are not included here. New illustrations have been included in this fourth edition to further illustrate important terms.

■ **Glossary/Index**

The index is also a glossary—a quick reference with a simplified definition of the term—along with the page number if needed. This feature makes the book even more convenient to use.

Coverage and Organization

Part 1 contains 14 chapters on terminology, in which word parts, prefixes, suffixes, and root words are introduced in a logical manner. Some important medical words that are not composed of these common parts are also included. Two comprehensive chapters on abbreviations and laboratory terms are followed by a brief introduction to medications and using the *Physicians' Desk Reference*.

Part 2 contains 12 chapters focusing on body systems. Each chapter opens with the function of that particular system, offers a brief outline of anatomy and physiology, and then moves into the system's pathophysiology. The pathophysiology section includes terms describing diseases and disorders and related surgical, diagnostic, and treatment terms followed by pertinent abbreviations.

Semester Syllabus

The sequence in which the book is studied can be altered by the instructor as desired. The instructor may choose to follow the book sequentially chapter by chapter. Another method would be to pair one or two chapters from Part 1 with a chapter from Part 2. For example, Chapters 1 and 2 can be used with 15, Chapter 3 with 16, and so on, with a total of two or three chapters assigned at one time. This is feasible for a class that meets once a week for three hours. Classes that meet for shorter periods two to three times per week may set up a different structure for assignments.

Students will find that besides its value as a text/workbook *Medical Terminology* will be a useful reference book after the course has been completed.

Course Objectives

At the completion of this course, the student will be able to:

- Analyze numerous medical terms and have a solid base on which to build a larger vocabulary.
- Spell medical terms correctly.
- Recognize medical terms in dictation and understand the context in which that word will be applied.
- Identify normal and abnormal functions of the human body and understand what medical terms mean in specific contexts and which terms are appropriate in professional practice.
- Enjoy working within a health-related field due to increased understanding of medical terminology.

Acknowledgments

We wish to express our gratitude to all Addison Wesley Longman personnel who were instrumental in the publishing of this book, with special thanks to Erin Mulligan, Kim Crowder, and Michele Mangelli.

Our thanks are also extended to the instructors who reviewed the manuscript and offered suggestions for improvement: Lucinda Campbell, West Virginia Career College; Sue Christensen, Rock Valley College; Melisse Gross, Langley College; Pat Hassel, De Anza College; Patti F. Nicks, Angelina College; and Karen Tilly, Rock Valley College. Appreciation is extended to those people who gave permission for the use of illustrations and other materials.

Our family, friends, and teachers are greatly appreciated for their continual love and support throughout this endeavor. Frances Fulton dedicates her work to Eme Fulton-Kemp, Lee Kemp, and Read Fulton with love.

Throughout our teaching careers we have found our students to be a great motivating factor. Their enthusiasm and questions inspired us to continue learning.

Alice V. Prendergast

Frances L. Fulton

Instructions for Workbook Use

Welcome to *Medical Terminology: A Text/Workbook,* Fourth Edition. To help you get the most out of this innovative text, the authors offer the following advice based on their years of teaching.

Concentrate on one chapter at a time; your instructor may wish to go over new words in class, pronouncing the words so you will become familiar with their sound. As you use this book:

1. Be sure you have mastered each chapter before going on to the next, regardless of the order in which they are presented.

2. Practice saying each word out loud.

3. Memorize all unfamiliar word parts.

4. Learn all example words given.

5. Work and rework worksheets and self-tests.

6. Continue to review as often as necessary to ensure that you retain what you have learned.

Pronunciation

You may not be called on to pronounce medical words often, but you will be required to recognize medical terms when you hear them and you must be able to spell them correctly. Unless you have heard the words many times, you will have difficulty recognizing them. This means that to learn useful medical terminology, you must also learn to pronounce the words.

Phonetic pronunciation guides, new in this edition, provide help with featured words. See the Pronunciation Key inside the front cover for what the symbols in these pronunciations mean. Many other words and word parts are shown with boldface type to show you which syllable to emphasize. For instance, electroencephalogram looks difficult, but if you separate the word parts and if you know which letters to emphasize, it becomes less formidable: electro/en **ceph** alo/gram.

Dictating words to yourself on audiocassette or to another student for spelling practice is a good way to become familiar with pronouncing terms. Additionally, many libraries provide computers and computer programs that provide terminology learning support. To further your understanding, there are also videos available of medical conditions and surgical procedures. Making flashcards to review the terms you find most challenging to define and pronounce may also be beneficial.

Medical Dictionary

A medical dictionary is essential to success. There are a number of good ones on the market varying in price and size from inexpensive paperbacks to very expensive volumes. If you plan to work in medical records, you may wish to purchase a more comprehensive dictionary at the outset. For some allied health careers, an inexpensive dictionary is adequate.

Worksheets and Self-Tests

Worksheets are provided to help you target the areas with which you are having difficulty. The answer keys for most are located in Appendix A. Do not refer to the answers until you have honestly tried to complete the worksheet. Self-tests are provided as an overview of the chapter you have been working on. Most self-tests have an answer key, also located in Appendix A. Do not refer to the key until after you have completed the test.

Review

Check Your Progress sections appear in Chapters 5, 9, 14, 21, and 24. Each corresponds with a review exam in Appendix F.

Appendix F also contains chapter tests, a midterm, and final exam. Your instructor will decide how the various exams are to be used, or may choose to provide different tests. Do not write on these tests until you are instructed to do so, but you are welcome to study them to see how well you have learned the material.

Good luck in your study of this course.

Contents

Preface v
Instructions for Workbook Use x

Part 1
Basic Medical Terminology and Word Structure 1

Chapter 1   Introduction and Basic Medical Words   3

Chapter 2   Surgical Procedures   15

Chapter 3   Medical Conditions and Diseases   20

Chapter 4   Medical Instruments and Machines   26

Chapter 5   Medical Specialists and Specialties   33

Chapter 6   Plural Endings   46

Chapter 7   Additional Prefixes   49

Chapter 8   Additional Suffixes and Root Words   58

Chapter 9   Bacteria, Colors, and Review   68

Chapter 10   Directional, Positional, and Numerical Terms   76

Chapter 11   Additional Terms   86

Chapter 12   General Abbreviations   91

Chapter 13   Diagnostic and Laboratory Abbreviations   99

Chapter 14   Basic Pharmacology   112

Part 2
Body Systems Terminology 119

Chapter 15   Structure of the Body   121

Chapter 16   Integumentary System   127

Chapter 17   Musculoskeletal System   137

Chapter 18   Cardiovascular System   152

Chapter 19   Respiratory System   168

Chapter 20   Gastrointestinal System   179

Chapter 21   Urinary System   194

Chapter 22   Female Reproductive System, Neonatology, and Genetics   202

Chapter 23   Male Reproductive System and Sexually Transmitted Diseases   212

Chapter 24   Nervous System and Psychiatric Terms   218

Chapter 25   Sense Organs: Eyes, Ears, and Mouth   232

Chapter 26   Endocrine System and Stress Response   251

Appendices

Appendix A   Answer Keys   261

Appendix B   Disease Report Outline   273

Appendix C   Using Your Medical Dictionary   274

Appendix D   Organizations Offering Literature and Information   275

Appendix E   Brief Introduction to Diagnostic Microbiology   277

Appendix F   Chapter Tests and Review Exams   279

Appendix G   Medications   379

Appendix H   Abbreviations   390

Glossary/Index   409

List of Case Histories

Chapter 16   Case History 1   Discharge Summary: Cellulitis of penis   135

Chapter 17   Case History 2   Discharge Summary: Torn medial meniscus   150

               Case History 3   Report of Operation: Herniated nucleus pulposus   150

Chapter 18   Case History 4   Discharge Summary: Chest pain   166

Chapter 19   Case History 5   Radiology Report: Posteroanterior, lateral chest   177

               Case History 6   Discharge Summary: Bronchitis   177

               Case History 7   Report of Operation: Bronchoscopy   177

Chapter 20   Case History 8   Admission Note: Diverticulitis   192

               Case History 9   Radiology Report: Barium enema   192

               Case History 10   Report of Operation: Cholecystectomy   193

Chapter 21   Case History 11   Radiology Report: Intravenous pyelogram   200

               Case History 12   Discharge Summary: Transitional cell carcinoma of the bladder   200

Chapter 22   Case History 13   Report of Operation: Hysterectomy with salpingo-oophorectomy   209

                    Case History 14   Report of Operation: Vaginal hysterectomy   210

                    Case History 15   Discharge Summary: Premature infant   210

Chapter 23   Case History 16   Report of Operation: Circumcision   217

Chapter 24   Case History 17   Radiology Report: Skull radiograph   229

                    Case History 18   Radiology Report: Cervical spine radiograph   230

                    Case History 19   Radiology Report: Myelogram   230

                    Case History 20   Radiology Report: Brain scan   230

                    Case History 21   Report of EEG: Electroencephalogram   230

Chapter 25   Case History 22   Report of Operation: Cataract extraction   248

                    Case History 23   Report of Operation: Tympanoplasty   248

                    Case History 24   Consultation: Dental examination   249

Chapter 26   Case History 25   Admission Note: Cataract and vitreous hemorrhage   258

List of Figures

Figure 1.1   Gyne (woman). Anterior view.   9

Figure 1.2   Andro (man). Anterior view.   10

Figure 10.1   Anatomical planes and directional terms.   77

Figure 10.2   Body movements and positions.   78

Figure 10.3   Abdominal quadrants.   79

Figure 13.1   Hematology laboratory form.   101

Figure 13.2   Chemistry laboratory form.   102

Figure 13.3   Urinalysis laboratory form.   103

Figure 13.4   Microbiology laboratory form.   104

Figure 13.5   Cytology laboratory form.   105

Figure 13.6   Laboratory form for flexible profiles and individual tests.   106

Figure 15.1   Body cavities.   121

Figure 16.1   Cross section of normal skin.   127

Figure 16.2   Primary and secondary lesions of the skin.   129

Figure 17.1   Shoulder dissection from rear.   137

Figure 17.2   Anterolateral aspect of the knee.   138

Figure 17.3   Anterior and posterior views of the skeleton.   139

Figure 17.4   Spinal column and vertebra.   140

Figure 17.5   Examples of fractures.   143

Figure 17.6   Spinal column showing hernia of intervertebral disk.   144

Figure 18.1   Cross section of the heart.   152

Figure 18.2   Capillary bed.   153

Figure 18.3   Coronary arteries.   154

Figure 18.4   Circulation in the normal heart.   155

Figure 18.5   Triple coronary artery bypass graft.   159

Figure 18.6   Examples of ECGs.   161

Figure 19.1   Lungs and airways.   169

Figure 19.2   CAT scan.   172

Figure 20.1   Gastrointestinal organs.   180

Figure 20.2   Gallbladder.   181

Figure 20.3   Areas of abdomen.   182

Figure 20.4   Indirect and direct inguinal hernias.   184

Figure 21.1   Normal urinary tract.   194

Figure 21.2   Foley catheter.   196

Figure 21.3   24-hour intake and output chart.   197

Figure 22.1   Female reproductive system.   202

Figure 22.2   Sonograms of a fetus.   205

Figure 23.1   Median sagittal section of the male pelvis.   212

Table 23.1   Sexually Transmitted Diseases (STDs).   215

Figure 24.1   Brain and spinal cord.   219

Figure 24.2   The meninges that surround the spinal cord.   220

Figure 25.1   Normal eye.   232

Figure 25.2   Detached retina.   235

Figure 25.3   The ear.   238

Figure 25.4   Structure of teeth.   242

Figure 25.5   Dental claim form.   243

Figure 26.1   Endocrine glands.   252

Figure 26.2   Stress and the adrenal gland.   256

Basic Medical Terminology and Word Structure

OVERVIEW

Beginning with basic medical concepts, terms, and structures, this part concentrates on building a basic foundation and framework.

OBJECTIVES

1. To correctly identify and understand word parts consisting of suffixes, prefixes, and root words found in each chapter.

2. To build medical terms using word parts.

3. To appropriately spell, define, and pronounce all medical terminology presented.

4. To apply medical terminology properly in context.

CHAPTER 1

Introduction and Basic Medical Words

Introduction to Word Parts

Define:

1. prefix _a word part, at the beginning of a word_ _____

2. suffix _____

3. root word _____

4. compound word _____

5. combining form _____

Examples of various combinations of word parts follow. Start your new vocabulary by trying to define the indicated medical words.

Words using a prefix and root word:

Prefix	Root	Example/Pronunciation	Define
semi-	final	semifinal	
mis-	interpret	misinterpret	
uni-	form	uniform	
pre-	mature	premature (prē-mă-**tŭr**)	6. _____
hyper-	active	hyperactive (hī-pĕr-**ăk**-tĭv)	7. _____

Words using a root and a suffix:

Root	Suffix	Example/Pronunciation	Define
care	-less	careless	
violin	-ist	violinist	
psych	-ology	psychology (sī-**kŏl**-ō-gē)	8. _____
tonsil	-ectomy	tonsillectomy (tŏn-sĭl-**lĕk**-tō-mē)	9. _____
bronch	-itis	bronchitis (brŏn-**kī**-tĭs)	10. _____

Words made up of two root words (compound words):

Root	Root	Example/Pronunciation		Define
head	ache	headache (**hĕd**-āk)		
news	paper	newspaper		
micro	scope	microscope (**mī**-krō-skōp)	11.	_____
hydr/o	therapy	hydrotherapy (hī-drō-**thĕr**-ăp-ē)	12.	_____
bronch/o	pneumonia	bronchopneumonia (brŏn-kō-nū-**mō**-nē-ă)	13.	_____

Words using combining form (adding o to the root word):

cardiovascular (kăr-dē-ō-**văs**-kū-lăr)   14. _____

gastrointestinal (găs-trō-ĭn-**tĕs**-tĭ-năl)   15. _____

Words using prefix and suffix only:

Prefix	Suffix	Example/Pronunciation	Define	
an-	-emia	anemia (ă-**nē**-mē-ă)	16.	_____
ex-	-cise	excise (**ĕk**-sīz)	17.	_____
poly-	-uria	polyuria (pŏl-ē-**ūr**-ē-ă)	18.	_____
ana-	-tomy	anatomy (ă-**năt**-ō-mē)	19.	_____

Words using prefix, root, and suffix:

Prefix	Root	Suffix	Example/Pronunciation	Define	
super-	nature	-al	supernatural		
un-	friend	-ly	unfriendly		
peri-	card	-itis	pericarditis (pĕr-ē-kăr-**dī**-tĭs)	20.	_____

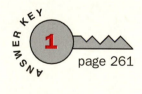

ANSWER KEY 1 page 261

Worksheet

-ec tomy (from *ektome;* Greek for "to cut out") to excise or cut out surgically. The accent is always on the *ec* syllable in **-ec** *tomy* (**ĕk**-tō-mē).

With this information, write a definition for the following words. Do not worry about whether the word makes sense to you or that you have never heard of it. These are obvious.

1. tonsillectomy (tŏn-sĭl-**lĕk**-tō-mē) _excision of the tonsils_

2. appendectomy (ăp-pĕn-**dĕk**-tō-mē) _____

3. adenoidectomy (ăd-nŏyd-**ĕk**-tō-mē) _____

4. thyroidectomy (thī-rŏy-**dĕk**-tō-mē) _____

5. splenectomy (splĕ-**nĕk**-tō-mē) _____

These are more difficult, but they are fairly common operations.

6. hysterectomy (hĭs-tĕ-**rĕk**-tō-mē) _____

7. cholecystectomy (kōl-ĕ-sĭs-**tĕk**-tō-mē) _____

8. hemorrhoidectomy (hĕm-ōr-rŏy-**dĕk**-tō-mē) _____

9. gingivectomy (dental) (jĭn-jĭ-**vĕk**-tō-mē) _____

10. mastectomy (măs-**tĕk**-tō-mē) _____

These are less commonly performed operations. Some are quite obvious.

11. adrenalectomy (ă-drē-năl-**ĕk**-tō-mē) _____

12. pancreatectomy (păn-krē-ă-**tĕk**-tō-mē) _____

13. colectomy (kō-**lĕk**-tō-mē) _____

14. neurectomy (nū-**rĕk**-tō-mē) _____

15. duodenectomy (dūō-dĕ-**nĕk**-tō-mē) _____

16. laryngectomy (lăr-ĭn-**jĕk**-tō-mē) _____

17. ureterectomy (ū-rē-tĕr-**ĕk**-tō-mē) _____

18. gastrectomy (găs-**trĕk**-tō-mē) _____

19. cervicectomy (sĕr-vĭ-**sĕk**-tō-mē) _____

20. tympanectomy (tĭm-pă-**nĕk**-tō-mē) _____

21. oophorectomy (ō-ŏ-fŏ-**rĕk**-tō-mē) _____

22. cystectomy (sĭs-**tĕk**-tō-mē) _____

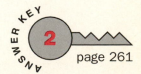

ANSWER KEY

2

page 261

Suffix -*ectomy*

Notice that all -ectomy words are not formed in exactly the same way. In fact, there are four ways of forming -ectomy words that may be categorized as follows:

1. Some -*ectomy* words are formed by simply adding -*ectomy* to a familiar word (body part or organ), for example:

    > adenoid = adenoid **ec** tomy

2. Some -*ectomy* words are formed by using an unfamiliar or foreign root word, for example:

    > gastr- = gas **trec** tomy (stomach)
    > hyster- = hyste **rec** tomy (uterus)

3. Some -ectomy words have a letter added, a letter dropped, or a letter changed, for example:

    > tonsil **lec** tomy (tonsils)
    > sple **nec** tomy (spleen)
    > pancrea **tec** tomy (pancreas)
    > laryn **gec** tomy (larynx)

4. In some -ectomy words, the last syllable of the root is dropped, for example:

    > **co** lon = co **lec** tomy (large intestine)
    > duo **de** num = duode **nec** tomy (first part of small intestine)
    > ap **pen** dix = appen **dec** tomy (small appendage on cecum)

Go back to the preceding worksheet and look at the words. Select the category that each word belongs in and write that word in the correct column of the following chart. Then check your answers with the numbers in the footnote below.*

1 word unchanged	2 unfamiliar or foreign root	3 letter changed added, or dropped	4 last syllable dropped
adenoidectomy	hysterectomy	tonsillectomy	appendectomy

*Category 1: 3, 4, 8, 11, 17, and 22; category 2: 6, 7, 9, 10, 14, 18, 21, and 22; category 3: 1, 5, 12, 16, and 19; category 4: 2, 13, 15, and 20.

Self-Test

You know what *-ectomy* means: to excise or cut out surgically. The spelling of *-ectomy* is always the same, and the accent is always on the *-ec* syllable.

Write a word that means:

1. Tonsils removed surgically ____________________
2. Adenoids removed surgically ____________________
3. Thyroid gland removed surgically ____________________
4. Adrenal gland removed surgically ____________________

Spell: Have someone dictate these words to you from Answer Key 3.

5. ____________________
6. ____________________
7. ____________________
8. ____________________
9. ____________________
10. ____________________
11. ____________________
12. ____________________
13. ____________________
14. ____________________
15. ____________________
16. ____________________
17. ____________________
18. ____________________
19. ____________________
20. ____________________

Define:

21. ex **cis** ion ____________________
22. in **cis** ion ____________________

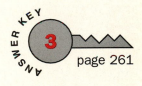

ANSWER KEY 3 page 261

If your score is not 100%, review and try again.

You will be using these and other less familiar root words in the following lessons. Gradually you will learn all of them, if you continue to use them. You must review or you will forget what you have learned. Remember to pronounce the words as you write them. The accented syllable is shown in boldface type.

■ **Assignment:** Go back and study the *-ectomy* words. Do not worry, at this point, if you do not fully understand what some of the root words mean. (For instance, you may not exactly know what a ureter or duodenum is, but you can still define *urete **rec** tomy* and *duode **nec** tomy*.) Work with a partner if possible. Dictate to each other for spelling and pronunciation practice.

Notice the addition of *o* to most root words. This means that the *o* may be used in some words but may be dropped in others. In general, the *o* (combining form) is used when two or more root words are combined, as in *gastro/enter **ol** ogy,* and the *o* is dropped when adding a suffix that begins with a vowel, as in *gas **tr/i** tis.*

List of Root Words

An alphabetical list of root words, most of which appear in Figures 1.1 and 1.2, is given here. A few that do not appear are also given. Most of these words will have to be memorized because they are derived from foreign languages. Cover the meaning column and see if you know some of them.

Word part	Meaning	Example	Pronunciation
abdomin/o (see *laparo*)	abdomen (general region of)	1. abdominopelvic	(ăb-dŏm-ĭn-ō-**pĕl**-vĭk)
aden/o	gland	2. adenectomy	(ădĕ-**nĕk**-tō-mē)
an/o	anus	3. anal	(**ā**-năl)
andr/o	man	4. androgen	(**ăn**-drō-jĕn)
angi/o (see *vas/o*)	vessel (lymph, blood)	5. angiogram	(**ăn**-jē-ō-grăm)
append	appendix	6. appendectomy	(ăp-pĕn-**dĕk**-tō-mē)
appendic/o	appendix	7. appendicitis	(ăp-pĕnd-ĭ-**sī**-tĭs)
arteri/o	artery	8. arteriosclerosis	(ăr-tĕr-ē-ō-sklĕ-**rō**-sĭs)
arthr/o	joint	9. arthritis	(ăr-**thrī**-tĭs)
bronch/o	bronchus	10. bronchitis	(brŏn **kī**-tĭs)
cardi/o	heart	11. electrocardiogram	(ē-lĕk-trō-**kăr**-dē-ō-grăm)
carp/o	wrist	12. carpal	(**kăr**-păl)
cephal/o	head	13. cephalic	(sĕ-**făl**-ĭk)
cerebr/o	cerebrum (part of brain)	14. cerebral	(sĕ-**rē**-brăl)
cervic/o	cervix (opening to and bottom neck of uterus)	15. cervical	(**sĕr**-vĭ-kăl)
cheil/o	lip	16. cheiloplasty	(**kī**-lō-plăs-tē)
cholecyst/o	gallbladder	17. cholecystectomy	(kōl-ĕ-sĭs-**tĕc**-tō-mē)
choledoch/o	common bile duct	18. choledochostomy	(kōl-ĕ-dŏ-**kŏs**-tō-mē)
chondr/o	cartilage	19. chondrectomy	(kŏn-**drĕk**-tō-mē)
col/o	colon (large intestine)	20. colostomy	(kō-**lŏs**-tō-mē)
colp/o	vagina	21. colposcope	(**kŏl**-pō-skōp)
cost/o	rib	22. costal margin	(**kŏs**-tăl măr-jĭn)
crani/o	cranium (skull)	23. cranial	(**krā**-nē-ăl)
cyst/o	bladder	24. cystitis	(sĭs-**tī**-tĭs)
dent/o, odont/o	tooth	25. dentist	(**dĕn**-tĭst)
derm/o	skin	26. dermabrasion	(dĕr-mă-**brā**-zhŭn)
dermat/o	skin	27. dermatologist	(dĕr-mă-**tŏl**-ō-jĭst)
duoden/o	duodenum (small intestine)	28. duodenectomy	(dū-ō-dĕ-**nĕk**-tō-mē)
encephal/o	brain	29. encephalitis	(ĕn-sĕf-ă-**lī**-tĭs)
enter/o	small intestine	30. enteritis	(ĕn-tĕr-ī-tĭs)
esophag/o	esophagus	31. esophagitis	(ē-sŏf-ă-**jī**-tĭs)
gastr/o	stomach	32. gastrectomy	(găs-**trĕk**-tō-mē)
gingiv/o	gums	33. gingivitis	(jĭn-jĭ-**vī**-tĭs)
gloss/o (see *lingua*)	tongue	34. glossitis	(glŏ-**sī**-tĭs)

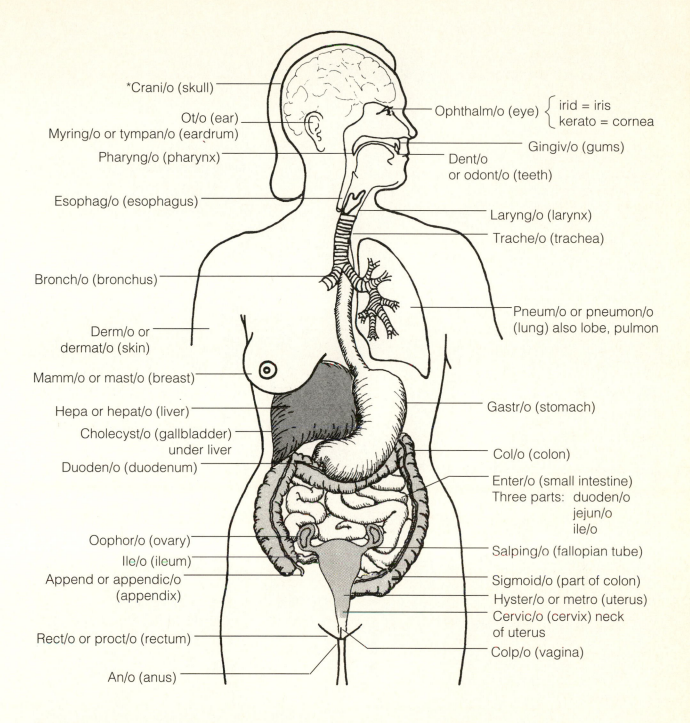

*Crani/o (skull)

Ot/o (ear)

Myring/o or tympan/o (eardrum)

Pharyng/o (pharynx)

Esophag/o (esophagus)

Bronch/o (bronchus)

Derm/o or dermat/o (skin)

Mamm/o or mast/o (breast)

Hepa or hepat/o (liver)

Cholecyst/o (gallbladder) under liver

Duoden/o (duodenum)

Oophor/o (ovary)

Ile/o (ileum)

Append or appendic/o (appendix)

Rect/o or proct/o (rectum)

An/o (anus)

Ophthalm/o (eye) { irid = iris
kerato = cornea

Gingiv/o (gums)

Dent/o or odont/o (teeth)

Laryng/o (larynx)

Trache/o (trachea)

Pneum/o or pneumon/o (lung) also lobe, pulmon

Gastr/o (stomach)

Col/o (colon)

Enter/o (small intestine) Three parts: duoden/o
jejun/o
ile/o

Salping/o (fallopian tube)

Sigmoid/o (part of colon)

Hyster/o or metro (uterus)

Cervic/o (cervix) neck of uterus

Colp/o (vagina)

Figure 1.1 *Gyne* is the root meaning "woman." Anterior view, no bony structure shown. Showing intestinal tract, female reproductive organs, lung, and airway. *Note:* There is a word in this figure that refers to a part of the head (indicated by *).

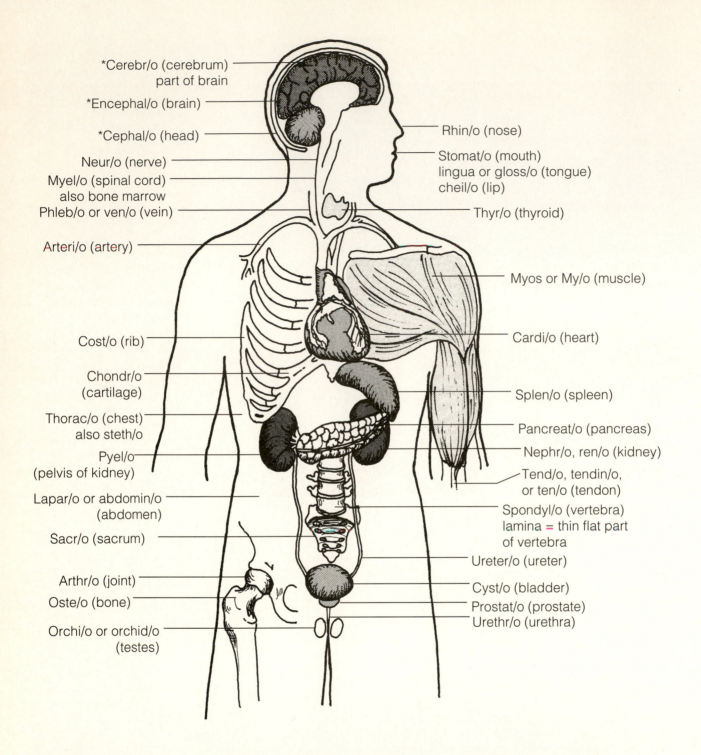

*Cerebr/o (cerebrum) part of brain
*Encephal/o (brain)
*Cephal/o (head)
Neur/o (nerve)
Myel/o (spinal cord) also bone marrow
Phleb/o or ven/o (vein)
Arteri/o (artery)
Cost/o (rib)
Chondr/o (cartilage)
Thorac/o (chest) also steth/o
Pyel/o (pelvis of kidney)
Lapar/o or abdomin/o (abdomen)
Sacr/o (sacrum)
Arthr/o (joint)
Oste/o (bone)
Orchi/o or orchid/o (testes)

Rhin/o (nose)
Stomat/o (mouth)
lingua or gloss/o (tongue)
cheil/o (lip)
Thyr/o (thyroid)
Myos or My/o (muscle)
Cardi/o (heart)
Splen/o (spleen)
Pancreat/o (pancreas)
Nephr/o, ren/o (kidney)
Tend/o, tendin/o, or ten/o (tendon)
Spondyl/o (vertebra)
lamina = thin flat part of vertebra
Ureter/o (ureter)
Cyst/o (bladder)
Prostat/o (prostate)
Urethr/o (urethra)

Figure 1.2 *Andro* is the root meaning "man." Anterior view, partial skeleton shown; abdominal viscera not shown. Showing male reproductive organs, urinary tract, heart, spleen, pancreas, hip joint, and some shoulder muscles. *Note:* There are three words in this figure that refer to part of the head (indicated by *).

Word part	Meaning	Example	Pronunciation
gyne	woman	35. gynecology	(gī-ně-**kŏl**-ō-jē)
hepa, hepat/o	liver	36. hepatitis	(hěp-ă-**tī**-tǐs)
hyster/o	uterus	37. hysterectomy	(hǐs-tě-**rěk**-tō-mē)
ile/o	ileum (small intestine)	38. ileostomy	(ǐlě-**ŏs**-tō-mē)
irid/o	iris (eye)	39. iridectomy	(ǐr-ǐ-**děk**-tō-mē)
jejun/o	jejunum (small intestine)	40. jejunitis	(jě-jū-**nī**-tǐs)
kerat/o*	cornea of eye;	41. keratoplasty	(**kěr**-ăt-ō-plăs-tē)
	horny substance	42. keratosis	(kěr-ă-**tō**-sǐs)
lamina	thin, flat part of vertebra	43. laminectomy	(lăm-ǐ-**něk**-tō-mē)
lapar/o	abdomen	44. laparotomy	(lăp-ă-**rŏt**-ō-mē)
(see *abdomin/o*)			
laryng/o	larynx (voice box)	45. laryngitis	(lăr-ǐn-**jī**-tǐs)
lingua (see *gloss/o*)	tongue	46. sublingual	(sŭb-**lǐng**-wăl)
lobe	lobe, as of lung	47. lobectomy	(lō-**běk**-tō-mē)
mast/o, mamm/o	breast	48. mastectomy	(măs-**těk**-tō-mē)
		49. mammoplasty	(**măm**-ō-plăs-tē)
metr/o	uterus	50. metrorrhagia	(mět-rōr-**rā**-jē-ă)
(see *hyster/o*)			
my/o, myos	muscle	51. myositis	(mī-ō-**sī**-tǐs)
myel/o*	bone marrow;	52. osteomyelitis	(ŏs-tē-ō-mī-ě-**lī**-tǐs)
	spinal cord	53. myelogram	(**mī**-ěl-ō-grăm)
myring/o	eardrum	54. myringotomy	(mī-rǐn-**gŏt**-ō-mē)
(see *tympan/o*)			
nephr/o	kidney	55. nephrectomy	(něf-**rěk**-tō-mē)
(see *ren/o*)			
neur/o	nerve	56. neuritis	(nŭ-**rī**-tǐs)
oophor/o	ovary	57. oophorectomy	(ō-ŏ-fŏ-**rěk**-tō-mē)
ophthalm/o	eye	58. ophthalmologist	(ŏf-thăl-**mŏl**-ō-jǐst)
orchi/o	testicle	59. orchitis	(ŏr-**kǐ**-tǐs)
orchid/o	testicle	60. orchidoplasty	(**ŏr**-kǐd-ō-plăs-tē)
oste/o	bone	61. osteochondritis	(ŏs-tē-ō-kŏn-**drī**-tǐs)
ot/o	ear	62. otoscope	(**ō**-tō-skōp)
pancreat/o	pancreas	63. pancreatectomy	(păn-krē-ă-**těk**-tō-mē)
pharyng/o	pharynx (throat)	64. pharyngitis	(făr-ǐn-**jī**-tǐs)
phleb/o	vein	65. phlebitis	(flě-**bī**-tǐs)
(see *ven/o*)			
pneum/o	lungs	66. pneumonia	(nŭ-**mō**-nē-ă)
(see *pulmon/o*)			
pod/o	foot	67. podiatry	(pŏ-**dī**-ăt-rē)
proct/o	rectum, anus	68. proctoscope	(**prŏk**-tō-skōp)
(see *rect/o*)			
prostat/o	prostate gland	69. prostatectomy	(prŏs-tă-**těk**-tō-mē)
pulmon/o	lung	70. pulmonary	(**pŭl**-mō-ně-rě)
(see *pneum/o*)			
pyel/o	pelvis of kidney	71. pyelitis	(pī-ě-**lī**-tǐs)
rect/o	rectum	72. rectal	(**rěk**-tăl)
(see *proct/o*)			
ren/o (see *nephr/o*)	renal (kidney)	73. renal failure	(rē-năl **fāyl**-ūr)

**Important: In a few cases, *one* word part can refer to two entirely different organs. Examples: *myelo* and *kerato*.*

Word part	Meaning	Example	Pronunciation
rhin/o	nose	74. rhinoplasty	(**rī**-nō-plăs-tē)
sacr/o	sacrum	75. sacroiliac	(să-krō-**ĭl**-ē-ăk)
salping/o	fallopian tube	76. salpingectomy	(săl-pĭn-**jĕk**-tō-mē)
sigmoid/o	lower portion of colon	77. sigmoidoscopy	
splen/o	spleen	78. splenectomy	(splĕ-**nĕk**-tō-mē)
spondyl/o	vertebra	79. spondylitis	(spŏn-dĭ-**lī**-tĭs)
steth/o	chest	80. stethoscope	(**stĕth**-ō-skōp)
(see *thorac/o*)			
stomat/o	mouth	81. stomatitis	(stō-mă-**tī**-tĭs)
ten/o, tend/o,	tendon	82. tendinitis	(**tĕn**-dĭ-**nī**-tĭs)
tendin/o		83. tenoplasty	(**tĕn**-ō-plăs-tē)
thorac/o	thorax (chest)	84. thoracic	(thŏ-**răs**-ĭk)
(see *steth/o*)			
thyr/o	thyroid gland	85. thyroidectomy	(thī-rŏy-**dĕk**-tō-mē)
trache/o	trachea	86. tracheotomy	(trā-kē-**ŏt**-ō-mē)
tympan/o	eardrum	87. tympanectomy	(tĭm-pă-**nĕk**-tō-mē)
(see *myring/o*)			
ureter/o	ureter	88. ureterectomy	(ūr-ē-tĕ-**rĕk**-tō-mē)
urethr/o	urethra	89. urethritis	(ūr-ĕ-**thrī**-tĭs)
vas/o (see *angi/o*)	vessel	90. vasoconstriction	(văs-ō-kŏn-**strĭk**-shŭn)
ven/o (see *phleb/o*)	vein	91. venogram	(**vē**-nō-grăm)

■ **Note:** You will have noticed that more than one word may pertain to certain structures:

Brain and head
cranio = skull only
cephalo = head
cerebro = part of brain
encephalo = entire brain

Kidneys
nephro = entire kidney
reno = entire kidney
pyelo = pelvis of kidney

This also applies to words for the abdomen, rectum, eardrum, vessels, and chest.

Use the preceding alphabetical listing of body parts and organs as a study guide. Cover the meanings and see if you can define the word part. Then cover the word part column and see if you know the root words. Pronounce the example words. Dictate them to a friend, then write them until you are sure of the spelling.

When you think you know the *-ectomy* words given, proceed to the self-test.

Self-Test

Spell: Have someone dictate the words from Answer Key 4.

Define any eight:

1. _____
2. _____
3. _____
4. _____
5. _____

6. _____   _____

7. _____   _____

8. _____   _____

9. _____   _____

10. _____   _____

11. _____   _____

12. _____   _____

Build a word:

13. Excision of the thyroid gland   _____

14. Excision of the adrenal gland   _____

15. Excision of the uterus   _____

16. Excision of the tonsils   _____

17. Excision of the hemorrhoids   _____

18. Excision of the appendix   _____

Extra: What is a T & A?   _____

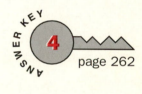

ANSWER KEY 4 page 262

If your score was not 100%, review and try again.

Worksheet

Fill in the meaning of each root word. At another time, cover the first column root word and see if you can look at the meaning and write in the root word and an example of its use in a word. You may not be able to use all of the roots in a word now, but you can add others as you learn more.

Root word	Meaning	Root word	Use root in a word
aden/o	gland	aden/o	adenoid
arteri/o	_____	_____	_____
appendic/o or append/o	_____	_____	_____

Root word	Meaning	Root word	Use root in a word
arthr/o	_____	_____	_____
bronch/o	_____	_____	_____
cardi/o	_____	_____	_____
carp/o	_____	_____	_____
cerebr/o	_____	_____	_____
cervic/o	_____	_____	_____
cholecyst/o	_____	_____	_____
chondr/o	_____	_____	_____
col/o	_____	_____	_____
colp/o	_____	_____	_____
cost/o	_____	_____	_____
crani/o	_____	_____	_____
cyst/o	_____	_____	_____
dent/o	_____	_____	_____
derm/o, dermato	_____	_____	_____
encephal/o	_____	_____	_____
gastr/o	_____	_____	_____
hepa, hepat/o	_____	_____	_____
hyster/o	_____	_____	_____
mast/o	_____	_____	_____
my/o	_____	_____	_____
neur/o	_____	_____	_____
nephr/o	_____	_____	_____
oste/o	_____	_____	_____
ot/o	_____	_____	_____
pneum/o	_____	_____	_____
proct/o	_____	_____	_____
pyel/o	_____	_____	_____
rhin/o	_____	_____	_____
spondyl/o	_____	_____	_____
thyr/o	_____	_____	_____
trache/o	_____	_____	_____

No Answer Key

This drill should be periodically reviewed orally, working from the root and from the meanings.

Test p. 281

CHAPTER 2

Surgical Procedures

List of Suffixes

You have learned to use the suffix *-ectomy*. Here are some other surgical procedure suffixes. Many of the root words you know can be used with these endings.

Recall *-ectomy*: "to excise or cut out surgically." The following endings have *specific meanings* other than to "excise." These are other kinds of surgical procedures. Define the following example words and try to think of some others using root words you know:

Suffix	Meaning	Example/Pronunciation	Define
-os tomy	a new permanent opening (to outside of body)	colostomy (kō-**lŏs**-tō-mē)	*new opening in colon*
		tracheostomy (trā-kē-**ŏs**-tō-mē)	
	(reunited inner structures)	gastroduodenostomy (găs-trō-dū-ō-dĕ-**nŏs**-tō-mē)	
		colocolostomy (kōl-**ŏs**-tō-mē)	
-ot omy	cutting into (making an incision)	laparotomy (lăp-ă-**rŏt**-ō-mē)	
		tracheotomy (trāk-ē-**ŏt**-ō-mē)	
-or rhaphy	surgical repair	herniorrhaphy (hĕr-nē-**ŏr**-răf-ē)	
		nephrorrhaphy (nĕf-**rŏr**-răf-ē)	
-o **pex** y	fixation or suturing (a type of repair)	nephropexy (nĕf-**rō**-pĕk-sē)	
		salpingopexy (săl-**pĭng**-ō-pĕk-sē)	

Suffix	Meaning	Example/Pronunciation	Define
-o **plas** ty	plastic surgery (surgical reforming or molding to improve function; to relieve pain; for cosmetic reasons)	rhinoplasty (**rī**-nō-plăs-tē)	_____
		arthroplasty (**ăr**-thrō-plăs-tē)	_____
		angioplasty (**ăn**-jē-ō-plăs-tē)	_____
-o **trip**sy	crushing, destroying	neurotripsy (**nūr**-ō-trĭp-sē)	_____
		lithoptripsy (**litho** = stone) (**lĭth**-ō-trĭp-sē)	_____
-o **cen**tesis	surgical puncture to remove fluid	abdominocentesis (ăb-dŏm-ĭn-ō-sĕn-**tē**-sĭs)	_____
		thoracentesis (thŏr-ă-sĕn-**tē**-sĭs)	_____
		paracentesis (păr-ă-sĕn-**tē**-sĭs)	_____
		amniocentesis (ăm-nē-ō-sĕn-**tē**-sĭs)	_____
		arthrocentesis (ăr-thrō-sĕn-**tē**-sĭs)	_____

■ **Note:** Watch the spelling of **-or** rhaphy. It is difficult but quite common in medical words. It may help if you pronounce the *h* (which is actually silent) when you study these words. Other words using *-orrh:* **hem** orrhage, menor **rha** gia, diar **rhe** a. But sometimes *rh* appears at the beginning of a word, as in rheu **mat** ic.

The spelling of these endings is always the same, regardless of how they may sound: for example, *trache* **ot** *omy* may sometimes sound like *trache* **od** *omy*, but it is always **-ot** *omy*.

No Answer Key

Worksheet

Define:

-os tomy

1. co **los** tomy *new permanent opening into the colon*
2. gas **tros** tomy _____
3. ile **os** tomy _____
4. trache **os** tomy _____
5. cys **tos** tomy _____
6. ente **ros** tomy _____
7. jeju **nos** tomy _____

-ot omy

8. lapa **rot** omy _____
9. trache **ot** omy _____
10. phle **bot** omy _____
11. gas **trot** omy _____
12. cys **tot** omy _____
13. lo **bot** omy _____

The preceding words are some of the more commonly seen words with **-os** *tomy* and **-ot** *omy* endings. *Learn all of them.*

Also, study the example words given for the other surgical procedure suffixes (pp. 15–16). Write them here. Add others as you discover them.

14. **-or** rhaphy

 herniorrhaphy
 _____
 _____
 _____
 _____
 _____
 _____

15. -o **pex** y

 _____
 _____
 _____
 _____
 _____
 _____

16. -o **plas** ty

 _____
 _____
 _____
 _____
 _____
 _____

17. -o **trip** sy

18. -cen **te** sis

_____

_____

_____

_____

_____

_____

Whenever you see these suffixes, you should recognize their meanings immediately. As you learn more root words, you will be able to add more words using these endings.

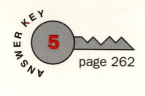

page 262

Worksheet

Write a specific word for:

1. Excision of the stomach _gastrectomy_ _____

2. A new permanent opening into the trachea _____

3. Incision into the bladder _____

4. Plastic surgery on a joint _____

5. Fixation of a kidney _____

6. Excision of an ovary _____

7. Surgical crushing of a nerve _____

8. New permanent opening in the ileum _____

9. New permanent opening into the colon _____

10. Excision of the gallbladder _____

11. Surgical puncture (tapping) of the chest cavity _____

12. Surgical repair of a hernia _____

13. "Tapping" a joint to remove fluid _____

Spell: Have someone dictate these words to you from Answer Key 6.

Define:

14. _____   _____

15. _____   _____

16. _____   _____

17. _____   _____

18. _____   _____

19. _____   _____

20. _____   _____

21. _____   _____

22. _____   _____

23. _____   _____

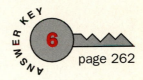

ANSWER KEY **6** page 262

Test p. 283

CHAPTER 3

Medical Conditions and Diseases

List of Suffixes

Define the following words. Later, starting with root words you have learned, make up words using **-o** *sis*, **-i** *tis*, and **-op** *athy* endings. Watch the pronunciation of **-op** *athy* words (the accent is always on *op*).
    Remember: The spelling of these suffixes never changes, regardless of how they may sound.

Suffix	Meaning	Example/Pronunciation	Define
-o sis	condition of	dermatosis (dĕr-mă-**tŏ**-sĭs)	*condition of the skin*
		neurosis (nŭ-**rŏ**-sĭs)	
		psychosis (sī-**kō**-sĭs)	
		sclerosis (sklĕ-**rō**-sĭs)	
		tuberculosis (tū-bĕr-kū-**lō**-sĭs) (tubercle = little swelling)	
		diverticulosis (dī-vĕr-tĭk-ū-**lō**-sĭs) (diverticulum = out-pouching or sac)	
		endometriosis (ĕn-dō-mē-trē-**ō**-sĭs)	
-i asis	condition of	cholelithiasis (kō-lĕ-lĭ-**thī**-ăs-ĭs)	
		amebiasis (ăm-ē-**bī**-ăs-ĭs)	
-i tis	inflammation of	appendicitis (ăp-pĕn-dĭ-**sī**-tĭs)	
		spondylitis (spŏn-dĭ-**lī**-tĭs)	
		tonsillitis (tŏn-sĭl-**lī**-tĭs)	
		peritonitis (pĕr-ĭt-ō-**nī**-tĭs)	
		arthritis (ăr-**thrī**-tĭs)	
		myositis (mī-ŏ-**sī**-tĭs)	
		pericarditis (pĕr-ĭ-kăr-**dī**-tĭs)	
-op athy	any disease of	hysteropathy (hĭs-tĕ-**rŏp**-ă-thē)	

Suffix	Meaning	Example/Pronunciation	Define
		adenopathy (ăd-ē-**nŏp**-ā-thē)	_____
		cardiomyopathy (kăr-dē-ō-mī-**ŏp**-ă-thē)	_____
		spondylopathy (spŏn-dĕ-**lŏp**-ă-thĕ)	_____
-al gia or -o **dyn** ia	pain	neuralgia or (nū-**răl**-jē-ă) neurodynia	_____
		myalgia (mī-**ăl**-jē-ă)	_____
		coccygodynia (kŏk-sĭg-ō-**dĭn**-ē-ă) (coccyx is the tailbone)	_____
		dentalgia (dĕn-**tăl**-jē-ă)	_____
		otalgia (ō-**tăl**-jē-ă)	_____
-cele	hernia or rupture or swelling	cystocele (**sĭs**-tō-sēl)	_____
		rectocele (**rĕk**-tō-sēl)	_____
		meningocele (mĕn-**ĭng**-ō-sēl) (meninges are membranes covering brain and spinal cord)	_____
-o/r**rha**gia	hemorrhage (blood bursting forth)	menorrhagia (mĕn-ŏr-**rā**-jē-ā)	_____
		metrorrhagia (mĕt-rōr-**rā**-jē-ă)	_____
-ectasis or **-ect**asia	stretching or dilating	bronchiectasis (brŏn-kē-**ĕk**-tă-sĭs)	_____
		atelectasis (ăt-ĕ-**lĕk**-tă-sĭs)	_____
		gastrectasia (găs-trĕk-**tā**-zē-ă)	_____

No Answer Key

■ **Note:** Learn to spell in*flam* **ma** *tion* (but note that in **flamed** has only one *m*). The cardinal signs of inflammation are redness, heat, swelling, and pain. Inflammation can occur without infection. Look up *inflammation* and *infection* in your dictionary.

Learn the word **her** *nia*. It is a projection of a part from its natural place and also may be called a rupture. Examples of common hernias: um **bil** ical hernia (the um **bil** icus or umbi **li** cus is the navel or belly button); **ing** uinal hernia (in the groin area); hi **a** tal hernia, also called diaphrag **mat** ic (in the diaphragm). (See Figure 20.4 on page 185 of direct and indirect inguinal hernias.)

Learn the words **di** *late*, *di* **la** *tion*, and *dila* **ta** *tion*. When something is dilated, it is made larger or opened up. Dilators are instruments that may be used to dilate an opening. Dilatation can also occur spontaneously.

Look up the definitions for con **ta** *gious* and com **mu** *nicable* and learn them.

Worksheet

Fill in the first column only. At another time, cover the definition column and see if you can remember all of the meanings. Write them in column three. This worksheet should be used for review as often as necessary.

Definition	*Suffix*	*Definition*	*Suffix*
excision of	*-ectomy*		
new permanent opening			
incision into			
surgical repair of			
surgical fixation			
plastic surgery			
crushing			
puncture (tapping)			
stretching (dilating)			
condition of			
inflammation of			
any disease of (general)			
pain			
hernia			
excessive bleeding			
The four signs of inflammation are			

No Answer Key

Self-Test

Give a word for:

1. A condition of the "mind" *psychosis* _____

2. Inflammation of the appendix _____

3. Pain along a nerve _____

4. Hernia of the bladder _____

5. Any disease of the glands _____

6. A condition of the "nerves" _____

7. Very heavy bleeding during the menstrual period _____

8. Inflammation of the skin _____

9. A toothache (pain in a tooth) _____

10. A "condition of" acidity _____

Spell: Have someone dictate these words to you from Answer Key 7.   **Define:**

11. _____   _____

12. _____   _____

13. _____   _____

14. _____   _____

15. _____   _____

16. _____   _____

17. _____   _____

18. _____   _____

19. _____   _____

20. _____   _____

21. _____   _____

22. _____   _____

23. _____   _____

24. _____   _____

25. What are the symptoms of inflammation? _____
_____
_____

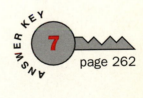

ANSWER KEY **7** page 262

List of Prefixes

Some of these word elements, such as *an-*, *ad-*, and *ab-*, look and sound similar but have different meanings. Define the example words.

Prefix	Meaning	Example/Pronunciation	Define
a- an- ar-	without or not	1. aseptic (septic = (ā-**sĕp**-tĭk) contaminated, dirty)	*without sepsis; sterile*
		2. afebrile (febrile = fever) (ā-**fĕb**-rīl)	_____

Prefix	Meaning	Example/Pronunciation	Define
		3. anemic (ă-**nē**-mĭk)	_____
		4. anesthesia (ăn-ĕs-**thē**-sē-ă)	_____
		5. arrhythmic (ār-**rĭth**-mĭk)	_____
ad-	near, toward	6. adduction (ăd-**dŭk**-shŭn)	_____
ab-	away from	7. adhesion (ăd-**hē**-shŭn)	_____
		8. abduction (ăb-**dŭk**-shŭn)	_____
		9. abnormal (ăb-**nŏr**-măl)	_____
ante-	before, forward	10. anteflexion (ăn-tē-**flĕk**-shŭn)	_____
anti-	against	11. antibiotic (ăn-tē-bī-**ŏt**-ĭk)	_____
		12. antiseptic (ăn-tĭ-**sĕp**-tĭk)	_____
		13. anticonvulsive (ăn-tē-kŏn-**vŭl**-sĭv)	_____
		14. antineoplastic (ăn-tē-nē-ō-**plăs**-tĭk)	_____
contra	against or not	15. contraindicated (kŏn-tră-**ĭn**-dĭ-kā-tĕd)	_____
dis-	from	16. disease (dĭ-**zēz**)	_____
dys-	painful or difficult	17. dysuria (dĭs-**ū**-rē-ă) (-uria = urinating)	_____
		18. dysmenorrhea (dĭs-mĕn-ŏr-**rē**-ă) (meno = menses)	_____
		19. dysentery (**dĭs**-ĕn-tăr-ē)	_____
		20. dyspnea (**dĭsp**-nē-ă) (-pnea = breathing)	_____
hemi-	half (one side)	21. hemiplegia (hĕm-ĭ-**plē**-jē-ă) (-plegia = paralysis)	_____
hyper-	too much, high	22. hypertension (hī-pĕr-**tĕn**-shŭn)	_____
		23. hypertrophy (hī-**pĕr**-trō-fē) (-trophy = growth)	_____
hypo-	not enough, low or under	24. hypoactive (hī-pō-**ăk**-tĭv)	_____
		25. hypodermic (hī-pō-**dĕr**-mĭk)	_____
inter-	between	26. intercostal (ĭn-tĕr-**kŏs**-tăl)	_____
intra-	within	27. intramuscular (ĭn-tĕr-**mŭs**-kū-lăr)	_____
		28. intravenous (ĭn-tră-**vē**-nŭs)	_____
		29. intrathecal (ĭn-tră-**thē**-kăl) (sheath of spinal canal)	_____

These terms need extra study for clear understanding. (See your dictionary.) Define:

30. sepsis _____

31. bladder _____

32. hernia _____

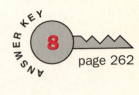
ANSWER KEY
8
page 262

Worksheet

Fill in only column one (definition). Later, see if you can fill in the word part column and give an example of a word using the prefix or suffix. This type of review will help you to retain what you have learned.

Word part	Define	Word part	Example
anti-	against	prefix	antiseptic
a- an- ar-			
ad-			
ab-			
dys-			
hemi-			
hyper-			
hypo-			
-ec tomy			
-os tomy			
-ot omy			
-o sis			
-i tis			
-al gia			
-cele			
-or rhaphy			
hyster-			
nephro-			

No Answer Key

Test p. 285

CHAPTER 4

Medical Instruments and Machines

List of Suffixes

Suffix	Meaning	Example/Pronunciation	Define
-o/**scope**	instrument for looking into	arthroscope (**ăr**-thrō-scōp)	instrument for looking into joint
		cystoscope (**sĭst**-ō-skōp)	_____
		otoscope (**ō**-tō-skōp)	_____
-o/s copy	procedure using a scope	colonoscopy (kō-lŏn-**ŏs**-kŏ-pē) (coloscopy)	_____
		cystoscopy (sĭs-**tŏs**-kŏ-pē)	_____
		otoscopy (ō-**tŏs**-kŏ-pē)	_____

■ **Note:** There is a difference in accented syllables between -o **scope** and **-os** copy. The scope instruments usually have a light at the end. The scope is inserted into an opening, and the light allows the physician to see deep into the cavity or organ. Look up the word **en** doscope. The following are exceptions:

> **Spec** ulum: instrument for looking into (but not a scope)
>
> **Steth** oscope: instrument used for listening, not looking, but is called a scope
>
> **Fe** toscope: instrument for listening to fetal heart tones

Suffix	Meaning	Example/Pronunciation	Define
-tome	instrument for cutting thin section	dermatome (**dĕr**-mă-tōm)	_____
		microtome (**mī**-krō-tōm)	_____
		osteotome (**ŏs**-tē-ō-tōm)	_____

■ **Note:** Recall that all of the suffixes that mean "cutting" have the letters tom in them: **ec** tomy, **ot** tomy, **os** tomy (also a **nat** omy).

Suffix	Meaning	Example/Pronunciation	Define
-(o)graph	instrument (or machine) that records	electroencephalograph (EEG) (ē-lĕk-trō-ĕn-**sĕf**-ăl-ō-grăf)	_____
		electrocardiograph (ECG, EKG) (ē-lĕk-trō-**kăr**-dē-ō-grăf)	_____
		myograph (**mī**-ō-grăf)	_____
		radiograph (**rā**-dē-ō-grăf)	_____

■ **Note:** There is not a special machine for all procedures that record. An X-ray machine is used for many, such as mye **log** raphy, which produces a **my** elogram. Look up these words in your dictionary: **an** giogram, **py** elogram, hysterosal **ping** ogram, **mam** mogram.

Suffix	Meaning	Example/Pronunciation	Define
-(o)g raphy	diagnostic procedure	angiography (ăn-jē-**ŏg**-ră-fē)	_taking pictures of vessels_
		cholecystography (kōl-ĕ-sĭs-**tŏg**-ră-fē)	_____
		cystography (sĭs-**tŏg**-ră-fē)	_____
		electrocardiography (ē-lĕk-trō-kăr-dē-**ŏg**-ră-fē)	_____
		electroencephalography (ē-lĕk-trō-ĕn-sĕf-ă-**lŏg**-ră-fē)	_____
		mammography (măm-**ŏg**-ră-fē)	_____
		myelography (mī-ĕ-**lŏg**-ră-fē)	_____
		myography (mī-**ŏg**-ră-fē)	_____
		radiography (rā-dē-**ŏg**-ră-fē)	_____
		*thermography (thĕr-**mŏg**-ră-fē)	_____
		ultrasonography (ŭl-tră-sŏ-nŏg**-ră-fē)	_____
		urography (ū-**rŏg**-ră-fē)	_____
-(o) gram	recording or "picture" produced by above procedure	angiogram (**ăn**-jē-ō-grăm)	_____
		electrocardiogram (ē-lĕk-trō-**kăr**-dē-ō-grăm)	_____

---

* Video camera process using infrared sensors to produce image of body's temperature (pain spots), used to prove or disprove disability claims.

** Used to detect a variety of internal changes noninvasively (such as aneurysms in aorta, structural changes in abdominopelvic organs, cancers, cysts, eye disorders; in obstetrics, to determine fetal size and placental position).

Suffix	Meaning	Example/Pronunciation	Define
-(o) **gram**		electrodynogram (ē-lĕk-trō-**dī**-nō-grăm)	_____
		electroencephalogram (ē-lĕk-trō-ĕn-**sĕf**-ă-lō-grăm)	_____
		myelogram (**mī**-ĕl-ō-grăm)	_____
		myogram (**mī**-ō-grăm)	_____
		roentgenogram (**rō-ĕnt**-jĕn-ō-grăm) (Roentgen was a German physicist who discoverd X rays)	_____
		ultrasonogram (ŭl-tră-**sŏn**-ō-grăm)	_____

■ **Note:** As there is for **-oscope** and **-os** _copy_, there is a difference in accented syllables between -o **graph** and **-og** _raphy_.

Suffix	Meaning	Example/Pronunciation	Define
-o/m eter	instrument that measures or counts	cytometer (sī-**tŏm**-ĕt-ĕr)	_____
		pelvimeter (pĕl-**vĭm**-ĕt-ĕr)	_____
		spirometer (spī-**rŏm**-ĕt-ĕr)	_____
		thermometer (thĕr-**mŏm**-ĕt-ĕr)	_____
		tonometer (tō-**nŏm**-ĕt-ĕr)	_____
-om etry, **-im** etry	procedure using the instrument	pelvimetry (pĕl-**vĭm**-ĕ-trē)	_____
		spirometry (spī-**rŏm**-ĕ-trē)	_____

No Answer Key

Self-Test

Which organs can the doctor look into with an instrument? Write the instrument and procedure names then pronounce them.

		Instrument	Procedure
1.	ear	otoscope	otoscopy
2.	stomach	_____	_____
3.	sigmoid	_____	_____
4.	bronchi	_____	_____

	Instrument	Procedure

5. eye _____ _____

6. rectum _____ _____

7. anus _____ _____

8. abdomen _____ _____

Write a word for:

9. Excision of a gland ___adenectomy_____

10. Inflammation of the appendix _____

11. Pain in the heart _____

12. Hernia of the bladder _____

13. Any disease or condition of the uterus _____

14. Instrument for looking into a joint (Example: knee) _____

15. Instrument for cutting thin sections of skin _____

16. Condition of the "nerves" _____

17. Inflammation of the gallbladder _____

18. Instrument that records electric impulses of the heart _____

19. X-ray picture of the spinal cord _____

20. Excision of the thyroid gland _____

21. X-ray procedure of the breasts _____

22. Inflammation of the kidney _____

23. Pain in the head _____

24. Recording or picture of brain waves _____

25. Tracing of muscle contractions _____

26. New permanent opening of the colon _____

27. X-ray picture of the kidney pelvis _____

28. Excision of a part or all of the stomach _____

Spell: Have someone dictate these words to you from Answer Key 9.   **Define:**

29. _____ _____

30. _____ _____

31. _____ _____

32. _____ _____

33. _____ _____

34. _____ _____

Spell: **Define**

35. _____   _____

36. _____   _____

37. _____   _____

38. _____   _____

39. Define *speculum:* _____

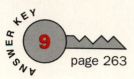

ANSWER KEY **9** page 263

Worksheet

Write a word for:

1. Instrument or device for measuring temperature *thermometer* _____

2. Inflammation of a gland _____

3. Pain in a nerve _____

4. Excision of the tonsils _____

5. New permanent opening into the ileum _____

6. Procedure of using a bronchoscope to examine the bronchi _____

7. Machine that records brain waves _____

8. Excision of the stomach _____

9. Inflammation of joints _____

10. Picture or recording of electrical impulses of the heart _____

11. Instrument for looking into the vagina _____

12. Excision of the uterus _____

13. Inflammation of the gallbladder _____

14. Incision into the abdomen _____

15. Condition of the kidney _____

True/False: Circle the number of the *true* statements only. Defend your answers. Explain what is "untrue" in the false statements.

16. A dermatome cuts a thin section of skin.

17. The physician uses an otoscope to look into the eye.

18. The electroencephalograph is a machine for recording electrical impulses of the heart.

19. A stethoscope is used to amplify sounds in the chest.

20. A bladder is a hollow organ (sac) that usually holds some fluid.

21. Sepsis is the opposite of asepsis.

22. Hemorrhage means internal bleeding.

23. Tuberculosis literally means a condition of having tubercles.

24. Hyperactive means too active.

25. ECG and EKG are both abbreviations for electrocardiogram.

Define: (See your dictionary.)

26. dilator _____

27. speculum _____

28. bougie (dilating) _____

29. sound (*not* the sound you hear!) _____

Extra: Look up the word *radiograph.* What is irregular about this word? _____

_____

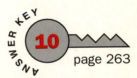

ANSWER KEY **10** page 263

Worksheet

Without looking back, make a list of suffixes you have learned and write a word with each.

Cutting or surgery of some kind:

Suffix   *Word*

-ectomy   cholecystectomy

_____   _____

_____   _____

_____   _____

_____   _____

_____   _____

Diseases or conditions:

Suffix   *Word*

_____   _____

_____   _____

_____   _____

_____   _____

_____   _____

_____   _____

Medical instruments and machines and their use:

Suffix   *Word*

_____   _____

_____   _____

_____   _____

_____   _____

_____   _____

No Answer Key (See chapter for review.)

Test p. 287

CHAPTER 5

Medical Specialists and Specialties

Suffixes

You have often heard the ending *-ol ogy*. It means "the study or science of." Recall the following words:

Bi **ol** ogy   Bacteri **ol** ogy
Psy **chol** ogy   Physi **ol** ogy
Hema **tol** ogy   Termi **nol** ogy

Now you will learn the words for the persons who study these sciences: the people who practice the art or science. They are bi **ol** ogist, bacteri **ol** ogist, psy **chol** ogist, physi **ol** ogist, hema **tol** ogist, and termi **nol** ogist. These people are not all "doctors" in the common usage of the word, although they may have doctorate degrees. In other words, they are not necessarily physicians.

Now consider the *exceptions* to the *-ol ogist* rule. These endings mean the same as *-ol ogist*:

-ist	internist (internal medicine)	(ĭn-**tĕrn**-ĭst)
	orthopedist (orthopedics)	(ŏr-thō-**pē**-dĭst)
-i atrist	psychiatrist (psychiatry)	(sī-**kī**-ă-trĭst)
	podiatrist (podiatry)	(pŏ-**dī**-ă-trĭst)
-i cian	pediatrician (pediatrics)	(pē-dē-ă-**trĭsh**-ăn)
	obstetrician (obstetrics)	(ŏb-stĕ-**trĭsh**-ăn)
	physician	(fĭ-**zĭsh**-ŭn)
-er (**-i** tioner)	practitioner (someone who practices, a doctor or nurse for example)	(prăk-**tĭ**-shŭn-ĕr)

Note the root word *iatro* in examples given here. It means "related to medicine or to physicians." *Iatro* **gen** *ic* means "any condition arising from treatment by a physician," for example: as a result of prescribed antibiotic, a patient may develop a skin reaction, a vaginal infection, diarrhea, or anemia.

Because the subject of specialists and specialties seems difficult for most students, a rather lengthy description and explanation follows.

Education of a Physician

MD (Doctor of Medicine) or DO (Doctor of Oste *op* athy)

The student must get a bachelor's degree at an undergraduate school (or spend at least three years in a premed program) and then spend four years in a medical school or an osteopathic school connected with a hospital. The student receives an MD or DO degree upon graduation.

To obtain a state license to practice, the individual must have the degree plus at least one year's internship in a hospital (an intern cares for patients in the absence of the resident or attending physicians, helps out in emergencies, and assists with operations). The term *intern* is being replaced with *first-year resident.*

To Become a Specialist   (in addition to the preceding requirements)   Two to five years of residency (during which time the physician is called a resident) and two years of practice are required for the physician to apply for certification. Then, if the physician passes boards (tests), he or she is board certified and is a specialist (also known as a diplomate).

License to Practice   Each state requires licensure. However, most grant reciprocity, meaning if a physician is licensed in one state, others will automatically grant a license to practice, for a certain fee. The license must be renewed yearly. In some states one may be required to pass a licensing exam.

Continued Education   Once physicians are licensed, they still take postgraduate courses throughout their lives to stay current on new developments. This is becoming mandatory for renewal of license. (CEUs = continuing education units).

General Practice (GP)   *General practitioner* is a term applied to the nonspecialist, generally a "family doctor." Depending on the area in which he or she practices (rural or urban), this person may prescribe medications, perform surgery, deliver babies, give various treatments, and perform a variety of other services. The general practitioner usually refers complicated cases to a specialist.

Although both MD and DO practitioners may specialize, the MD is more likely to do so, and the DO is more likely to remain in general practice.

■ **Note:** What is the difference between a medical doctor and an osteopathic doctor? They both attend school for the same amount of time, but at different and separate schools. In philosophy and treatment the osteopath places more emphasis on the interrelationship of the body's muscles, bones, and joints, but he or she treats all kinds of illnesses.

Specialists and Specialties (MD or DO)

There are two organizations that recognize special training by awarding the title of "fellow." Thus, upon qualifying, a physician may use the designation FACP (Fellow of the American College of Physicians), or FACS (Fellow of the American College of Surgeons).

administrative medicine   the administrator of a medical center (but in some centers, the administrator is not a physician).

anesthesiology, anesthesiologist (ăn-ĕs-thēs-ē-**ŏl**-ō-jē)   administers anesthesia during surgery; other persons administer anesthesia in certain limited situations (dentists, nurse anesthetists).

bariatrics, bariatrician (băr-ē-**ăt**-rĭks)   treats obesity; science of weight reduction and nutrition.

cardiovascular diseases, cardiologist (kăr-dē-ō-**văs**-kū-lăr dĭ-**zēz**-ĕz)   treats diseases of the heart and blood vessels; cardiovascular surgery.

dermatology, dermatologist (dĕr-mă-**tŏl**-ō-jē)   deals with diseases of the skin.

embryology, embryologist (ĕm-brē-**ŏl**-ō-jē)   monitors prenatal development between the stages of ovum and fetus (through 8th week in humans).

emergency medicine, traumatologist (trăw-mă-**tŏl**-ō-jĭst)   deals with injury, accidental or physiological (emergency room [ER] medicine).

endocrinology, endocrinologist (ĕn-dō-krĭn-**ŏl**-ō-jē) treats disorders of the ductless or endocrine glands: sterility, diabetes, thyroid and obesity disorders, for example.

epidemiology, epidemiologist (ĕp-ĭ-dē-mē-**ŏl**-ō-jē) studies factors regarding how to prevent, control, and/or contain communicable diseases.

family practice specialty, family practice specialist similar to general practice, but qualified as a specialty; also similar to internal medicine, internist.

gastroenterology, gastroenterologist (găs-trō-ĕn-tĕr-**ŏl**-ō-jē) deals with diseases of the digestive system.

geriatrics or **gerontology, geriatrician** or **gerontologist** (jĕr-ē-**ăt**-rĭks), (jĕr-ŏn-**tŏl**-ō-jē) deals with all aspects of aging and disorders thereof.

hematology, hematologist (hēm-ă-**tŏl**-ō-jē) treats disorders of the blood and blood-forming organs.

internal medicine, internist focuses on medical conditions; often sees patients referred by the general practitioner or family practice specialist for consultation and diagnostic help. Performs no surgery or obstetrics. Not an intern.

medical examiner performs investigative examinations of bodies to determine the cause of death in suspicious or questionable circumstances.

neonatology, neonatologist (nē-ō-nă-**tŏl**-ō-jē) treats infants in first 6 weeks of life (high-risk, premature infants).

neurology or **neurosurgery, neurologist** or **neurosurgeon** (nū-**rŏl**-ō-jē), (nū-rō-**sŭr**-jĕr-ē) deals with diseases and/or injuires to the brain, spinal cord, and nerves.

nuclear medicine (**nū**-klē-ăr **mĕd**-ĭ-sĭn) makes diagnostic and therapeutic use of radionuclides.

obstetrics-gynecology, obstetrician and gynecologist (ŏb-**stĕt**-rĭks), (gī-nĕ-**kŏl**-ō-jē) concerned with female reproductive tract disorders; prenatal, delivery, postpartum care; gyneco **log** ic surgery; sterility and insemination; some urinary tract infections.

oncology, oncologist (ŏn-**kŏl**-ō-jē) uses radiation, surgery, and chemotherapy in the treatment of tumors, cancers.

ophthalmology, ophthalmologist (ŏf-thăl-**mŏl**-ō-jē) deals with eye diseases, eye surgery; also prescribes glasses and does eye examinations. Many specialize further: retinas, cataract extractions, corneal transplants, and so on.

orthopedics, orthopedist, orthopedic surgeon, or **orthopod** (ŏr-thō-**pēd**-ĭks) treats disorders of musculoskeletal system, joint diseases (literally means "straight child" and is often confused with osteopathy).

otology, otologist (ō-**tŏl**-ō-jē) deals with ear surgery, hearing problems, hearing aids.

otorhinolaryngology, otorhinolaryngologist (ō-tō-rīn-ō-lăr-ĭn-**gŏl**-ō-jē) treats ear, nose, and throat (ENT) disorders and performs surgery.

pathology, pathologist (păth-**ŏl**-ō-jē) diagnoses morbid changes in tissues from biopsy or postmortem. A medical examiner (coroner) usually is a pathologist.

pediatrics, pediatrician (pēd-ē-**ăt**-rĭks) deals with disease prevention, diagnosis, and treatment of children, usually to age 16. Many specialties within pediatrics: pediatric hematology, oncology, etc.

physiatry, physiatrist (fĭz-ē-**ăt**-rē) deals with physical medicine and rehabilitation (R).

proctology, proctologist (prŏk-**tŏl**-ō-jē) treats diseases of the rectum, sigmoid colon.

psychiatry, psychiatrist (sī-**kī**-ă-trē) diagnoses and treats mental disorders; may prescribe medications.

psychoneuroimmunology, psychoneuroimmunologist (sī-kō-nū-rō-ĭm-mū-**nŏl**-ō-jē) explores the relationship between the immune system and psychological factors.

public health, administrative medicine   is concerned with epidemiology and control of communicable disease; prevention.

radiology, radiologist also **roentgenology, roentgenologist** (rād-ē-ŏl-ō-jē)   uses radiant energy, X-rays, radium, and cobalt in diagnosis and treatment.

sports medicine   concerned with injuries peculiar to participants in sports activities; prevention and treatment.

surgery, surgeon (sŭr-jĕr-ē)   performs general surgery. Specialties: neurosurgery, orthopedic surgery, plastic surgery, thoracic and heart surgery, etc.

trauma (trăw-mă)   see *emergency medicine.*

urology, urologist (ŭ-rŏl-ō-jē)   treats urinary tract diseases; male reproductive organs.

Define:

Specialist _____

Intern "first-year resident" _____

Internist _____

Resident _____

Attending physician _____

Medical examiner _____

Coroner _____

Forensic medicine _____

Worksheet

Name the specialists: What kind of physicians (specialists), other than general practitioners and family practice specialists, could treat a patient with the following health problems?

1. Upper respiratory infection (URI) _internist, pediatrician_____

2. Vaginal infection _____

3. Urinary tract infection (UTI) _____

4. Fractured wrist _____

5. Deep laceration (cut) _____

6. Hay fever, asthma _____

7. Severe sunburn _____

8. Ear infection _____

9. Severe indigestion or food poisoning _____

10. Obesity _____

11. Object embedded in the eyeball _____

12. Bleeding during pregnancy _____

13. Depression _____

14. Heart attack _____

15. Arthritis _____

16. Diabetes _____

17. Cancer _____

18. Mumps _____

19. Epilepsy _____

20. Blurred vision _____

Define:

21. intern _physician still in training, doing practical work_

22. resident _____

23. practitioner _____

24. osteopath _____

25. What does a radiologist do? _____

26. Does an internist treat children? _____

27. Who usually refers a patient to a medical specialist? _____

28. What types of practitioners do acupuncture? _____

29. Patients with leukemia are usually treated by a _____

30. Physician who examines biopsy tissue _____

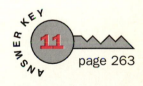

ANSWER KEY **11** page 263

Related Professions

Some confusing terms relate to other physicians and specialists who do not hold the degree of Doctor of Medicine (MD) or Doctor of Osteopathy (DO). They are also called "Doctor" (for example, someone who earns a doctorate in fine arts may be referred to as "Doctor"). Not all "doctors" have an MD.

chiropractor (kī-rō-prăk-tĕr) DC, Doctor of Chiropractic; treats with manipulation only. (chiro = hand)

naturopath (nă-tŭr-ō-păth) treats with "natural" forces or substances, such as vitamins, diets, light, heat, air, and water.

optometrist (ŏp-tŏm-ĕ-trĭst) OD, Doctor of Optometry; treats refractive errors; fits eyeglasses.

pharmacist (făr-mă-sĭst) Pharm. D., Doctor of Pharmacy; licensed to prepare and dispense drugs.

podiatrist (pŏ-**dī**-ă trĭst) DPM, Doctor of Podiatric Medicine; specialist in care of feet, including X-ray, surgery, various therapies, and medication.

psychologist (sī-**kŏl**-ŏ-jĭst) PhD, Doctor of Philosophy, or Psy. D., Doctor of Psychology; group and individual counseling and testing; treats emotional disorders but cannot prescribe medication.

Notice the phone book listings in the Yellow Pages under "Physicians, MD" and "Physicians, DO." Look in the Yellow Pages and make a list of other specialists you find. Note that acupuncture is used by some MDs, DOs, and some DCs.

_____   _____

_____   _____

_____   _____

_____   _____

Worksheet

Name "specialists" who are *not* MDs or DOs:

1. One who tests vision and prescribes eyeglasses _____

2. One who treats with manipulation only _____

3. One who treats *foot* disorders only (including taking X-ray films and surgery) _____

4. One who counsels, tests, and provides therapy for emotional problems _____

True/False: Circle the number of the *true* statements only. Defend your answers. Explain what is "untrue" in the false statements.

5. Doctors, nurses, and physical therapists may all be called practitioners.

6. A resident doctor (after the first year) is working toward or at least considering specialization in one particular field of medicine.

7. An osteopath is the same as a chiropractor.

8. A family doctor is usually a general practitioner (MD or DO).

9. All doctors must renew their license to practice every year.

10. Surgeons may perform general surgery or specialize in one area such as thoracic surgery.

11. All "doctors" are physicians.

12. An intern is still a student (not yet licensed to practice).

Name ten* specialists and their specialty. Define the kinds of patients or conditions each treats.

13. _internist, internal medicine: all nonsurgical cases; no obstetrics_ _____

_____

_____

14. _____

_____

_____

15. _____

_____

_____

16. _____

_____

_____

17. _____

_____

_____

18. _____

_____

_____

19. _____

_____

_____

20. _____

_____

_____

21. _____

_____

_____

22. _____

_____

_____

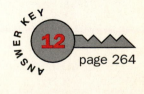

ANSWER KEY **12** page 264

_____

*These are ten of many possibilities.

Allied Health (Paramedical) Personnel

certified medical technologist, CMT   formerly laboratory technician; performs all laboratory procedures; may specialize in one area, such as bacteriology (American Society of Clinical Pathologists).

certified nursing assistant, CNA   one who helps nursing staff perform uncomplicated, routine tasks.

emergency medical technician, EMT   emergency specialist.

licensed practical nurse, LPN/LVN   (vocational) graduate of a one-year program; may perform some duties similar to RN in limited hospital settings. More likely to work in a nursing home or extended care facility.

medical transcriptionist   technician who transcribes medical data.

nurse midwife   RN with additional training; delivers in uncomplicated births.

nurse practitioner, NP   RN with additional preparation, especially in pediatrics, obstetrics; does examinations and some treatment.

nursing unit clerk   assistant to nurses on a nursing unit.

occupational therapist—registered, OTR   similar to RPT but accent on *fine motor* skills, activities of daily living, and job skills.

paramedic   ambulance attendant.

physical therapist   see *registered physical therapist.*

physician's assistant, PA   usually has served an internship with a physician; may also have medical corpsman experience; does examinations, simple suturing, and so on.

public health nurse, PHN   RN with at least a BS degree; works for health departments, schools, or health agencies.

radiologic technologist, RT   takes X-ray films, prepares patient for X-ray films (American Registry of X-ray Technicians).

records technician, MRT   (also called a medical records clerk or librarian) collects, files, organizes, and retrieves medical data

registered nurse, RN   nurse (from two- to four-year program); may work in hospitals, clinics, or offices; may specialize. Often has a BSN, Bachelor of Science in Nursing (four-year program)

registered physical therapist, RPT   performs treatments by physical means such as heat, cold, and exercise; accent on *gross motor* skills.

respiratory therapist or pulmonary therapist, ARRT   treats patients with breathing difficulties; uses machines to facilitate breathing; teaches breathing exercises; conducts postural drainage and nebulizer treatments.

Dental Practitioners and Specialists

endodontist (ĕn-dō-**dŏn**-tĭst)   endodont = inside tooth; treats diseases of pulp, root canal work.

general dentist, DDS and **DMD**   Doctor of Dental Surgery; Doctor of Medical Dentistry; usually treats all ages but may restrict practice to adults only.

gerodontist, gerodon tol ogist (jĕr-ō-**dŏn**-tĭst)   specializes in dental problems of aged.

oral surgeon   extractions, especially complicated ones; maxillofacial trauma cases, congenital defects such as cleft palate.

orthodontist (ŏr-thō-**dŏn**-tĭst)   treats maloc **clu** sion with braces, retainers.

pedodontist (pēd-ō-**dŏn**-tĭst)   specializes in treating children.

periodontist (pĕr-ē-ō-**dŏn**-tĭst)   periodont = around teeth; treats gum diseases such as gingivitis; performs surgery and deep cleaning, gingivectomy.

prosthodontist (prŏs-thō-**dŏn**-tĭst)   prosthesis = false part; dentures, bridgework, artificial appliances.

Paradental Personnel

dental hygienist   does prophylactic dental care; cleaning, teaching patients proper prophylactic care; takes X-rays.

chairside dental assistant   assists dentist with fillings, suction, instruments, etc.

The educational requirements for the preceding personnel vary considerably, from one year for LPN and dental assistant to four years or more for others (eight or more for dental specialties).

There are many other kinds of assistants and technicians with varying years of training. It is often difficult to know "who's who". Other technicians include: surgical technologist, central service aide, psychiatric aide, cardiac technician, biomed technician, EEG technician, pharmacist assistant, nuclear medicine technician, phlebotomist, and those nursing assistants or aides (who are not certified).

Self-Test

Give the meaning for the following word parts. Later, cover word part (first column) and fill in remainder.

Word part	Meaning	Word part	Example word
-oscope	lighted instrument inserted into organ	-oscope	cytoscope
-oscopy			
-tome			
-ograph			
-ography			
-meter			
-ogram			
-ologist			
-ist			

Word part	Meaning	Word part	Example word
-iatrist	_____	_____	_____
	_____		
-ician	_____	_____	_____
	_____		
-iatro	_____	_____	_____
	_____		

Give the meaning of the following abbreviations. Later, cover the abbreviations (first column) and fill in the last column.

	Meaning	Abbreviation
MD	_doctor of medicine_	_____
DO	_____	_____
DDS	_____	_____
RN	_____	_____
LPN	_____	_____
RPT	_____	_____
RT	_____	_____
CMT	_____	_____
OTR	_____	_____

Fill in the blanks:

1. An internist is a specialist in (name the specialty). _____

2. The specialist who interprets X-ray films is a _____

3. The specialist who treats bone injury or disease is _____

4. The specialist who studies tissues after death as well as organs removed during surgery is a _____

    _____

5. The "combined" specialty that treats women only is _____

6. Define _prophy_ **_lac_** _tic:_ _____

7. Define _paramedical:_ _____

8. Is a _technician_ the same as a _technologist?_ _____

No Answer Key
(If you had difficulty, review the chapter.)

Test p. 289

By this time you should be feeling a sense of accomplishment. If you find that certain words are especially difficult for you, look them up in a medical dictionary. Practice writing and rewriting them. Make and use flash cards. Discuss your problem with the instructor.

You may now be given a **review test** for Chapters 1–5, which can be found on page 291 in Appendix F. Before taking the review test, you may want to complete the following review exercise. So far you have learned how to construct words that describe surgical procedures, medical conditions and diseases, medical instruments and machines, and medical specialists and specialties.

You will now move on to learn additional word parts, plural endings, and terms for bacteria and colors. Remember to continue to review the completed chapters so that you do not forget what you have learned.

Review

Below is an alphabetical listing of example words formed from the root words listed in Chapter 1. Write the definition for each word.

1. abdominopelvic — *pertaining to the abdomen and pelvis*
2. adenectomy _____
3. anal _____
4. androgen _____
5. angiogram _____
6. appendectomy _____
7. appendicitis _____
8. arteriosclerosis _____
9. arthritis _____
10. bronchitis _____
11. electrocardiogram _____
12. cephalic _____
13. cerebral _____
14. cheiloplasty _____
15. cholecystectomy _____
16. choledochostomy _____
17. chondrectomy _____
18. colostomy _____

19. colposcope   _____

20. costal   _____

21. cranial   _____

22. cystitis   _____

23. dentist   _____

24. dermabrasion   _____

25. dermatologist   _____

26. duodenectomy   _____

27. encephalitis   _____

28. esophagitis   _____

29. gastrectomy   _____

30. glossitis   _____

31. gynecology   _____

32. hepatitis   _____

33. hysterectomy   _____

34. ileostomy   _____

35. iridectomy   _____

36. jejunitis   _____

37. keratoplasty   _____

38. keratosis   _____

39. laminectomy   _____

40. laparotomy   _____

41. sublingual   _____

42. lobectomy   _____

43. mastectomy   _____

44. mammoplasty   _____

45. myositis   _____

46. osteomyelitis   _____

47. myelogram   _____

48. myringotomy   _____

49. nephrectomy   _____

50. neuritis   _____

51. oophorectomy   _____

52. ophthalmologist   _____

53. orchitis   _____

54. orchidoplasty   _____

55. osteochondritis _____

56. otoscope _____

57. pancreatectomy _____

58. pharyngitis _____

59. phlebitis _____

60. pneumonia _____

61. podiatry _____

62. proctoscope _____

63. prostatectomy _____

64. pyelitis _____

65. rectal _____

66. renal failure _____

67. rhinoplasty _____

68. sacroiliac _____

69. salpingectomy _____

70. splenectomy _____

71. spondylitis _____

72. stethoscope _____

73. stomatitis _____

74. tendinitis _____

75. tenoplasty _____

76. thoracic _____

77. thyroidectomy _____

78. tracheotomy _____

79. tympanectomy _____

80. ureterectomy _____

81. urethritis _____

82. vasoconstriction _____

83. venogram _____

No Answer Key (Review the chapter)

CHAPTER 6

Plural Endings

List of Plural Endings

Study the following examples. Write the plural form and define the example word:

Singular	Plural	Example/Pronunciation	Give plural form and define
a	ae (pronounced ī, ē, or ā*)	vertebra (**věr**-tě-brǎ)	vertebrae; bones of spine
		bursa (**bŭr**-sǎ)	_____
		gingiva (**jĭn**-jĭv-ǎ)	_____
		fascia (**făs**-sē-ǎ)	_____
		petechia (pě-**tě**-kē-ǎ)	_____
		sequela (sē-**kwě**-lǎ)	_____
um	a	memorandum (měm-ō-**rǎn**-dŭm)	_____
		speculum (**spěk**-ū-lŭm)	_____
		diverticulum (dī-věr-**tĭk**-ū-lŭm)	_____
		ovum (**ō**-vŭm)	_____
		datum (**dǎ**-tŭm)	_____
		serum (**sě**-rŭm)	_____
		medium (**mē**-dē-ŭm) (culture medium)	_____
		bacterium (băk-**tēr**-ē-ŭm)	_____
us	i	coccus (**kŏk**-kŭs)	_____
		bacillus (bă-**sĭl**-lŭs)	_____

---

* Dictionaries do not agree on pronunciation, and many do not give *any* pronunciation for the plural form.

Singular	Plural	Example/Pronunciation	Give plural form and define
		focus (**fō**-kŭs)	_____
		nucleus (**nū**-klē-ŭs)	_____
		thrombus (**thrŏm**-bŭs)	_____
		uterus (**ū**-tĕr-ŭs)	_____
		fungus (**fŭn**-gŭs)	_____
is	es	diagnosis (dī-ăg-**nō**-sĭs)	_____
		urinalysis (ūr-ĭ-**năl**-ĭ-sĭs)	_____
		crisis (**krī**-sĭs)	_____
		testis (**tĕs**-tĭs)	_____
ex, ix	ices	apex (**ā**-pĕks)	_____
		cervix (**sĕr**-vĭks)	_____
		appendix (ăp-**pĕn**-dĭks)	_____
ma	mata	enema (**ĕn**-ĕm-ă)	_____
		carcinoma (kăr-sĭ-**nō**-mă)	_____
inx	inges	meninx (**mĕn**-ĭnks)	_____
anx	anges	phalanx (**fā**-lănks)	_____
ur	ora	femur (**fē**-mŭr)	_____
en	ina	lumen (**lū**-mĕn)	_____
an	a	protozoan (prō-tō-**zō**-ăn)	_____

No Answer Key

![ ] **Self-Test**

Write the plural form:

1. vertebra _vertebrae_____
2. ovum _____
3. diagnosis _____
4. thrombus _____
5. apex _____

6. enema _____
7. coccus _____
8. medium _____
9. nucleus _____
10. bursa _____

Write the singular form:

11. bacteria _____

12. data _____

13. crises _____

14. prognoses _____

15. uteri _____

16. specula _____

17. carcinomata _____

18. gingivae _____

19. foci _____

20. appendices _____

Fill in the blank:

21. The medical laboratory uses many different kinds of culture _____ (on which to grow bacteria).

22. Many books have an appendix. Some large reference books have many _____

23. Tiny pinpoint hemorrhages are called _____

24. Diverticula is the plural of _____

25. Protozoan is the singular of _____

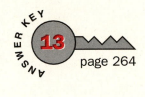

ANSWER KEY 13 page 264

Test p. 295

CHAPTER 7

Additional Prefixes

List of Prefixes

Study the prefix and meaning, then define the examples. (Use a dictionary if needed.) Some of these have been presented earlier, and will serve as a review.

Prefix	Meaning	Example/Pronunciation	Define
a-, an-	without, not	afebrile (ā-**fĕb**-rīl)	1. _without fever_
		anesthesia (ăn-ĕs-**thē**-sē-ă)	2.
		apnea (**ăp**-nē-ă)	3.
bio-	life	bioavailability (bī-ō-ă-vāl-ă-**bĭl**-ĭ-tē)	4.
		bioethics (bī-ō-**ĕth**-ĭks)	5.
brady-	slow	bradycardia (brā-dē-**kăr**-dē-ă)	6.
tachy-	fast	tachycardia (tăk-ĕ-**kăr**-dē-ă)	7.
de-	take away, remove	dehydrate (dē-**hī**-drāt)	8.
re-	put back	rehydrate (rē-**hī**-drāt)	9.
		recurrence (rē-**kŭr**-ĕns)	10.

Prefix	Meaning	Example/Pronunciation	Define
dia-	through (as in running through)	diarrhea (dī-ă-**rē**-ă)	11. _____
		diuresis (dī-ū-**rē**-sĭs)	12. _____
hemi-	one side, half	hemiplegia (hĕm-ĭ-**plĕ**-jē-ă)	13. _____
hemo-	blood	hematemesis (hĕm-ăt-**ĕm**-ĕ-sĭs)	14. _____
hydro-	water	hydrate (**hī**-drāt) also dehydrate	15. _____
hyper-	high; too much	hypertension* (hī-pĕr-**tĕn**-shŭn)	16. _____
		hyperactive (hī-pĕr-**ăk**-tĭv)	17. _____
hypo-	low; not enough; under	hypotension (hī-pō-**tĕn**-shŭn)	18. _____
		hypodermic (hī-pō-**dĕr**-mĭk)	19. _____
		hypothyroid (hī-pō-**thī**-rōyd)	20. _____
lip-	fat	lipoma (lĭ-**pō**-mă)	21. _____
poly-	many, much	polyuria (pŏl-ē-**ŭ**-rē-ă)	22. _____
		polycystic (pŏl-ē-**sĭs**-tĭk)	23. _____
pre-	before	preoperative (prē-**ŏp**-ĕr-ă-tĭv)	24. _____
		prenatal (prē-**nā**-tăl)	25. _____
pro-	preceding, coming	prognosis (prŏg-**nō**-sĭs)	26. _____

---

*Does not mean "tension" in this word.

Prefix	Meaning	Example/Pronunciation	Define
		prodromal (prō-**drō**-măl) (-drome = running)	27._____
post-	following, after	postoperative (pōst-**ŏp**-ĕr-ă-tĭv)	28._____
		postpartum (-partus = birth) (pŏst-**păr**-tŭm)	29._____

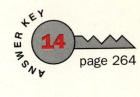

ANSWER KEY **14** page 264

Worksheet

a-, an-: Remember that this little prefix completely changes the meaning of a word.

Define: Learn these words for future use!

1. a **feb** rile   without fever (normal temperature)_____
2. apy **rex** ia   _____
3. a **typ** ical   _____
4. a **pha** sia   _____
5. **ap** nea   _____
6. **at** rophy   _____
7. anes **the** sia   _____
8. anal **ge** sia   _____
9. anaer **o** bic   _____
10. ar **rhyth** mia   _____
11. a **sep** sis   _____
12. asympto **mat** ic   _____
13. amenor **rhe** a   _____
14. a **nox** ia   _____
15. atrau **mat** ic   _____

16. a **pha** gia _____

17. a **vas** cular _____

18. ano **rex** ia _____

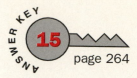

ANSWER KEY 15 page 264

Make a list of words using these prefixes and define the words. Some words with these prefixes were introduced in Chapter 3. Use the dictionary if necessary.

	Word	Define
hyper-	_____	_____
	_____	_____
	_____	_____
	_____	_____
	_____	_____
hypo-	_____	_____
	_____	_____
	_____	_____
	_____	_____
dys-	_____	_____
	_____	_____
	_____	_____
	_____	_____
pre-	_____	_____
	_____	_____
	_____	_____
	_____	_____

	Word	*Define*
anti-	_____	_____
	_____	_____
	_____	_____
	_____	_____
	_____	_____
post-	_____	_____
	_____	_____
	_____	_____
	_____	_____
poly-	_____	_____
	_____	_____
	_____	_____
	_____	_____
	_____	_____

▦ Self-Test

True/False: If a word is misspelled, the statement is false. (Remember, one letter can change the meaning of the word.) Circle the number of the *true* statements only. Explain why the statement is false.

1. If *febrile* means "fever," *afebrile* means "without fever."

2. *Bioavailability* means "amount of drug actually reaching body tissues."

3. *Hyper-* is the opposite of *hypo-*.

4. Dyspnea is the same as apnea.

5. *Postpartum* means "following childbirth."

6. If *esthesia* means "feeling," *anethesia* means "without feeling."

Correct spelling: Mark an X after the *correctly* spelled word.

7. antehistamine _____ antihistamine _____

8. hypodermic _____ hypadermic _____

9. tackycardia _____ tachycardia _____

10. prenatel   _____   prenatal   _____

11. hemiplegia   _____   hemoplegia   _____

12. anemia   _____   aremia   _____

Define:

13. anaer **o** bic   *without air (oxygen)*

14. a **ne** mia

15. **at** rophy

16. anal **ge** sic

17. bio **eth** ics

18. bio **feed** back

19. de **hy** drate

20. hyper **ten** sion

21. hypo **thy** roid

22. prog **no** sis

23. post **op** erative

24. poly **u** ria

25. tachy **car** dia

26. pre **men** strual

27. pro **dro** mal

28. hyper **ther** mia

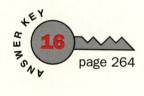

ANSWER KEY **16** page 264

More Prefixes

Define the following example words. In analyzing the example words, it will help if you separate the word parts. For example:

     acro = extremities
     derma = skin
     itis = inflammation

     Meaning: Skin on the extremities is inflamed.

Prefix	Meaning	Example/Pronunciation	Define	
acro-	extremities, top or extreme point	acrodermatitis (ăk-rō-dĕr-mă-**tī**-tĭs)	1.	*skin inflammation of extremities*
		acrocephaly (ăk-rō-**sĕf**-ăl-ē)	2.	
aero-	air	aerobic (ăyr-**ō**-bĭk)	3.	
		anaerobic (ăn-ăyr-**ō**-bĭk)	4.	
aniso- (see *iso-*)	unequal	anisocytosis (ăn-ī-sō-sī-**tō**-sĭs)	5.	
dys-	bad, painful, difficult	dystocia (dĭs-**tō**-shă)	6.	
		dysphoria (dĭs-**fŏr**-ē-ă)	7.	
		dysplasia (dĭs-**plā**-zē-ă)	8.	
eu-	good, easy	eutocia (ū-**tō**-shă)	9.	
		euphoria (ū-**fŏr**-ē-ă)	10.	
		euthanasia (ū-thă-**nā**-zē-ă)	11.	
hetero-	different	heterosexual (hĕt-ĕr-ō-**sĕk**-shū-ăl)	12.	
		heterogeneous (hĕt-ĕr-ō-**jē**-nē-ŭs)	13.	
homo-	same	homosexual (hō-mō-**sĕk**-shū-ăl)	14.	
		homophobia (hō-mō-**fō**-bē-ă)	15.	
		homogeneous (hō-mō-**jē**-nē-ŭs)	16.	
		homeostasis (hō-mē-ō-**stā**-sĭs) (statis = standing still)	17.	
iso-	equal, same	isocytosis (ī-sō-sī-**tō**-sĭs)	18.	
		isotonic (ī-sō-**tŏn**-ĭk)	19.	
		isothermal (ī-sō-**thĕr**-măl)	20.	
mal-	bad, poor	malaise (mă-**lāz**)	21.	
		malocclusion (măl-ō-**klū**-zhŭn)	22.	
megalo-, -megaly	large (enlarged)	acromegaly (ăk-rō-**mĕg**-ă-lē)	23.	
		megalocardia (mĕg-ă-lō-**kăr**-dē-ă) cardiomegaly (kăr-dē-ō-**mĕg**-ă-lē)	24.	
meno-	menses (menstruation)	menopause (**mĕn**-ō-păws)	25.	
		dysmenorrhea (dĭs-mĕn-ŏr-**rē**-ă)	26.	
noct-, nyct-	night	nocturia (nŏk-**tū**-rē-ă), nycturia (nĭk-**tū**-rē-ă)	27.	

Prefix	Meaning	Example/Pronunciation	Define
pan-	all, every	pandemic (păn-**děm**-ĭk)	28. _____
sym-	going together, united	symptom (**sĭmp**-tŏm)	29. _____
syn-	going together, united	syndrome (**sĭn**-drōm)	30. _____

Check a medical dictionary for specific syndromes. Make a list and define.

<u>Down syndrome*</u>

_____

_____

_____

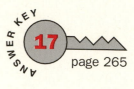

ANSWER KEY **17** page 265

Review

Define each of the prefixes listed below. At another time, cover the first column and see if you can look at the definition and give an example word.

Prefix	Define	Example
a-, an-	_____	_____
acro-	_____	_____
aero-	_____	_____
aniso-	_____	_____
anti-	_____	_____
brady-	_____	_____
de-	_____	_____
dia-	_____	_____
dys-	_____	_____

_____

*Formerly Down's syndrome

Prefix	Define	Example
eu-	_____	_____
hemi-	_____	_____
hemo-	_____	_____
hetero-	_____	_____
homo-	_____	_____
hyper-	_____	_____
hypo-	_____	_____
hydro-	_____	_____
lip-	_____	_____
mal-	_____	_____
megalo-	_____	_____
meno-	_____	_____
noct-	_____	_____
nyct-	_____	_____
pan-	_____	_____
pre-	_____	_____
pro-	_____	_____
post-	_____	_____
poly-	_____	_____
sym-	_____	_____
syn-	_____	_____
tachy-	_____	_____

No Answer Key

Test p. 297

CHAPTER 8

Additional Suffixes and Root Words

List of Suffixes

Study the structure of and define the following example words. Some of these should be familiar to you, as they have been used in examples in preceding lessons.

Suffix	Meaning	Example/Pronunciation	Define
-o/lysis	destruction, to separate out	hemolysis (hē-**mŏl**-ĭ-sĭs)	*destruction of blood*
		osteolysis (ŏs-tē-**ŏl**-ĭ-sĭs)	
		chemonucleolysis (kē-mō-nū-klē-**ŏl**-ĭ-sĭs)	
-o/lytic		hemolytic* (hē-mō-**lĭt**-ĭk)	
-o/lyzed		hemolyzed (**hē**-mō-līzd)	
-oma	tumor (new growth), neoplasm, space-occupying lesion	carcinoma (kăr-sĭ-**nō**-mă)	
		sarcoma (săr-**kō**-mă)	
	swelling	hematoma (hē-mă-**tō**-mă)	
-oid	like, similar to	lipoid (**lĭp**-ŏyd)	
		polypoid (**pŏl**-ē-pŏyd)	
		mucoid (**mū**-kŏyd)	
		sesamoid (**sĕs**-ă-mŏyd)	
		thyroid (**thī**-rŏyd)	
		xiphoid (**zī**-fōyd)	
-plasia	growth (cells)	hyperplasia (hī-pĕr-**plā**-zē-ă)	
-trophy	development	hypertrophy (hī-**pĕr**-trŏ-fē) (note pronunciation)	
-malacia	softening	osteomalacia (ŏs-tē-ō-mă-**lā**-shē-ă)	

---

*Hemolytic streptococcus is an organism that destroys red blood cells.

Suffix	Meaning	Example/Pronunciation	Define
		encephalomalacia (ĕn-sĕf-ă-lō-mă-**lā**-shē-ă)	_____
-orrhea	flow or discharge	pyorrhea (py = pus) (pī-ŏr-**rē**-ă)	_____
		diarrhea (dī-ăr-**rē**-ă)	_____
-pnea	breathing, air, lungs	dyspnea (**dĭsp**-nē-ă)	_____
(also pneumo-)		pneumonia (nū-**mō**-nē-ă)	_____
		pneumonitis (nū-mō-**nī**-tĭs)	_____
-plegia	paralysis	hemiplegia (hēm-ĭ-**plē**-jē-ă)	_____
		paraplegia (pă-ră-**plē**-jē-ă)	_____
		quadriplegia (kwă-drĭ-**plē**-jē-ă)	_____
		tetraplegia (tĕ-tră-**plē**-jē-ă)	_____
-paresis	weakness (less than paralysis)	hemiparesis (hĕm-ĭ-**păr**-ĕ-sĭs)	_____

No Answer Key

An Important Word

Genesis: the origin or coming into being of something; production; birth. Many words are derived from *genesis:*

gene (jēn) the unit of heredity (Greek *gennin* = to produce)

genetics (jĕ-nĕt-ĭks) branch of biology that deals with heredity (beginnings)

pathogen (păth-ō-jĕn) bacterium (or virus) that causes disease (from which disease begins)

genitals (jĕn-ĭt-ăls) organs of reproduction (from which life begins)

homogenous or **homogeneous** (hō-mŏj-ĕn-ŭs) derived from like source; uniform; the same throughout, as in homogenized milk.

Gen may come at the beginning of a word, in the middle of a word, or at the end of a word. Whenever you see it, think of *genesis* and see if you can figure out the meaning of the word. (*Gen* comes from the Greek; similar word from the French means something different.)

![pink bar] **Worksheet**

Define the following *-oma* words. The accent pattern is always **-o** *ma.* You will need a dictionary.

1. ade **no** ma   *tumor of a gland (epithelial tissue)* _____

2. carci **no** ma _____

3. fi **bro** ma _____

4. gli **o** ma (glia cells = supporting tissue of brain and spinal cord) _____

5. hepa **to** ma _____

6. lym **pho** ma _____

7. granu **lo** ma _____

8. mye **lo** ma _____

9. my **o** ma _____

10. sar **co** ma _____

11. hema **to** ma _____

12. glau **co** ma (not a tumor) _____

Define the following -*pnea* words. The accent pattern is usually -*p* **ne** *a.* The adjective form is shown in parentheses.

13. **dysp** nea, also dysp **ne** a (dysp **ne** ic) _____

14. **ap** nea, also ap **ne** a (ap **ne** ic) _____

15. or **thop** nea (orthop **ne** ic) _____

16. tachyp **ne** a (tachyp **ne** ic) _____

17. bradyp **ne** a (bradyp **ne** ic) _____

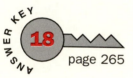

ANSWER KEY **18** page 265

■ **Note:** *-oma* at the end of a word means "a tumor or swelling." Tumors are neoplasms—new "things" formed; new growths. Tumors may be benign (innocent) or malignant (deadly, cancerous). Malignant tumors me **tas** tasize (spread to other parts of the body). A cancerous tumor that has not metastasized or infiltrated surrounding tissue is called *in situ* (ĭn-**sī**-tū, meaning "in position"). An in situ tumor is a primary tumor. A secondary tumor is a *meta* **stat** *ic* tumor. Benign lesions do not metastasize, but many grow large enough to cause obstruction.

Carcinoma and sarcoma always mean malignancy; for example, adenocarci **no** ma, lymphosar **co** ma.

■ **Note:** *-pnea* words are often used in the adjectival form. For example, we usually say "the patient is *dysp* **ne** *ic*" (instead of "the patient has dyspnea") or "the patient is *orthop* **ne** *ic*" (instead of "the patient has orthopnea"). Therefore, the spelling of the adjective is important.

▨ **Self-Test**

Give the correct word for the following definitions:

1. A tumor of fat ___lipoma___

2. A tumor of blood (clot) _____

3. Resembling mucus _____

4. Overdeveloped (as with muscles) _____

5. Difficult breathing _____

6. Very rapid breathing _____

7. Paralysis on one side of the body _____

8. Paralysis of the lower half of body (waist down) _____

9. Flow of pus _____

10. "Running through" of stool or feces (bowel movement) _____

11. Softening of the bones _____

12. Destruction of blood (cells) _____

13. Cancerous or malignant tumor _____

14. Without breathing (adjective) _____

15. Able to breathe only when sitting upright _____

Define:

16. ho **mog** enized   *same throughout; particles dispersed evenly* _____

17. quadri **ple** gia _____

18. **lip** oid _____

19. gene _____

20. hemi **par** esis _____

21. **gen** itals _____

22. ade **no** ma _____

23. pneumo **ni** tis _____

24. hyper **pla** sia _____

25. **path** ogen _____

26. Is a meta **stat** ic tumor a malignant tumor? (yes or no) _____

27. in **si** tu _____

28. secondary tumor _____

29. **ne** oplasm _____

30. li **pol** ysis _____

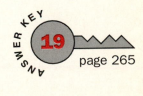

page 265

Suffix Review

Some of these suffixes have been used in preceding lessons in example words. This will serve as a review. Define the examples:

Suffix	Meaning	Example/Pronunciation	Define
-orrhexis	break open	hysterorrhexis (**hǐs**-tĕr-ŏr-x-ǐs)	*rupture of the uterus*
		angiorrhexis (ăn-jē-ŏr-**rĕk**-sǐs)	
-spasm	spasm, contraction, twitching	neurospasm (**nŭ**-rō-spăzm)	
		laryngospasm (lă-**rǐnj**-ō-spăzm)	
-gnos	knowledge	prognosis (prŏg-**nō**-sǐs)	
		diagnosis (dī-ăg-**nō**-sǐs)	
-drome	running	syndrome (**sǐn**-drōm)	
		prodromal (prō-**drō**-măl)	
-opia	vision	myopia* (mī-**ō**-pē-ă)	
		diplopia (dǐ-**plō**-pē-ă)	

Some word parts can be used at the beginning or at the end of a word, such as in the following examples:

Word part	Meaning	Example/Pronunciation	Define
megalo-, mega-, megaly	large	acromegaly (ăk-rō-**mĕg**-ă-lē)	
		megalomania (mĕ-gă-lō-**mā**-nē-ă)	
		cardiomegaly (kăr-dē-ō-**mĕg**-ă-lē)	
		megalocardia (mĕg-ă-lō-**kăr**-dē-ă)	
		megacolon (mĕg-ă-**kō**-lŏn)	
		organomegaly (ŏr-găn-ō-**mĕg**-ă-lē)	
phago-, -phagia	eat	dysphagia (dǐs-**fā**-jē-ă)	
		phagocytosis (făg-ō-sī-**tō**-sǐs)	
therm-, -thermy	heat	thermometer (thĕr-**mŏm**-ĕt-ĕr)	
		diathermy (**dī**-ă-thĕr-mē)	
		thermotherapy (thĕr-mō-**thĕr**-ă-pē)	

---

*my does not mean "muscle" in this word. It means "to squint," which is a tendency for nearsighted people.

Some prefixes and suffixes that are not entirely similar have the same meaning. Note these examples.

Meaning	Prefix	Suffix	Example/Pronunciation	Define
urine	ur-, uro-	-uria	uremia (ū-**rē**-mē-ă)	_____
			urogenital (ū-rō-**jĕn**-ĭ-tăl)	_____
			urinalysis (ū-rĭ-**năl**-ĭ-sĭs)	_____
			nocturia (nŏk-**tŭ**-rē-ă)	_____
			polyuria (pŏl-ē-**ū**-rē-ă)	_____
			hematuria (hē-mă-**tū**-rē-ă)	_____
			pyuria (pī-**ū**-rē-ă)	_____
			diuresis (dī-ū-**rē**-sĭs)	_____
			diuretic (dī-ū-**rĕt**-ĭk)	_____
blood	hem/o, hema, hemat/o	-emia	hemorrhage (**hĕm**-ĕ-rĭj)	_____
			hematology (hē-mă-**tŏl**-ō-jē)	_____
			hemoglobin (**hē**-mō-glō-bĭn)	_____
			hemarthrosis (hĕm-ăr-**thrō**-sĭs)	_____
			hemoptysis (hē-**mŏp**-tĭ-sĭs)	_____
			hematemesis (hĕm-ă-**tĕm**-ĕ-sĭs)	_____
			hemangioma (hē-măn-jē-**ō**-mă)	_____
			anemia (ă-**nē**-mē-ă)	_____
			leukemia (lū-**kē**-mē-ă)	_____
			azotemia (ăz-ō-**tē**-mē-ă)	_____

No Answer Key

List of Root Words

Study the structure of the following examples, then define them. One of the more difficult ones has been done for you.

Root word	Meaning	Example/Pronunciation	Define
ankylo	stiffening (with adhesion formation) or fusion by surgery	ankylosis (ăn-kĭ-**lō**-sĭs)	_condition of stiffening_
bio	life	biology (bī-**ŏl**-ō-jē)	_____
		bioethics (bī-ō-**ĕth**-ĭks)	_____
carcino	cancer (malignancy)	carcinoma (kăr-sĭ-**nō**-mă)	_____

Root word	Meaning	Example/Pronunciation	Define
cryo	cold	cryosurgery (krī-ō-**sŭr**-jĕr-ē)	_____
		cryoextraction (krī-ō-ĕks-**trăk**-shŭn) (of lens)	_____
cyt/o	cell	cytometer (sī-**tŏm**-ĕt-ĕr)	_____
		cytoplasm (**sī**-tō-plăzm)	_____
		leukocyte (**lū**-kō-sīt)	_____
crypt	hidden (small, hidden sacs, especially anal)	cryptitis (krĭp-**tī**-tĭs)	_____
		cryptorchidism (krĭpt-**ŏr**-kĭd-ĭzm)	_____
esthesia	feeling	anesthesia (ăn-ĕs-**thē**-sē-ă)	_____
gravid	pregnant	primigravida (prī-mĭ-**grăv**-ĭ-dă)	_____
hem/o	blood	hemostat (**hēm**-ō-stăt)	_____
		hemolysis (hē-**mŏl**-ĭ-sĭs)	_____
hydr/o	water	hydrophobia (hī-drō-**fō**-bē-ă)	_____
		hydrotherapy (hī-drō-**thĕr**-ă-pē)	_____
laryng/o	larynx (voice box)	laryngitis (lăr-ĭn-**jī**-tĭs)	_____
lip	fat	lipoma (lĭ-**pō**-mă)	_____
also adipo		adipoma (ăd-ĭ-**pō**-mă)	_____
also steato		steatoma (stē-ă-**tō**-mă)	_____
		lipectomy (lĭ-**pĕk**-tō-mē)	_____
lith	stone	cholelithiasis* (kō-lĕ-lĭ-**thī**-ă-sĭs)	_____
		lithoptripsy (**lĭth**-ō-trĭp-sē)	_____
necro	dead (decayed)	necrosis (nĕ-**krō**-sĭs)	_____
onych/o	nail	paronychia (păr-ō-**nĭk**-ē-ă)	_____
orchid/o	testes	orchidoplasty (**ŏr**-kĭd-ō-plăs-tē)	_____
par/o	to bear (children)	multipara (mŭl-**tĭp**-ă-ră)	_____
path	disease	pathology (pă-**thŏl**-ŏ-jē)	_____
		pathogenic (păth-ŏ-**jĕn**-ĭk)	_____
pelvi	pelvis	pelvimeter (pĕl-**vĭm**-ĕt-ĕr)	_____
phago-, -phagia	eating, swallowing	phagocytosis (făg-ō-sī-**tō**-sĭs)	_____
		dysphagia (dĭs-**fā**-jē-ă)	_____
phasia	speech	aphasia (ă-**fā**-zē-ă)	_____

*-_iasis_ means the same as -_osis_, but is only used in certain words.

Root word	Meaning	Example/Pronunciation	Define
phonia	voice	aphonia (ă-**fō**-nē-ă)	_____
psych/o	mind	psychology (sī-**kŏl**-ō-jē)	_____
pub/o	pubic bones	supra pubic (sū-pră **pū**-bĭk) (supra = above)	_____
pyo	pus	pyogenic (pī-ō-**jĕn**-ĭk)	_____
		pyorrhea (pī-ŏr-**rē**-ă)	_____
schizo	split	schizophrenia (skĭz-ō-**frĕ**-nē-ă) (phren = mind)	_____
sclero	hardening	arteriosclerosis (ăr-tēr-ē-ō-sklĕ-**rō**-sĭs)	_____
soma, somat/o	body	psychosomatic (sī-kō-sō-**mă**-tĭk)	_____
stasis	slowed down (sluggish)	hemostasis (hē-mō-**stā**-sĭs)	_____
tars/o	ankle	metatarsal (mĕt-ă-**tăr**-săl)	_____
therapy	treatment (to cure or alleviate symptoms)	sclerotherapy (sklĕr-ō-**thĕr**-ă-pē)	_____
		chemotherapy (kē-mō-**thĕr**-ă-pē)	_____
		therapeutic (thĕr-ă-**pū**-tĭk)	_____
therm	heat	diathermy (**dī**-ă-thĕr-mē)	_____
		hyperthermia (hī-pĕr-**thĕr**-mē-ă)	_____
		thermometer (thĕr-**mŏm**-ĕt-ĕr)	_____
thrombo	clot	thrombosis (thrŏm-**bŏ**-sĭs)	_____
trauma	injury	traumatic (trăw-**mă**-tĭk)	_____

No Answer Key

Worksheet

Fill in the meaning of the given root word and check your answers. After you feel you know them, cover the given root word and complete the drill using the meaning you have given. Do this as many times as necessary until you are familiar with the material.

Root word	Meaning	Root word	Example word
ankyl/o	*stiffening*	*ankyl/o*	*ankylosis*
gravid	_____	_____	_____
par/o	_____	_____	_____

Root word	Meaning	Root word	Example word
esthesia	_____	_____	_____
lith/o	_____	_____	_____
necr/o	_____	_____	_____
cryo	_____	_____	_____
lip/o	_____	_____	_____
crypt	_____	_____	_____
path/o	_____	_____	_____
megalo-	_____	_____	_____
-megaly	_____	_____	_____
phag/o	_____	_____	_____
cyt/o	_____	_____	_____
hydr/o	_____	_____	_____
-phagia	_____	_____	_____
phasia	_____	_____	_____
schizo-	_____	_____	_____
scler/o	_____	_____	_____
stasis	_____	_____	_____
therapy	_____	_____	_____
therm/o	_____	_____	_____
thromb/o	_____	_____	_____
trauma	_____	_____	_____
hem/o	_____	_____	_____
ur/o	_____	_____	_____
hetero-	_____	_____	_____
aero-	_____	_____	_____

Write the word endings that pertain to surgical procedures and some words using them.

Word ending	Example	Word ending	Example
-ectomy	tonsillectomy	_____	_____
_____	_____	_____	_____
_____	_____	_____	_____
_____	_____	_____	_____

Word ending	Example	Word ending	Example
-itis	_pneumonitis_		
___	___	___	___
___	___	___	___
___	___	___	___

No Answer Key

Test p. 299

CHAPTER 9

Bacteria, Colors, and Review

Bacteria

Bacteria is a plural word. The singular is *bacterium*. The study of bacteria is a complex and fascinating one, but beyond the scope of this course. However, some basic concepts and terms are essential. *Micro* means small, and because of the size of bacteria, they are called microorganisms. The two terms *microbi* **ol** ogy and *bacteri* **ol** ogy mean essentially the same thing—the study of small life. Related subjects are *my* **col** ogy, *parasi* **tol** ogy, and *vi* **rol** ogy. (What do these terms mean?)

Characteristics of Microorganisms

Shape

cocci (**kŏk**-sī)   round or spherical shape (singular = coccus (**kŏk**-ŭs)

Some formations and examples:

diplo   in pairs; diplococcus, as in gonococcus

strepto   in chain formation, as in streptococcus

staphylo   in clusters or bunches, as in staphylococcus

bacilli (bă-**sĭl**-ī)   rod shape (singular = bacillus [bă-**sĭl**-ŭs])

How They Grow

colonies   vary in size, shape, color, consistency; may be smooth, moist, glistening, pearly, raised, translucent, white or colored, irregular or even

Food and Air Requirements

aerobic   need oxygen

anaerobic   grow in absence of oxygen

facultative   may grow either way

culture media   food; examples are plain agar, broth, blood agar, chocolate agar, meat extract

Special Characteristics

motile (able to move), nonmotile, spore forming, flagellated, encapsulated

Understanding the characteristics of microorganisms and their growth requirements enables the practitioner to distinguish organisms, to control their growth, reproduction, and spread; this is important in treating diseases.

Pathogenic Organisms

Pathogenic organisms are those that cause disease. They do this in a variety of ways: by attacking and destroying cells, producing poisons called toxins, competing with host tissue for available nourishment, and causing violent allergic reactions in some people. The factors involved in whether a person succumbs to a bacterial disease (or many other diseases) are:

the general health of the person; *resistance*
the numbers and strength of the *organisms; virulence*
the presence of *favorable conditions* of growth

The formula:

the resistance of the host (human being)
> *versus*
the virulence of the organism (bacteria, virus)

This is exactly what makes Acquired Immune Deficiency Syndrome (AIDS) so deadly. The AIDS virus renders the individual vulnerable by reducing the effectiveness of the body's immune system. This allows "opportunistic" organisms (OIs) to invade the body and in many cases cause death. OIs only affect a person whose resistance is low.

Important Differences Between Bacteria and Viruses

Bacteria are larger, easily grown in the laboratory (in vitro), and can be seen with regular microscopes. Generally they can be treated successfully with antibiotics however, many bacteria are now becoming resistant to antibiotics.

Viruses are so small that they can only be seen with an electron microscope, cannot be grown on artificial media, need a live medium such as embryonated egg yolk (in vivo), and are not successfully treated by antibiotics.

Colors

Study the structure of the following examples, then define them.

Root word	Meaning	Example/Pronunciation	Define
chromo-	color	chromosome (**krō**-mō-sōm)	(soma = body) "colored bodies," pieces of DNA
erythro-	red	erythrocyte (ĕ-**rĭth**-rō-sīt) abbreviated "RBC"	_____
(*also* rub-)		rubella (rū-**bĕl**-lă)	_____
leuko-	white	leukocyte (**lū**-kō-sīt) abbreviated "WBC"	_____
(*also* alb-)		albinism (**ăl**-bĭn-ĭzm)	_____
		leukocytosis (lū-kō-sī-**tō**-sĭs)	_____
		leukemia (lū-**kē**-mē-ă)	_____

Root word	Meaning	Example/Pronunciation	Define
melano-	black	melanoma (měl-ă-**nō**-mă)	_____
cyano-	blue	cyanosis (sī-ă-**nō**-sĭs)	_____
cirrh-	orange yellow	cirrhosis (sĭr-**rō**-sĭs)	_____
xanth/o	yellow	xanthoderma (zăn-thō-**děr**-mă)	_____
polio	gray	poliomyelitis (pō-lē-ō-mī-ě-**lī**-tĭs)	_____

No Answer Key

Worksheet

Fill in the meaning of the given root word and check your answers. After you feel you know them, cover the given root words and complete the drill using the meanings you have given. Do this as many times as necessary until you are familiar with the material.

Root word	Meaning	Root word	Example
coccus	round-shaped bacterium	_____	streptococcus
bacillus	_____	_____	_____
strept/o	_____	_____	_____
staphyl/o	_____	_____	_____
diplo	_____	_____	_____
chromo	_____	_____	_____
erythr/o	_____	_____	_____
leuk/o	_____	_____	_____
polio	_____	_____	_____
xanth/o	_____	_____	_____
melano	_____	_____	_____
cyan/o	_____	_____	_____
cirrh	_____	_____	_____

No Answer Key

Test p. 301

✔ Check Your Progress

You are now midway through Part 1 of *Medical Terminology*. You should be building a solid foundation in medical terminology. If you find that certain words are giving you trouble, look them up in a dictionary. Try using them in a sentence or find a word association for that term to help you remember it. Also, discuss your problem with the instructor.

You may now be given a review test for Chapters 6–9, which can be found on page 303 in Appendix F. In this section, you have learned plural endings, additional suffixes, prefixes, and root words, and information on bacteria and colors.

You will now move on to the last section in Part 1, which contains information on general abbreviations; diagnostic and laboratory abbreviations; directional, positional, and numerical terms; and basic pharmacology. Remember to continue to review the terminology you have previously studied in Chapters 1 through 9 so that you do not forget what you have learned.

Review

Fill in the correct word:

1. A red cell *erythrocyte (abbreviated RBC)* _____

2. Condition of blueness _____

3. "Black tumor" _____

4. "White blood" _____

5. Malignant tumor _____

6. Treatment with water _____

7. Fat tumor _____

8. Condition of clots or clotting _____

9. Science dealing with disease conditions _____

10. Round bacteria growing in clusters _____

11. Round bacteria growing in chain formation _____

12. Rod-shaped bacteria _____

Define:

13. pri **mip** ara _____

14. **trau** ma _____

15. arterioscle **ro** sis _____

16. hemo **sta** sis _____

17. choleli **thi** asis _____

18. ne **cro** sis _____

19. **di** athermy _____

20. anes **the** sia _____

21. hema **tol** ogy _____

22. u **re** mia _____

23. gravida III, para II _____

True/False: Circle the numbers of the *true* statements only.

24. A person who is aphasic cannot speak.

25. A leukocyte is a white blood cell, but the word means only white cell.

26. Schizophrenia is a mental illness, often incorrectly referred to as a split personality.

27. Pathogenic organisms are harmless.

28. Aerobic organisms do not require oxygen.

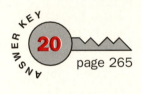
page 265

Define:

1. **leu** kocyte ___white blood cell (abbreviated WBC)_____

2. phagocy **to** sis _____

3. schizo **phre** nia _____

4. hydro **ther** apy _____

5. hemo **sta** sis _____

6. hemi **ple** gia _____

7. a **ne** mia _____

8. u **re** mia _____

9. megalo **ma** nia _____

10. hema **tol** ogy _____

11. carci **no** ma _____

12. my **o** pia _____

13. **neu** rospasm _____

14. mega **col** on _____

15. hema **tu** ria _____

Spell: Have someone dictate these words to you from Answer Key 21.

Define:

16. _____

17. _____

18. _____

19. _____

20. _____

21. _____

22. _____

23. _____

24. _____

25. _____

26. _____

27. _____

28. _____

29. _____

30. _____

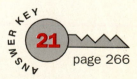

page 266

This review drill may be used in any manner that you find helpful in learning the material. A suggestion is to fill in the meaning for each word part, then to cover the given word part and complete the last two columns. This drill can be repeated as many times as necessary.

Word part	Meaning	Word part	Example words
-olysis	destruction of	suffix	hemolysis
-oma			
-oid			
-plasia			
-trophy			
-malacia			
-orrhea			
-pnea			
-plegia			
gen			
aero-			
hetero-			
homo-			
iso-			
mal-			
megalo-			
-megaly			
noct-			
syn-			
acro-			
meno-			
-itis			
-ectomy			
hem/o			
hemi-			

No Answer Key

Fill in the blank:

1. The physician examined the boy and made a tentative ___*diagnosis*___, based on the ___*symptoms*___, which consisted of a sore throat and fever.

2. A certain "round" bacterium that grows in chain formation and causes many different illnesses:

   _____

3. The physician prescribed a medication that would retard or kill bacterial life, an _____

4. He predicted that the recovery would be complete. In other words, the _____ was good.

5. The ophthalmologist prescribed glasses for Joe Smith because he was nearsighted. The medical word

   for nearsightedness is _____ . If a person is nearsighted, it means he

   (circle the correct word) can/cannot see very far.

6. In physical therapy many treatments are given: treatment with water is called _____; heat

   treatment is _____; treatment with cold is _____.

7. The laboratory technologist counted all of the *white cells* (_____) and the *red cell*

   (_____) in a sample of blood.

8. The abbreviation for these two procedures is _____ and _____.

9. Bacteria that cause disease are called. _____ The two main kinds of bacteria (by

   their shape or form) are _____ and _____.

10. A woman in her first pregnancy is called a _____ .

11. Gravida V, para II means _____ and

    two _____ .

12. A medication given before surgery to make the patient drowsy is called a _____

    medication; one given during surgery to remove all sense of feeling is called a general _____ .

    Medications given following surgery are called _____ medications.

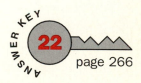

ANSWER KEY 22

page 266

CHAPTER 10

Directional, Positional, and Numerical Terms

List of Directional and Positional Terms

anterior (ventral) (ăn-**tēr**-ē-ŏr)	toward the front, or in front of; abbreviated A
posterior (dorsal) (pŏs-**tēr**-ē-ŏr)	toward the back, or in back of; abbreviated P; Example: AP of chest (X-ray order for a view from the front [toward the back])
lateral (**lăt**-ĕr-ăl)	side
bilateral (bī-**lăt**-ĕr-ăl)	both sides; Example: bilateral pneumonia
medial (mesial) (**mē**-dē-ăl)	middle
oblique (ō-**blēk**)	at an angle
superior (supra) (sū-**pēr**-ē-ŏr)	above; Example: superior vena cava, suprapubic
inferior (sub) (infra) (ĭn-**fēr**-ē-ŏr)	below; Example: inferior vena cava, substernal, infraorbital
cephalic (sĕ-**făl**-ĭk)	head (similar to superior)
caudal (**căw**-dăl)	"tail" or base of spine (similar to inferior)
proximal (**prŏk**-sĭm-ăl)	nearest to center; Example: PIP = proximal interphalangeal joint
distal (**dĭs**-tăl)	farthest from center; Example: DIP = distal interphalangeal joint (tip of finger)
peripheral (pĕr-**ĭf**-ĕr-ăl)	outer edges; Example: peripheral vision, peripheral vascular disease
transverse (trans-) (trăns-**vĕrs**)	horizontal body plane, divides body into top and bottom sections; across or through; Example: transvaginal hysterectomy, transurethral resection of prostate (TURP)
sagittal (**săj**-ĭt-tăl)	vertical body plane, through trunk of body; if exactly through middle, it is *mid*saggital, and divides the body into equal right and left sides
coronal (frontal) (kŏ-**rō**-năl)	vertical body plane, divides body into front and back sections (anterior and posterior) standing
upright (**ŭp**-rīt)	standing
decubitus (dē-**kū**-bĭ-tŭs)	lying down; Example: decubitus ulcers, caused by prolonged lying down
recumbent (rē-**kūm**-bĕnt)	lying down; Example: dorsal recumbent, lying face up

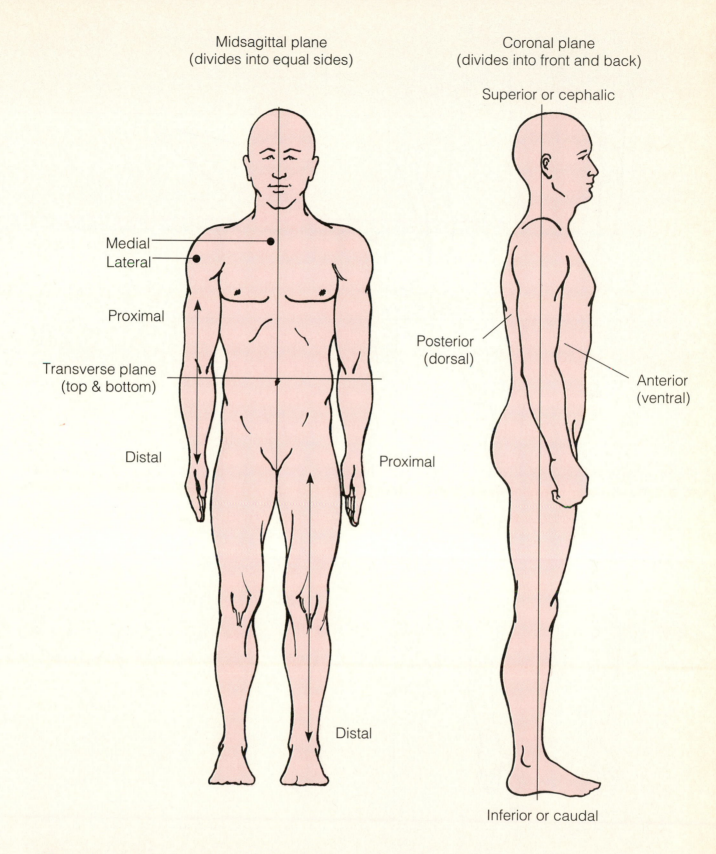

Midsagittal plane
(divides into equal sides)

Coronal plane
(divides into front and back)

Superior or cephalic

Medial

Lateral

Proximal

Transverse plane
(top & bottom)

Distal

Proximal

Posterior
(dorsal)

Anterior
(ventral)

Distal

Inferior or caudal

Figure 10.1 Anatomical planes and directional terms.

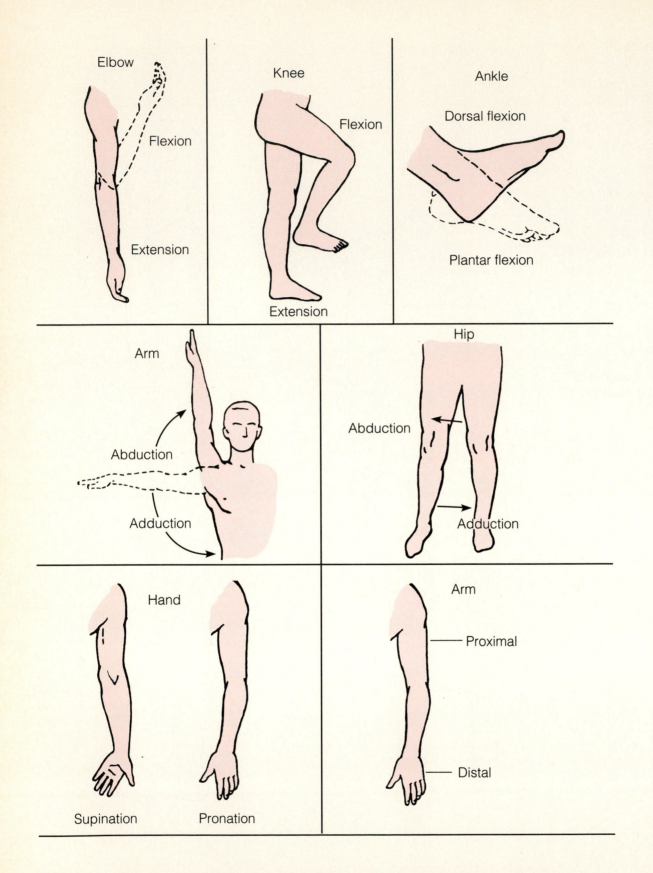

Figure 10.2 Illustration of some terms used to describe body movements and body positions.

supine, supination (sū-**pīn**), (sū-pĭ-**nā**-shŭn)	face up, or palm up
prone, pronation (prōn), (prō-**nā**-shŭn)	face down, or palm down
rotation (version) (rō-**tā**-shŭn)	turning
eversion (ĕ-**vĕr**-zhŭn)	turning outward, or inside out
flexion (flexing) (**flĕk**-shŭn)	bending
extension (extending) (ĕks-**tĕn**-shŭn)	straightening
internal (ĭn-**tĕr**-năl)	inside
external (ĕks-**tĕr**-năl)	outside
sinistro (**sĭn**-ĭs-trō)	to the left, or the left; OS = oculus sinister, left eye
dextro (**dĕks**-trō)	to the right, or the right; OD = oculus dexter, right eye
adduction (ăd-**dŭk**-shŭn)	toward the midline
abduction (ăb-**dŭk**-shŭn)	away from the midline
quadrants of abdomen (**kwă**-drănts)	right and left upper, right and left lower

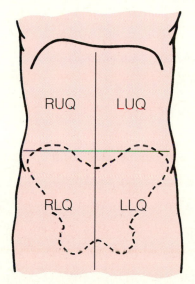

Figure 10.3 **The quadrants are labeled from the patient's point of view:** the right quadrants are on the patient's right side.

■ **Note:** The above terms are used in anatomical drawings, in doctors' orders for X-rays, physical therapy and other kinds of therapy, and in surgery/pathology reports.

Terms That Describe an Exact Position

These are positions used in surgery, examination, and so on. (Most medical dictionaries will list these under "positions.")

Tren *del* enburg   lying on back, face up, body straight on a bed tilted at 45 degrees with the head low.

lith ot omy   lying flat on back, legs in stirrups. (What does the word *lithotomy* mean literally?)

Sims'   lying on left side, right leg slightly forward, knees flexed.

knee-chest   kneeling, chest on table.

Fowler's   head of bed raised 1½ feet, knees elevated.

List of Directional and Positional Prefixes

Prefix	Meaning	Example/Pronunciation	Define
ab-	away from	1. abduction (ăb-**dŭk**-shŭn)	movement away from midline (of body)
ad-	toward	2. adduction (ăd-**dŭk**-shŭn)	
circum-	around	3. circumcision (sĭr-kŭm-**sĭ**-zhŭn)	
contra-	opposition, against	4. contraindicated (kŏn-tră-**ĭn**-dĭ-kā-těd)	
ecto-, -exo	outside	5. exogenous (ĕk-**sŏj**-ĕn-ŭs)	
		6. ectogenous (ĕk-**tŏj**-ĕn-ŭs)	
		7. ectopic (ĕk-**tŏp**-ĭk)	
		8. exocrine (**ĕk**-sō-krĭn)	
endo-	within	9. endocrine (**ĕn**-dō-krĭn)	
		10. endogenous (ĕn-**dŏj**-ĕn-ŭs)	
		11. endoscope (**ĕn**-dō-skōp)	
epi-	upon, over	12. epigastric (ĕp-ĭ-**găs**-trĭk)	
extra-	outside	13. extrauterine (**ĕk**-stră-ū-těr-ĭn)	
infra-, sub-	below, under	14. infrasternal (ĭn-fră-**stěr**-năl)	
		15. subnormal (sŭb-**nŏr**-măl)	
ipsi-	same	16. ipsilateral (ĭp-sĭ-**lăt**-ěr-ăl)	
meso-	middle, pertaining to mesentery	17. mesosternum (měs-ō-**stěr**-nŭm)	
		18. mesopexy (**měs**-ō-pěk-sē)	
meta-	after, beyond, over, change or transformation, following in a series	19. metastasis (mě-**tăs**-tă-sĭs)	
		20. metabolism (mě-**tăb**-ō-lĭzm)	
		21. metatarsus (mě-tă-**tăr**-sŭs)	

Prefix	Meaning	Example/Pronunciation	Define
para-	near, beside, past, beyond, opposite, abnormal, irregular, two like parts, similar to	22. paramedical (păr-ă-**mĕd**-ĭkăl)	_____
		23. paratyphoid (păr-ă-**tī**-fŏyd)	_____
		24. paraplegia (păr-ă-**plē**-jē-ă)	_____
peri-	around, about, surrounding	25. periodontal (pĕr-ē-ō-**dŏn**-tăl)	_____
		26. peritonsillar (pĕr-ĭ-**tŏn**-sĭl-lăr)	_____
		27. pericardium (pĕr-ĭ-**kăr**-dē-ŭm)	_____
		28. perineum (pĕr-ĭ-**nē**-ŭm)	_____
retro-	behind, backward	29. retroperitoneal (rĕt-rō-pĕr-ĭ-tō-**nē**-ăl)	_____
		30. retroversion (rĕt-rō-**vĕr**-zhŭn)	_____
trans-	across, through	31. transurethral (trăns-ū-**rē**-thrăl)	_____
		32. transvaginal (trăns-**văj**-ĭn-ăl)	_____

■ **Note:** These are difficult because, in some cases, they can mean so many different things. In addition to that, some may be used interchangeably: for instance, _peri_ **ton** _sillar_ and _para_ **ton** _sillar_ are both correct and synonymous.

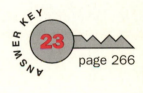

ANSWER KEY **23** page 266

Self-Test

Define:

1. upright _____

2. flexion _____

3. decubitus _____

4. extension _____

Fill in the blank:

5. The opposite of proximal is _____. A term that means "side" is _____; "both sides" _____

6. *Recumbent, decubitus, supine,* and *prone* are all terms that refer to the _____ position.

7. The terms that refer to the "head" are _____; "tail," _____

8. The position used for a pelvic exam (with legs in stirrups) is _____

9. *Internal* and *external* mean _____ and _____

10. Interpret this X-ray order and explain what it means: AP, PA, and left lat. of chest. _____
    _____

True/False: Circle the numbers of the *true* statements only. Defend your answers. Explain what is "untrue" in the false statements.

11. A transvaginal hysterectomy requires no abdominal incision.

12. A finger has three small bones—distal, medial, and proximal. The distal one is the tip of the finger.

13. Caudal anesthesia is injected into an arm vein.

14. The head is superior to the spine.

15. The abdomen is divided into quadrants to make describing an area easier and more exact.

16. An ectopic or extrauterine pregnancy is usually in the fallopian tube, but it could also be in the perineum.

17. A subnormal temperature is below 98.6 F.

18. When the gums are inflamed, a person has periodontal disease.

19. Paraplegia is paralysis of one side of the body.

20. Movement of the arm away from the body is called *abduction. Abduction* also means kidnapping (taking someone away).

21. *Addiction* and *adduction* both use the prefix *ad-* because they mean "drawing toward something."

22. Peripheral vision is vision out to the sides.

23. The peritoneal cavity is the abdominopelvic cavity.

24. *DIP* refers to the joint at the far end of the finger.

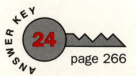

ANSWER KEY
24
page 266

List of Numerical Prefixes

Study the examples and their prefixes, then define them.

Prefix	Meaning	Example/Pronunciation	Define
uni-	one	unilateral (ū-nĭ-**lăt**-ĕr-ăl)	*one side*
bi-	two (double), twice	bilateral (bī-**lăt**-ĕr-ăl)	
		biweekly (bī-**wēk**-lē)	*once every 2 weeks (can also mean twice a week, in which case semi-weekly is the preferred term)*
		bicuspid (bī-**kŭs**-pĭd)	
tri-	three	tricuspid (trī-**kŭs**-pĭd)	
quadri-	four	quadriplegic (kwă-drĭ-**plē**-jĭk)	
multi-	many (more than one)	multipara (mŭl-**tĭp**-ă-ră)	
primi-	first	primipara (prī-**mĭp**-ă-ră)	
semi-	half (partially)	semicomatose (sĕm-ē-**kō**-mă-tōs)	
hemi-	half, also one side	hemiplegia (hĕm-ĭ-**plē**-jē-ă)	
ambi-	both or both sides	ambiopia (ăm-bē-**ō**-pē-ă)	
		ambidextrous (ăm-bĭ-**dĕks**-trŭs)	
		ambivalence (ăm-**bĭv**-ă-lĕns)	
ambly-	dull, dim, not clear	amblyopia (ăm-blē-**ō**-pē-ă)	
diplo-	double	diplopia (dĭp-**lō**-pē-ă)	
		diplococcus (dĭp-lō-**kŏk**-ŭs)	

No Answer Key

Worksheet

Word part	Meaning		Word part	Meaning
-orrhexis	*rupture*		ad-	
-spasm			ab-	
-gnos			endo-	
-drome			ecto-	
-opia			meso-	

Word part	Meaning	Word part	Meaning
extra-	_____	hemi-	_____
retro-	_____	ambi-	_____
peri-	_____	diplo-	_____
para-	_____	bi-	_____
epi-	_____	tri-	_____
infra-	_____	quadri-	_____
trans-	_____	multi-	_____
uni-	_____	sinistr/o-	_____
primi-	_____	dextr/o-	_____
semi-	_____	ipsi-	_____

Abbreviation	Meaning
AP	_____
RUQ	_____
LUQ	_____
OS or O.S.	_____

No Answer Key

Worksheet

Fill in the blank:

1. To be drawn toward a habit *addicted* _____

2. To move away from the midline _____

3. Arising or originating from outside of the organism (body) _____

4. Out of natural place _____ (as a tubal pregnancy)

5. Behind the peritoneum _____

6. Across (or through) the urethra _____

7. The four "areas" of the abdomen _____

8. Separate, conflicting emotions _____

9. A tooth or a heart valve with three cups _____

10. Position used for pelvic exam _____ (literal meaning: surgical incision for removal of a stone)

11. Both fallopian tubes excised: _____ salpingectomy

12. Pneumonia in both lungs: _____ pneumonia

Define:

13. semicomatose _____*partially in a coma*_____

14. multipara _____

15. diplopia _____

16. epigastric _____

17. endogenous _____

18. adduction _____

19. substernal _____

20. perineum _____

21. Sims' position _____

22. unilateral _____

23. periodontal _____

24. flexion _____

25. diplococcus _____

Write the abbreviation for the following:

26. right eye ___*O.D.*_____

27. X-ray picture taken from the front of chest _____

28. Draw or describe:

    a. midsagittal plane _____

    b. coronal plane _____

    c. transverse plane _____

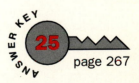

ANSWER KEY **25** page 267

Test p. 305

CHAPTER **11**

Additional Terms

Organ Transplant Terms

anti-rejection drugs	cyclosporine (sī-klō-**spŏr**-ēn), azathioprine (ā-ză-**thī**-ō-prēn), and steroids are given to try to prevent rejection of transplanted organ
artificial heart	mechanical heart to sustain a person waiting for a transplant organ
"beating heart" cadaver (kă-**dăv**-ĕr)	body maintained on a respirator in order to "harvest" a usable organ
cadaver organ	donor organ from a deceased person
cardiectomy (kăr-dē-**ĕk**-tō-mē)	surgical excision of donor heart
immunosuppressant	suppression (as by drugs) of natural immune responses
harvest or **retrieve**	terms for taking an organ (neither term seems to be satisfactory)
perfusion, perfusionist (pĕr-**fū**-zhŭn)	heart/lung machine, and operator
pneumocystis (nū-mō-**sĭst**-ĭs)	type of pneumonia that recipients often develop due to suppression of immune system
PPH	primary pulmonary hypertension; candidate for heart-lung transplant
procurement coordinator	person responsible for obtaining donor organ, getting permission, arranging transportation, etc.
retrieve	see *harvest*
sternotomy (stĕr-**nŏt**-ō-mē)	incision for heart and heart-lung transplant
xenograft (**zĕ**-nō-grăft)	organ from an animal for transplant

General Information on Organ Transplants

Organs that have been successfully transplanted include the heart, heart-lung, kidney, and liver. Donor age limit for these organs is approximately 45 years. Skin, cornea, bone, and bone-marrow donors have no age limit. Skin, bone and corneas can be stored, but the other organs must be rushed to the recipient.

Although television and news media portray the recipient of a transplanted organ as a person who will thereafter live a "normal" life, nothing is further from the truth. Even when the surgery is successful, the recipient must take immunosuppressant drugs for the rest of his or her life. These drugs are very expensive and often generate side effects that may be devastating. Organ recipients and their families may have difficulty financing the surgery and aftercare, and adults may discover they are no longer considered "employable." The strain these problems put on a marriage often leads to divorce. There is also the possibility that another transplant may be necessary if the organ fails, with all the stress of the first operation: the need to be "on call" (available at a moment's notice), often in a strange city, the long surgical procedure, and the postoperative rejection problems that may start all over.

There are, of course, successful transplants, especially for corneas and kidneys. Medical research continues to make progress in this area, and organ recipients and their families are willing to take the risks involved. Many support groups, such as Mended Hearts, are available for transplant patients.

Worksheet

Define the following words: Think before you look them up. Pronounce the words as you work with them. Later, cover the words and pronunciations and rewrite each word in the last column using only the definition.

Word/Pronunciation   *Define*   *Word*

1. abortion (ă-**bŏr**-shŭn)   *termination of pregnancy* _____

2. abdomen (**ăb**-dō-mĕn)   _____   _____

3. abdominal (ăb-**dŏm**-ĭ-năl)   _____   _____

4. abscess (**ăb**-sĕs)   _____   _____

5. acute (ă-**kūt**)   _____   _____

6. adhesion (ăd-**hē**-zhŭn)   _____   _____

7. adnexa (ăd-**nĕk**-să)   _____   _____

8. auscultation (ăws-kŭl-**tā**-shŭn)   _____   _____
   (combined with percussion)

9. autoclave (**ăw**-tŏ-klāv)   _____   _____

10. axilla (axillary) (ăk-**sĭl**-lă)   _____   _____

11. anomaly (ă-**nŏm**-ăl-ē)   _____   _____

12. biopsy (**bī**-ŏp-sē)   _____   _____

13. catgut (**kăt**-gŭt)   _____   _____

14. catheter (**kăth**-ĕ-tĕr)   _____   _____

15. cervical (**sĕr**-vĭ-kăl)   _____   _____

16. chronic (**krŏn**-ĭk)   _____   _____

17. chromic (**krō**-mĭk)   _____   _____

18. coccyx, coccygeal   _____   _____
    (**kŏk**-sĭx), (kŏk-sĭ-**gē**-ăl)

19. congenital (kŏn-**gĕn**-ĭ-tăl)   _____   _____

Word/Pronunciation	Define	Word
20. dilatation, dilation (dĭ-lă-**tā**-shŭn), (dī-**lā**-shŭn)		
21. edema (ĕ-**dē**-mă) (swelling that leaves pitting when depressed with finger)		
ascites, anasarca (ăs-**sī**-tēz, ăn-ă-**săr**-kă)		
22. embolism, embolus (**ĕm**-bō-lĭzm), (**ĕm**-bō-lŭs)		
23. emesis (**ĕm**-ĕs-ĭs)		
24. enema (**ĕn**-ĕm-ă)		
25. excretion (ĕk-**krē**-shŭn)		
26. exacerbation (ĕg-zăs-ĕr-**bā**-shŭn)		
27. fascia (**făsh**-ē-ă)		
28. febrile (**fĕb**-rīl)		
29. fibrilliation, defibrillate (fĭ-brĭ-**lā**-shŭn), (dē-**fĭ**-brĭ-lāt)		
30. hemorrhage (**hĕm**-ĕ-rĭj)		
31. icterus (**ĭk**-tĕr-ŭs)		
32. immunization, immunity (ĭm-mū-nī-**zā**-shŭn)		
33. incontinence, incontinent (ĭn-**kŏn**-tĭn-ĕns)		
34. inflammation, inflamed (ĭn-flăm-**mā**-shŭn), (ĭn-**flāmd**)		
35. ischemia (ĭs-**kē**-mē-ă)		
36. jaundice (**jŏn**-dĭs) (related terms: bilirubin, Coombs')		
37. metastasis, metastasized (mĕ-**tăs**-tă-sĭs) (mĕ-**tăs**-tă-sīzd)		
38. mucus, mucous, mucosa (**mū**-kŭs), (mū-**kō**-să)		
39. obese, obesity (ō-**bēs**), (ō-**bēs**-ĭt-ē)		
40. palpable (**păl**-păb-l)		
41. paralyzed, paralysis (**păr**-ă-līzd), (pă-**răl**-ĭ-sĭs)		
42. parietal (pă-**rī**-ĕt-ăl)		
43. percussion (pĕr-**kŭsh**-ŭn)		

Word/Pronunciation	Define	Word
44. perineum, perineal (pĕr-ĭ-**nē**-ŭm), (pĕr-ĭ-**nē**-ăl)	_____	_____
45. peritoneal, peritoneum (pĕr-ĭ-tō-**nē**-ăl), (pĕr-ĭ-tō-**nē**-ŭm)	_____	_____
46. pleural (**plĕr**-ăl)	_____	_____
47. prolapse (**prō**-lăps)	_____	_____
48. prophylaxis (prō-fĭ-**lăk**-sĭs)	_____	_____
49. purulent (**pūr**-ū-lĕnt)	_____	_____
50. remission (rē-**mĭsh**-ŭn)	_____	_____
51. rheumatic (rū-**măt**-ĭk)	_____	_____
52. serous, serum (**sĕ**-rŭs) (**sĕ**-rŭm)	_____	_____
53. sputum (**spū**-tŭm)	_____	_____
54. suture (**sū**-chŭr)	_____	_____
55. triage (**trē**-ăzh)	_____	_____
56. virus (**vī**-rŭs)	_____	_____
57. viscera (**vĭs**-sĕr-ă)	_____	_____
58. void (voided) (vŏyd)	_____	_____

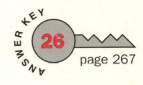

ANSWER KEY 26 page 267

Self-Test

True/False: Circle the number of the *true* statements only. Defend your answers. Explain what is "untrue" in the false statements.

1. A disease that is severe and comes on suddenly is a chronic disease.

2. A person who is afebrile has a normal temperature.

3. A congenital anomaly is one that appears late in life.

4. P & A is the abbreviation for percussion and auscultation; this means tapping and listening.

5. A person who cannot void is said to be incontinent.

6. Normal bodily excretions are urine and stool.

7. An exacerbation is an acute onset of symptoms.

8. The autoclave is one device for sterilizing medical supplies; it is used only for articles that can withstand steam under pressure.

9. A biopsy is the examination of dead tissues.

10. Mucous membranes secrete mucus.

Write a word that means:

11. Vomiting _____emesis_____

12. Excessive fluid in body tissues _____

13. Introduction of fluid into the rectum _____

14. The armpit _____

15. Redness, heat, swelling, pain _____

Spell: Have someone dictate these words to you from Answer Key 27.

16. _____

17. _____

18. _____

19. _____

20. _____

Define:

21. voided _____expelled urine_____

22. purulent _____

23. prolapse _____

24. palpable _____

25. prophylaxis _____

26. ascites _____

27. anasarca _____

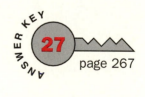
page 267

Test p. 307

CHAPTER 12

General Abbreviations

Introduction to Abbreviations

The number of abbreviations used in medicine is overwhelming to most students. As with medical words, many abbreviations are derived from foreign words, which compounds the problem.

This chapter will introduce you to some more of the most commonly used abbreviations. Your need to know these will depend on your choice of work. For instance, if you choose to work as an unit secretary, it would be important to know the abbreviations used in physicians' orders. Laboratory abbreviations and terms would be essential in this kind of job as in many other medically related jobs. It is generally difficult to read physicians' handwriting; therefore, if you are trying to decipher scrawled handwriting and you are unsure about what words or abbreviations are being used, the task of reading orders may be difficult. Learning these words and abbreviations will help you.

This chapter will only scratch the surface on abbreviations; you will gradually learn others as you are exposed to them. Along with standard abbreviations, you will find that each department or office may have their own shortcuts for writing terms they use frequently. In a new situation, try to figure out what initials stand for, and if you cannot, ask! *Warning:* Abbreviations may have more than one meaning. Each must therefore be considered in context (the best "abbreviations" book I have found is *Medical Abbreviations* by Edward B. Steen, published by the F.A. Davis Company). You will find some abbreviations listed alphabetically in medical dictionaries, and you may also find a separate section of abbreviations.

An alphabetical list of abbreviations is given in Appendix H, with separate sections for physical therapy, pulmonary function, and cancer.

Physicians' Orders

Activity, Toileting

CBR, ABR   complete bedrest, absolute bedrest
ambulate   walk
OOB   out of bed
BRP   bathroom privileges; may get up only to go to bathroom
commode   bedside toilet
ROM   range of motion (exercise)

Diet Orders

NPO (NBM) nothing by mouth

I & O intake and output (measured for 24-hour period or longer)

liq liquids only (clear, full)

   clear liquids liquid you can see through

   full liquids all types of liquids

lo salt, low NA (sodium)

salt free

reg, full soft, bland, and so on types of diets

FF (force fluids), push fluids strongly encourage intake of fluid

DAT diet as tolerated

hypo hypoglycemic diet

ADA American Dietetic Association diet

Other Routine Procedures

TPR temperature, pulse, respirations

B/P blood pressure

V/S vital signs: TPR and B/P

ECG, EKG electrocardiogram (record of heart waves)

EEG electroencephalogram (record of brain waves)

X-Ray, Laboratory

AP and **Lat** routine X-ray picture of chest (front to back and side view)

up upright X-ray picture

decub de **cu** bitus (lying down)

IVP intravenous pyelogram (kidney)

BE barium enema (colon)

GI series gastrointestinal X-ray upper (barium swallow), lower (same as BE)

GB series gallbladder X-ray picture

RADS radiation dose

RAI, RAIU radioactive iodine (uptake), thyroid function

Scan CT, CAT computerized (axial) to **mog** raphy

S & A sugar and acetone

CBC complete blood count

UA urinalysis

VC vital capacity (lungs)

Scans

Scans can detect changes in size, shape, and position; changes in density, as happens in edema, hemorrhage, inflammation, neoplasms, clots, calcium deposits, cysts, and abscesses. CAT, CT, MRI, PET (position emission tomography) are names of machines used.

CAT, CT Computerized (axial) tomography is the analysis of multiple X-ray films in successive layers to provide a three-dimensional view. Images are projected onto a television screen and photographed; the result is a series of sections of an organ such as the brain. Dye may be used to highlight certain areas, but if dyes are used there may be some unpleasant sensations or side effects. A scan is noninvasive and painless if no contrast dye is used.

MRI Magnetic resonance imaging uses a diagnostic system that includes a scanner, computer, display screen, and recorder. MRI uses a powerful magnetic field and radio-frequency energy (that can "see" through bone) to produce images. It is used to scan abdomen, bone marrow, brain, spinal cord, chest, extremities, pelvis, orbit/face/neck.

   Organs that can be "scanned" include:

head and neck brain, skull, ear, sinuses

thorax lungs, heart

vessels aorta, vena cava

abdomen pancreas, liver, gallbladder, adrenals, kidneys, spleen, and peritoneum

pelvis reproductive organs, male and female; urinary tract

extremities, spinal canal, and flat bones

The advantage of scans is that scans are more sensitive than X-ray procedures and sharper pictures are produced; therefore, earlier diagnosis is possible. The disadvantages are their relatively high cost and inability to show such tiny detail (as vascular damage).

Ultrasonography

Noninvasive technique using ultrasound is useful in obtaining "pictures" of the heart, aneurysms of the aorta, and changes in size and structure in the abdominopelvic organs; tumors, foreign bodies, and retinal detachment in the eye; fetal size and maturity in prenatal development, as well as placental placement. It is not useful for diagnosing lung cancers because ultrasound waves do not pass through structures that contain air.

Routine Immunizations

DTP (DPT)   diph **ther** ia, per **tus** sis, **tet** anus

TD (DT)   diph **ther** ia, **tet** anus (over age seven)

rube o la   hard measles (red measles)

ru bell a   German (three-day, measles)

OPV   oral poliomye **lit** is vaccine

paro ti tis   mumps

MMR   combined measles, mumps, rubella

HiB (HbCV)   hemophilus b conjugate vaccine

Varivax (Merck)   expected to be recommended for all healthy children ages 12 to 18 months; may be given with other vaccines

Other Immunizations (not routine)

variola (văr-ē-ō-lă)   smallpox, no longer required

influenza and **pneumonia** (ĭn-flū-ĕn-ză) recommended for the elderly and special groups

hepatitis B virus vaccine (hĕ-pă-tī-tĭs) recommended for high-risk medical professionals

typhoid, yellow fever, etc. (tī-fŏyd)   may be required for travel to some countries

Miscellaneous Abbreviations

qns   quantity not sufficient (Lab requires a larger specimen.)

c̄   with

s̄   without

dc   discontinue, discharge

TLC   tender loving care

stat   immediately (**ASAP:** as soon as possible)

EUA   examination under anesthesia

DOA   dead on arrival

OD   overdose (also means "right eye")

D   diopters, used for lenses of eye glasses

dB   decibels, used for level of sound (hearing tests)

degrees F or C   temperature, Fahrenheit or Celsius. The degree sign (°) is not used; as in 98.6 F

positive +   (may be 1 plus to 4 plus; may also be written 4+ or ++++)

negative −   (may be written −1 or −2, for example)

DRG   diagnostic-related groupings (determine average hospital stay)

CPT   current procedural terminology (code numbers)

ICD   International Classification of Diseases (code numbers)

prep   prepare

pre-op   preoperatively

post-op   postoperatively

H_2O   water

O_2   oxygen

CO_2   carbon dioxide

CPR   cardiopulmonary resusci **ta** tion

SOB   significant other at bedside or shortness of breath

1. Abbreviations are written with or without periods. (Periods are unnecessary on most abbreviations and are required only on those that may be confusing.)

2. Roman numerals are often used: I, II, III, IV, V, VI, VII, VIII, IX, and X.

3. For any patient in the hospital, the physician's orders should always include the following:

   a. diet order (NPO, for example)

   b. activity level (BRP or OOB, for example)

   c. prn (meaning "as needed") sleep medication and prn pain medication

   d. additional orders as necessary (X-ray or lab, for example)

4. Try to read the next prescription you receive before having it filled.

5. Preparations for tests vary; some are stringent, and usually printed instructions are given to the patient with an explanation.

Hospital or Clinic Departments

A & D   admitting and discharge

CCU or **ICU**   coronary care unit or intensive care unit

CS   central service or supply

dietary   food service

DOU   definitive observation unit (less than intensive care, but more than "floor" care)

ENT   ear, nose, and throat

ER, ED   emergency room, emergency department

GU   genitourinary

housekeeping   maintains cleanliness of hospital environment

lab   medical laboratory

med-surg   ward for medical and surgical patients (may be combined or separate)

morgue   place in which bodies of persons who have died are temporarily kept

MR   medical records

NP   neuropsychiatric

OB   obstetrics (includes labor and delivery rooms, postpartum ward, newborn nursery and **ICN** or intensive care nursery)

OPD   outpatient department

OR   operating room, surgery (**MOR**, minor surgery)

peds   pediatrics

pharmacy   drug dispensary

PT & OT   physical therapy and occupational therapy (may be under **PM & R**, physical medicine and rehabilitation)

RR   recovery room

SS   social service

X-ray   radiology

Insurance Abbreviations and Terms

HMO   health maintenance organization

AHCCCS   Arizona Health Care Cost Containment System, pronounced "access" (Arizona's substitute for Medicaid)

long-term care   Providing for custodial care in nursing homes and private homes

Medicaid   federal program providing health care to the indigent

Medicare   federal program providing health care to elderly and some disabled persons

Medigap insurance   Provides payment for the part of expenses not covered by Medicare

PPO   preferred provider organization. Patients may choose their health care providers.

Prescriptions

Time or Number of Times

qd   every day

od   once a day

qod   every other day

q_h   every ____3____ hours (for a 24 hour period)

bid   twice a day

tid   (*ter in die*) three times a day

qid   (*quater in die*) four times a day

hs   at bedtime

ac   before meals

pc   after meals

prn   (*pro re nata*) as needed

ad lib   as desired

stat   immediately

Units or Amounts

tabs.   tablets, pills

caps.   capsules

supp   sup **pos** itory

ss   one-half

mg   milligrams

g or **gm**   grams, 1 gm = 15 gr

gr   grains, 1 gr = 65 mg (5 gr = 325 mg.)

cc   cubic **cen** timeters

mL or **ml**   **mil** liliters

L   liter (1000 cc or mL [ml])

mEq   millie **quiv** alent

U   units. **TU:** tuberculin units

gtt   (*guttae*) drops

℥   ounces

ℨ   drams

Routes of Administration

PO   (*per os*) by mouth

par *en* **teral administration**   not by mouth

IV   intra **ve** nously, 5% **glu** (glucose) in **DW** distilled water

IM   intra **mus** cularly

H   hypo **der** mically

subcu, subq (SQ)   subcu **tan** eously

subling (SL)   sub **ling** ually

R   **rec** tally

ns   normal (iso **ton** ic) saline solution

cly sis   fluids given by needle, under skin (not in vein)

TKO   to keep open (vein)

KVO   keep vein open

Example of a Prescription

A.S.A., gr. V, (p.o.), Q4h., p.r.n. for back pain. Interpretation: Aspirin, 5 grains, by mouth (*per os*), every 4 hours, as needed for back pain

Worksheet

Interpret (spell out) these orders:

1. Procaine penicillin 600,000 U (IM) q8h   _600,000 units intramuscularly every eight hours_

2. Codeine 30 mg (PO) q4h prn for headache _____

3. Seconal gr Iss hs prn _____

4. Nembutal 100 mg (PO) hs _____

5. NPO after midnight _____

6. 1000 cc 5% glu in DW (IV) stat _____

7. OOB, BID _____

8. Push fluids; I & O _____

Write the abbreviation for the following:

9. three times a day _tid_____

10. grains _____

11. grams _____

12. with _____

13. without _____

14. discontinue _____

15. water _____

16. oxygen _____

17. before meals _____

18. may go to bathroom only _____

19. gastrointestinal _____

20. one-half _____

Identify:

21. IVP   _intravenous pyelogram_ _____

22. qid _____

23. U _____

24. qns _____

25. supp _____

26. ns _____

27. TLC _____

28. IV _____

29. EKG _____

30. TPR _____

31. What are the vital signs? _____

32. What is a CT scan? _____

33. Write the abbreviations for: cubic centimeter _____ positive _____ milligram _____

Extra:

What orders should always be included for a patient in hospital? _____

_____

What are the routine immunizations? _____

_____

_____

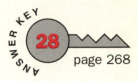

ANSWER KEY **28** page 268

Worksheet

Use abbreviations to fill in the blanks:

1. Before being admitted to the hospital as a patient, one must go through either ___ER_____

   or ___A & D_____

2. After surgery in the _____, a patient usually goes to the _____

   and then to the _____ unit.

3. If a fracture is suspected, the patient goes to _____ (for help in diagnosis).

4. For treatment only, not a hospital admission, a patient may go to the _____ or the

   _____

5. After a severe heart attack, a patient is usually sent to the _____ or_____

6. For delivery, a woman goes to the _____ department, _____

   room. After delivery, the newborn infant is taken to the _____ and the mother is

   taken to the _____ unit.

7. Children are cared for in _____

8. Most reusable supplies are cleaned and sterilized for the entire hospital in _____

9. Blood and urine samples are sent to the _____ for testing.

10. After recovery from a stroke, a patient may have treatment to restore weak muscles in the _____

    department.

11. After discharge from the hospital, a patient's file is sent to _____

12. After a patient dies, the body goes to the _____

13. If a patient needs help with child care or with family problems, the patient or the patient's family is referred to _____

14. Patients with psychological problems or mental illness are generally treated in _____

15. Tonsillectomies may be done in _____ or_____

16. A person who must learn a new skill because he or she is no longer able to perform on a previous job may be referred to _____

17. Intravenous fluids are generally stored in _____ and picked up or ordered from the units as needed.

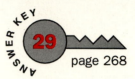

page 268

Test p. 309

CHAPTER 13

Diagnostic and Laboratory Abbreviations

Diagnostic Abbreviations

AAR	acute anxiety reaction
AIDS	acquired immune deficiency syndrome
ARC	AIDS-related complex
ASHD	arteriosclerotic heart disease (ăr-tēr-ē-ō-sclēr-**ŏt**-ĭk)
ASCVD	arteriosclerotic cardiovascular disease
CA	carci **no** ma (cancer)
CBS	chronic brain sydrome
CHD	coronary heart disease
CHF	congestive heart disease
COPD/ COLD	chronic obstructive pulmonary (lung) disease
CP	**cer** ebral palsy
CVA	cerebro **vas** cular accident (stroke)
CVD	cardio **vas** cular disease
DJD	degenerative joint disease (osteoarthritis)
FUO	fever of undetermined origin
GC	gonorrhea (gŏn-ŏr-**rē**-ă)

HBV	hepatitis B virus
HIV	human immunodeficiency virus
HPV	human papilloma virus (precancerous)
HTLV III	human T-lymphotropic virus type III
HTLV½	a new virus in addict populations, causes leukemia and neurologic disease
(S)LE	(systemic) lupus erythema **to** sus
MD	muscular dystrophy
MI	myo **car** dial in **farc** tion (coronary occlusion, coronary thrombosis
MS	multiple scle **ro** sis
NTD	neural tube defect
PID	pelvic inflammatory disease
RA	rheumatoid ar **thri** tis
STD	sexually transmitted disease(s)
T & A	tonsil **lec** tomy and adenoid **ec** tomy
TIA	transient is**che**mic attack (ĭs-**kē**-mĭk)
URI	upper respiratory infection
UTI	urinary tract infection

Do not let abbreviations "throw" you; recall your knowledge of terminology and use a little imagination. Often you will be able to figure out what the abbreviation stands for (in a medical history, for example) by the information given around it. In a particular work situation, you will soon learn the abbreviations pertinent to your job.

History-Taking and Physical Examination Abbreviations

Abbreviations used in taking a patient's medical history and giving a physical exam are numerous. The following are just a few:

CC	chief complaint	**Hx**	history
PI	present illness	**Sx** or **sm**	symptoms
et	etiology	**HEENT**	head, eyes, ears, nose, throat
sg	physical signs	**PE**	physical exam
lb	laboratory data	**PERLA**	pupils equal, react to light and accommodation (eyes)
xr	radiologic findings		
pa	pathology	**pt**	patient
PH	past history	**SOB**	shortness of breath, or significant other at bedside
FH	family history		
SR or **ROS**	systemic review or review of systems	**P & A**	percussion and auscultation
		A & P	auscultation and percussion
Rx	recipe, take, prescription	**R/O**	rule out
Dx	diagnosis	**m**	murmur
		c/o	complains of

Example of History and Exam Notes

Sx: Pt c/o RLQ discomfort, nausea, vomiting, and diarrhea. CC RLQ pain.

PH: Unremarkable

FH: Diverticulosis

PE: HEENT unremarkable

R/O: Appendicitis and gastroenteritis

Laboratory Abbreviations and Terms

The following material is a brief sketch of laboratory information. Although you may not understand all of it at this time, read through it; this outline contains many commonly used terms and abbreviations. Refer to lab forms on pp. 101–106 (Figures 13.1 to 13.6).

Hematology

Specimen   blood; this examination includes physical properties of blood such as:

Numbers of cells; blood counts

Size and shape: morphology

Microscopic appearance

Laboratory information continues on p. 107.

Figure 13.1 Hematology lab form (Courtesy of Sonora Laboratory Sciences).

SONORA
Laboratory Sciences
Professionals in Laboratory Medicine

PATIENT NAME			AGE
SONORA, TEST PATIENT			37Y
			M
IDENTIFICATION	ROOM	DATE OF BIRTH	SEX

COMPUTER TEST (PRINTS)

PHYSICIAN

COLLECTED: 04/21/96   RECEIVED: 04/21/96   REPORTED: 04/21/96 13:21

ADDITIONAL INFO:

TEST	ABNORMAL	RESULT NORMAL	UNITS	REFERENCE RANGE
CHEM PROFILE 30			COMPLETED	04/21/96
GLUCOSE	C HIGH 501		MG/DL	65-115
	** CRITICAL RESULT **			
BUN		15	MG/DL	5-25
CREAT		1.3	MG/DL	0.5-1.5
BUN/CRE		11.5		10.0-20.0
URIC ACID		4.0	MG/DL	2.2-6.5
SODIUM		140	MEQ/L	133-145
POTASS		4.0	MEQ/L	3.5-5.2
CHLORIDE		100	MEQ/L	95-112
CO2		25	MEQ/L	22-30
GAP		15		4-18
OSMO-CALC	HIGH 308		MOSM/K	275-295
T PROT	LOW 5.8		G/DL	5.9-8.4
ALBUMIN		3.6	G/DL	3.6-5.2
GLOBULIN		2.2	G/DL	1.9-3.4
ALB/GLOB		1.6		1.1-2.2
CHOL		100	MG/DL	0-200
TRIG		50	MG/DL	30-175
CALCIUM		9.0	MG/DL	8.5-10.5
ION CA-CAL		4.4	MG/DL	3.5-5.2
PHOS		3.0	MG/DL	2.5-4.5
GGT		40	IU/L	0-55
ALK PHOS		40	IU/L	30-130
SGPT (ALT)		20	IU/L	0-30
SGOT (AST)		20	IU/L	0-41
LDH		100	IU/L	95-250
CPK		50	IU/L	25-225
T BILI		0.5	MG/DL	0.2-1.2
D BILI		0.1	MG/DL	0.0-0.3
I BILI		0.4	MG/DL	0.0-1.2
IRON		100	MCG/DL	40-150

** FINAL **

Figure 13.2 Chemistry lab form (Courtesy of Sonora Laboratory Sciences).

SONORA
Laboratory Sciences

Professionals in Laboratory Medicine

PATIENT NAME			AGE
SONORA, TEST PATIENT			37Y
		02/20/59	F
IDENTIFICATION	ROOM	DATE OF BIRTH	SEX

COMPUTER TEST (PRINTS)

PHYSICIAN

COLLECTED: 04/01/96   RECEIVED: 04/01/96   REPORTED: 04/01/96 13:37

ADDITIONAL INFO:

		RESULT			
TEST	**ABNORMAL**		**NORMAL**	**UNITS**	**REFERENCE RANGE**
URINALYSIS ROUTINE					COMPLETED 04/01/96
COLL TIME: : 0					
COLOR			NORM		NORM
SP GRAV			1.015		1.002-1.030
ESTERASE	POS				NEG
NITRITE	POS				NEG
PH			7.5		5.0-8.0
BLOOD			NEG		NEG
PROTEIN			NEG	MG/DL	NEG
GLUCOSE			NEG	MG/DL	NEG
KETONES			NEG		NEG
UROBIL			NORM	EU/DL	NORM
BILE			NEG		NEG
MICRO					
MICROSCOPIC INDICATED					
URINALYSIS-MICROSCOPIC					COMPLETED 04/01/96
WBCS	HIGH	30		/HPF	0-10
RBCS			0	/HPF	0-10
BACTERIA	MODERATE			NEG	

** FINAL **

Figure 13.3 Urinalysis lab form (Courtesy of Sonora Laboratory Sciences).

Figure 13.4 Microbiology lab form (urine culture and sensitivity) (Courtesy of Sonora Laboratory Sciences).

SONORA Laboratory Sciences

096811 ACCOUNT INFORMATION

96811 96811
96811 96811
96811 96811

PATIENT I.D. ROOM NO.

REFERRING PHYSICIAN

COLLECTION DATE COLLECTION TIME ☐ AM ☐ PM

PATIENT LAST NAME (PLEASE PRINT) FIRST NAME MI

| ☐ PHYSICIAN CLIENT | ☐ PATIENT | ☐ INSURANCE | ☐ MEDICARE | ☐ AHCCCS |

BIRTH DATE AGE SEX PATIENT SOCIAL SECURITY NO.

I N S U R A N C E   I N F O

RESPONSIBLE PARTY RELATIONSHIP ☐ SELF ☐ SPOUSE ☐ DEPENDENT

ADDRESS (REQUIRED)

POLICY, I.D. OR MEDICARE # GROUP #

CITY STATE ZIP CODE PHONE

INSURANCE COMPANY

TOTAL DUE $ PAID AMOUNT DUE INITIAL

ADDRESS

CC TO: DR: ADDRESS CITY, STATE, ZIP

CITY STATE ZIP

CALL RESULTS TO ☐ FAX RESULTS TO ☐ **STAT** INDICATE TEST(S) NEEDED: DRAWING FEE ☐

EMPLOYER NAME:

☐ FASTING ☐ NON-FASTING CLINICAL DATA/COMMENTS

PHOTOCOPY BOTH SIDES OF INSURANCE CARD AND STAPLE TO REQUISITION DIAGNOSIS CODE ICD-9# REFERRAL/AUTHORIZATION #

CERTIFICATIONS: MEDICARE NO. 03L0008087 (3401 E. HARBOUR DR.) CAP NO. 22200-01 CAP NO. 22201-01 CHAMPUS NO. FS0030022824 CLIA (INTERSTATE) NO. 03L0000031 TAX I.D. NO. 86-0592349 AHCCCS NO. 05-1342-10

09 ***** PHYSICIAN'S DIAGNOSIS *****
10 ☐ 623.5 ABNORMAL DISCHARGE
11 ☐ 626.6 ABNORMAL BLEEDING
12 ☐ 795.0 ABNORMAL PAP
13 ☐ 285.90 ANEMIA
14 ☐ 627.3 ATROPHIC VAGINITIS
15 ☐ 611.72 BREAST MASS
16 ☐ 622.10 CERVICAL DYSPLASIA
17 ☐ 622.7 CERVICAL POLYP
18 ☐ 616.0 CERVICITIS
19 ☐ 634.92 COMPLETE ABORTION
20 ☐ 078.1 VIRAL WARTS
21 ☐ 625.30 DYSMENORRHEA

☐ 276.60 EDEMA
☐ V25.01 FAMILY PLANNING (ORAL CONTRACEPTIVES)
☐ 780.70 FATIGUE
☐ 616.9 FEMALE GENITAL INFLAMMATION, NOS
☐ 218.90 FIBROID
☐ 091.0 GENITAL SYPHILIS, PRIMARY
☐ 098.0 GONOCOCCAL INFECTIONS
☐ 054.9 HERPES
☐ 259.9 HORMON INBALANCE
☐ 626.10 HYPOMENORRHEA
☐ 628.90 INFERTILITY

☐ 626.9 MENSTRUAL DISORDER
☐ 765.0 NON-VIABLE FETUS
☐ V22.0 PREGNANT
☐ 627.0 PREMENOPAUSAL
☐ 626.2 MENORRHAGIA
☐ 627.1 POST-MENOPAUSAL BLEEDING
☐ 616.10 VAGINITIS
☐ 616.11 VULVITIS
☐ V72.3 ROUTINE PAP
☐ V76.2 SCR ANNUAL PAP
☐ V15.89 SCR ANNUAL PAP W/CERVICAL RISK

WE RETURN SPECIMENS WHICH ARE UNLABELED, OR DO NOT INCLUDE SOURCE, BIRTHDATE OR AGE, AND CLINICAL HISTORY

CYTOLOGY

CLINICAL HISTORY

☐ LMP __/__/__
☐ HYSTERECTOMY __/__/__
☐ SUPRACERVICAL
☐ HYSTERECTOMY __/__/__
☐ RADIATION __/__/__
☐ ESTROGEN THERAPY __/__/__
☐ CHEMOTHERAPY __/__/__
☐ POST CRYO
☐ POST LASER

☐ BIRTH CONTROL PILLS
☐ NORPLANT
☐ PERI MENOPAUSAL
☐ POST MENOPAUSAL
☐ PREGNANT
☐ POST PARTUM
☐ DISCHARGE
☐ IUD

PAP SMEAR SOURCE
☐ VAGINAL
☐ CERVICAL
☐ ENDOCERVICAL

☐ MATURATION INDEX

SEPARATE SLIDE LABELED WITH SOURCE AND NAME FROM LATERAL VAGINAL WALL

OTHER CYTOLOGY
☐ BREAST
☐ BRONCHIAL BRUSH
☐ BRONCHIAL WASH
☐ CSF
☐ GASTRIC BRUSH
☐ GASTRIC WASH
☐ FINE NEEDLE ASPIRATION

☐ PERITONEAL FLUID
☐ PLEURAL FLUID
☐ SPUTUM
☐ URINE
☐ OTHER

IMPORTANT INFORMATION FOR ACCURATE SCREENING
☐ HIGH RISK
HISTORY _____
CLINICAL DIAGNOSIS _____

PREVIOUS PAP HISTORY
☐ SONORA CASE NO. _____
☐ OTHER LAB
☐ NO INFORMATION AVAILABLE

NUMBER OF SLIDES SUBMITTED
☐ ONE
☐ TWO
☐ THREE
☐ OTHER _____
☐ BIOPSY ALSO SUBMITTED

SOURCE: _____
SEE REVERSE FOR DIAGRAM

☐ RIGHT
☐ LEFT
☐ SOLID MASS
☐ CYST

PATHOLOGIST'S COMMENTS:

CLIN PATH ASSOCIATES PC AFFILIATED WITH SONORA LABORATORY SCIENCES

CYTOTECHNOLOGIST'S INITIALS DATE

PATHOLOGIST'S SIGNATURE

DATE RECEIVED STAMP CA NO. SLIDES

Figure 13.5 Cytology lab form (Courtesy of Clin-Path Associates PC affiliated with Sonora Laboratory Sciences).

SONORA
Laboratory Sciences

2812552 2812552

2812552 2812552

2812552 2812552

2812552 ACCOUNT INFORMATION

PATIENT I.D.   ROOM NO.

REFERRING PHYSICIAN

COLLECTION DATE   COLLECTION TIME
                   ☐ A.M.
                   ☐ P.M.

PATIENT LAST NAME (PLEASE PRINT)   FIRST NAME   MI

☐ PHYSICIAN CLIENT ☐ PATIENT ☐ INSURANCE ☐ MEDICARE ☐ AHCCCS

BIRTH DATE   AGE   SEX   PATIENT SOCIAL SECURITY NO.

RESPONSIBLE PARTY   RELATIONSHIP
☐ SELF ☐ SPOUSE ☐ DEPENDENT

ADDRESS (REQUIRED)

POLICY, I.D. OR MEDICARE #   GROUP #

CITY   STATE   ZIP CODE   PHONE

INSURANCE COMPANY

TOTAL DUE $ PAID   AMOUNT DUE   INITIAL

ADDRESS

CC TO: DR:
ADDRESS
CITY, STATE, ZIP

CITY   STATE   ZIP

CALL RESULTS TO ☐   FAX RESULTS TO ☐   ☐ STAT INDICATE TEST(S) NEEDED:
DRAWING FEE ☐

EMPLOYER NAME:

☐ FASTING
☐ NON-FASTING   CLINICAL DATA/COMMENTS

INSURANCE INFO

PHOTOCOPY BOTH SIDES OF INSURANCE CARD AND STAPLE TO REQUISITION   DIAGNOSIS CODE ICD-9#   REFERRAL/AUTHORIZATION #

WRITTEN TESTS CUSTOM PROFILES - CONTACT LABORATORY FOR ADDITION OF CUSTOM PROFILES

PROFILES AND TEST COMBINATIONS ** SEE LAB USERS GUIDE OR FEE LIST FOR SEPARATELY BILLED CPT-4 CODES

☐ 2950 CHEM30 (80019, 82977, 83540)	S	☐ 2958 CHEM BASIC (80019)	S	☐ 2000 CALC CARDIAC RISK (CALC. LDL)	
☐ 2067 CHEM30, CBC	S,W	☐ 4794 CHEM BASIC, CBC	S,W	☐ 2002 CARDIAC RISK (CHOL, TRIG, HDL, DIRECT LDL, VLDL, CHOL/HDL RATIO)	2S
☐ 4849 CHEM30, CBC, UA	S,W,U	☐ 4855 CHEM BASIC, CBC, UA	S,W,U	☐ 6165 COCCI PANEL (COCCI IgM, IgG COMP FIX IF IND)	S
☐ 4736 CHEM30, CBC, SED RATE	S,W	☐ 4856 CHEM BASIC, CBC, SED RATE	S,W	☐ 2455 ELECTROLYTES (NA, K, CL, CO2, GAP)	S
☐ 2072 CHEM30, CBC, T7	S,W	☐ 4857 CHEM BASIC, CBC, T7	S,W	☐ 6006 EPSTEIN BARR-WITH INTERP (IgG, IgM, EBNA)	2S
☐ 4850 CHEM30, CBC, T7, UA	S,W,U	☐ 4858 CHEM BASIC, CBC, T7, UA	S,W,U	☐ 4750 HEPATITIS ABC (HAAB IgM, HBSAG, HBCAB IgM, HCAB)	3S
☐ 4851 CHEM30, CBC, T7, TSH	2S,W	☐ 4859 CHEM BASIC, CBC, T7, TSH	S,W	☐ 2164 HEPATITIS PANEL (HBSAG, HBSAB, HBCAB IgM, HAAB IgM)	3S
☐ 2022 CHEM30, CALC CARDIAC RISK CCR	2S	☐ 4681 CHEM BASIC, CALC CARDIAC RISK (CCR)	S	☐ 2165 HEPATITIS ACUTE (HBSAG, HBCAB IgM, HAAB IgM)	3S
☐ 2069 CHEM30, CCR, CBC	2S,W	☐ 4682 CHEM BASIC, CCR, CBC	2S,W	☐ 2254 HYPOTHYROID PROFILE (T7, TSH)	S
☐ 2214 CHEM30, CCR, CBC, UA	2S,W,U	☐ 4683 CHEM BASIC, CCR, CBC, UA	2S,W,U	☐ 2700 LH/FSH	S
☐ 4852 CHEM30, CCR, CBC, SED RATE	2S,W	☐ 4688 CHEM BASIC, CCR, CBC, SED RATE	2S,W	☐ 1017 PRENATAL 1 ABO/RH, AB SCR, CBC, RPR, RUBELLA, S,C,T,W	
☐ 2071 CHEM30, CCR, CBC, T7	2S,W	☐ 4684 CHEM BASIC, CCR, CBC, T7	2S,W	☐ 1018 PRENATAL 2 ABO/RH, AB SCR, CBC, RPR, RUBELLA, UA, S,C,T,W,U	
☐ 4853 CHEM30, CCR, CBC, T7, UA	2S,W,U	☐ 4686 CHEM BASIC, CCR, CBC, T7, UA	2S,W,U	☐ 1019 PRENATAL 3 ABO/RH, AB SCR, CBC, RPR, RUBELLA, HBSAG), S,C,T,W	
☐ 4954 CHEM30, CCR, CBC, T7, TSH	2S,W	☐ 4860 CHEM BASIC, CCR, CBC, T7, TSH	2S,W	☐ 2855 PSA/PAP	S

MICROBIOLOGY / VIROLOGY (★= COMPLETE VIROLOGY INFO SHEET)

☐ 6130 CHLAMYDIA CULTURE★	☐ 6016 CHLAMYDIA EIA★
☐ 6265 HERPES CULTURE★	☐ VIRUS CULTURE★
☐ 6240 GC GENPROBE	☐ 6375 OVA & PARASITES

CULTURES-ALWAYS INDICATE SOURCE WHEN ORDERING CULTURE†

☐ 6010 AFB CULTURE	☐ 6080 BETA STREP CULTURE
☐ 6225 FUNGUS CULTURE	☐ 6230 GC CULTURE
☐ 6570 ANAEROBIC CULTURE	☐ ROUTINE CULTURE

†SOURCE:

MANY TESTS AND PROFILES CONTAIN SEPARATE BILLABLE CPT-4 CODES. ALL TESTS BILLED TO PATIENTS AND THIRD PARTY PAYORS INCLUDING MEDICARE AND AHCCCS WILL BE BILLED ACCORDING TO THEIR RESPECTIVE CODES. SEE YOUR FEE LIST, LAB USER'S GUIDE OR THE REVERSE SIDE OF THIS PAGE FOR SEPARATE CODES.

INDIVIDUAL TESTS

☐ 1050 ABO/RH TYPE	CT	☐ 2465 GLUCOSE (FASTING)	S	☐ 6315 MONOTEST	S		
☐ 2220 AMYLASE	S	☐ 2510 GLUCOSE (RANDOM)	S	☐ 2790 POTASSIUM	S	☐ 4290 SED RATE (WEST)	W
☐ 6040 ANA	S	☐ 2030 GLUCOSE-2HR PP	S	☐ 2915 PREGNANCY, SERUM	S	☐ 2013 THEOPHYLLINE	CT
☐ 2250 BUN	S	☐ GLUCOSE TOL HRS	S	☐ 2102 PSA	S	☐ 2985 T3 (TOTAL)	S
☐ 4075 CBC (AUTO DIFF)	W	☐ GESTATIONAL TOL HRS	S	☐ 4255 PROTIME (INR)	P(F)	☐ 2023 T7 (T3U/T4/T7)	S
☐ 2305 CEA	S	☐ 2520 GLYCOHEMOGLOBIN	W	☐ 4020 PTT	P(F)	☐ 2043 T4	S
☐ 2395 CREATININE	S	☐ 2530 HDL CHOL	W	☐ 6415 RPR	S	☐ 2118 TSH	S
☐ 2430 DIGOXIN	CT	☐ 6260 HIV (SEE REVERSE *)	S	☐ 6440 RUBELLA IgG	S	☐ 4370 URINALYSIS	U

SPECIMEN REQUIREMENT CODES

SST					
S - SERUM OR SST		W - WHOLE BLOOD		U - RANDOM URINE	
CT - CLOTTED TUBE		- (LAVENDER TOP TUBE)		(F) - SPIN, FREEZE IN PLASTIC VIAL	
P - PLASMA (BLUE TOP)		U24 - 24 HOUR URINE		(R) - SUBMIT AT ROOM TEMPERATURE	

I AUTHORIZE SONORA LABORATORY SCIENCES TO BILL ME FOR CHARGES NOT COVERED BY MY INSURANCE.

DRAWN   OPEN   TR   LABEL   VERIFY   CHANGE   PATIENT SIGNATURE

SEND FIRST 2 COPIES TO LABORATORY

Figure 13.6 Flexible profiles and individual tests (Courtesy of Sonora Laboratory Sciences).

Routine Tests

CBC complete blood count (see Fig. 13.1)

RBC red cell count (erythrocytes)

WBC white cell count (leukocytes)

WBC & diff(erential) count number of each kind of white cell: neutrophils, eosinophils, and basophils, lymphocytes, and monocytes (see Notes on p. 108 for further discussion of neutrophils)

Hb, Hgb hemoglobin

Crit, Hct hematocrit

Platelet count

ESR, sed rate erythrocyte sedimentation rate

Biochemistry

SMA, SMAC sequential multiple analyzer computer: group of chemistry tests often called chemistry profile; in some areas these tests must be ordered separately.

Specimen blood serum; this examination includes tests for the following chemical elements:

Glucose; tests include **FBS**, fasting blood sugar, and **GTT**, glucose tolerance test

Sodium, potassium, chlorides, and so on

BUN, BSP, NPN, SGOT, and so on

See the explanation of blood chemistry tests on page 109.

Specimen urine may be collected by these methods: voided, midstream, or catheterized or cath spec. Routine urinalysis, UA may include testing for the following:

pH reaction (acid or alkaline)

Albumin or glucose

Specific gravity: weight as compared to water

Casts, bacteria, WBCs, RBCs (microscopic exam)

Serology

Specimen blood serum; the following are blood serum tests:

STD tests: STS (serological test for syphilis), VDRL (Venereal Disease Research Laboratory), Kahn, and others

Pregnancy tests: Pregnosticon and UCG (ultrasound cardiogram)

RA: rheumatoid arthritis

Landsteiner blood types: ABO (type and crossmatch done before transfusion)

Rh factor

Rubella

Antibody titer (titre): Rh, HIV

Bacteriology

Specimen   blood, sputum, spinal fluid, any excretion, feces (for presence of occult blood or parasites)

To isolate and identify pathogenic bacteria, the following test is ordered:

C & S culture and sensitivity; bacteria are grown from specimen and subjected to various antibiotics to determine the most effective one for treatment of bacterial diseases.

Other common terms:

gram stain   one of the basic stains used in classifying bacteria (gram neg. or pos.)

AFB   acid-fast bacillus (tuberculosis organism)

hanging drop culture   placing drop of culture medium containing microorganisms on coverslip and inverting over concave slide

Histology and Cytology

Histology is the study of tissues; cytology is the study of cells.

Specimen   tissues and cells; histologic and cytologic studies include the following:

Biopsy examination of living tissue (tests for abnormal cells such as cancer)

Pap smear cancer detection (Papanicolaou)

Miscellaneous tests may be done on bone marrow, gastric contents, and spinal fluid, depending on the size and scope of the lab.

■ **Note:** The term *neutrophil* is seldom used on lab forms. They may be called PMNs (polymorpho **nu** clear **leu** kocytes) or segs (segmented nuclei), meaning mature cells with the nucleus in segments. The term *stabs* and *bands* refer to immature cells. *Aniso* and *poik* are abbreviations for anisocy **to** sis (variation in size of red blood cells) and poikilocy **to** sis (variation in shape of RBCs).

Lab stix: Many simple lab procedures are now done with commercial *lab stix* of various kinds. For example, a treated paper stick need only be dipped into a urine sample to test for sugar and other substances. These are used in many offices and by patients who regularly test their urine at home (diabetics). Tablets are also used for simple, routine urine tests. Fecal occult blood test kits such as Hemoccult are used to test stool for blood.

Communication with the Laboratory

The laboratory is usually under the direction of a *pathologist*, with *medical technologists* performing the complicated laboratory tests and assistants the simpler tests. All hospitals and clinics have laboratories, and many lab tests can be performed in the physician's office. There are lab requisition slips for each laboratory division (every lab uses different forms, unfortunately) or tests are ordered by computer. You will become familiar with the various laboratory forms as you use them. Figures 13.1 to 13.6 contain sample lab requisition forms. Some labs use color coding and code numbers.

The following are some important points to remember in dealing with the laboratory:

1. Use care if directed to collect specimens (use gloves, don't stick self, dispose of needles properly, etc.).

2. Label specimens accurately and completely.

3. Use properly prepared containers (for example, some containers have a preservative added and some are color coded).

4. Use the right requisition form in ordering lab work (if not using a computerized request).

5. Refrigerate specimens if they must be held for a specified time (unless directed otherwise).

6. If your job involves instructing patients about specimen collection, explain clearly and make sure the patient understands.

Sample lab forms for hematology, chemistry, urinalysis, microbiology, cytology, and flexible profiles are presented in Figures 13.1 through 13.6. Look at the headings on the first three forms—hematology, chemistry, and urinalysis. The heading to the far right, Normals, gives the range of values considered to be healthy, or within the norm for a particular test. The patient's test values will be listed under the heading in the middle (Normal) if the test results fall within the range listed on the right, or under the heading Abnormal if the test results fall outside the normal range.

Blood Chemistry Tests (SMA)

Test	What it is
Calcium, phosphorus	Indicative of bone function and of the parathyroid hormones that influence bone function.
Glucose	Useful test for diabetes; varies with state of fasting and age.
BUN, creatinine, BUN/creatinine ratio	Detect the presence of kidney disease but are influenced by a number of other factors; BUN may be elevated in severe dehydration and is reduced in pregnancy. BUN = blood urea nitrogen; say it as the letters, B-U-N.
Uric acid	May be elevated in gout, but levels are variable; increased during periods of stress.
Cholesterol, triglycerides (fats)	Associated with increased probability of heart disease.
Total protein, albumin, globulin, albumin/globulin ratio	General index of overall health and nutrition. The globulin fraction of blood serum contains antibodies.
Bilirubin, direct bilirubin	Test of liver function; may be elevated because of disease of red blood cells. In circulation it may indicate liver disease, hemolysis, gout, increased risk of MI. Bilirubin is the orange pigment in bile seen as jaundice.
Alkaline phosphatase	Indicates possible liver or bone disorders. Elevated in adolescence when bones are growing.
LDH	Detects cell damage of various types; not specific for any certain disease. LDH = lactic dehy **drog** enase.
SGOT	May indicate possible liver disease or heart muscle damage; may also be elevated due to recent vigorous exercise. SGOT = serum glu **tam** ic oxaloa **ce** tic trans **am** inase.
SGPT	Test of liver function.
Iron	If low, may indicate presence of anemia.
Sodium, potassium, chloride	Blood electrolytes. May be abnormal due to a number of diseases.
Magnesium	Another electrolyte, required for normal neural and muscular function.

The suffix -ase indicates an enzyme. When a tissue or organ is damaged due to disease or trauma, enzymes are released into the blood.

■ Note: It is important to remember that most laboratory tests are not diagnostic in themselves. Along with other findings, they do aid the physician in making a diagnosis. Blood test results are known to fluctuate from day to day, owing to changes within an individual patient and/or laboratory variation. Sometimes a certain group of blood tests gives the physician a better overall picture of the patient's status better than a single test can give. These are called *profiles*. They are often done to aid the physician in establishing a diagnosis. Some examples are arthritis profile, cardiac profile, thyroid profile, and hepatitis profile; a prenatal profile is also done.

Self-Test

Identify:

1. CBC   *complete blood count (per cubic millimeter)* _____

2. WBC   _____

3. RBC   _____

4. Hb, Hgb   _____

5. Hct, Crit   _____

6. FBS   _____

Complete the following:

7. Explain what *diff* means in "WBC and diff":   *differential; it means counting each of the* _____
    different kinds of leukocytes or white blood cells in a sample _____

    _____

8. Name the five basic kinds of leukocytes: _____

    _____

9. What are the physical properties of blood, and which lab division works in this area? _____

    _____

10. Name three tests done in a routine UA: _____

    _____

    _____

11. What is the difference between a voided and a catheterized urine specimen (in how it is obtained)?

    _____

    _____

    _____

    Which of these would be least likely to contain contaminants? _____

    _____

12. Which lab division analyzes the STD tests results? _____ Name one such test: _____

13. To which lab division would a throat swab specimen be sent if strep sore throat was suspected?

    _____

    Which test would the doctor order to find out the best antibiotic to prescribe? _____

    _____

14.* What is a Pap smear and why and how is it done? _____

    _____

    In which lab department is it examined? _____

15. What is a biopsy? _____

    _____

    _____

16. List the six important points in collection of specimens: _____

    _____

    _____

    _____

    _____

    _____

17.* What is meant by a "fasting" kind of test? _____

    _____

18. What terms or abbreviations are used for neutrophils on laboratory forms (hematology)? _____

    _____

19.* What kinds of white cells (in a differential count) normally run less than (<) 1%? _____

    _____

20. An -ase suffix denotes an _____

21. What is the normal range of hemoglobin? (see lab form, hematology) _____

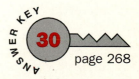

ANSWER KEY 30 page 268

Test p. 311

---

*The answers to questions 14, 17, and 19 are not found in your text. You may want to discuss them in class.

CHAPTER 14

Basic Pharmacology

Introduction to Pharmacology and the PDR*

In every medical situation where medications are prescribed, you will find a book called the PDR, *Physicians' Desk Reference*. It is published yearly and lists all prescription drugs and information about them. During the year, a supplement is published listing new additions and new information about drugs. You will find this book helpful, especially for the spelling of drug names. Get acquainted with it.

The PDR is divided into different color-coded sections to facilitate use. These are the usual sections:

Section 1	white	manufacturers' index, lists addresses and partial list of their products
Section 2	pink	brand and generic name index
Section 3	blue	product category index (what conditions are this drug used for?)
Section 4	gray glossy	product identification guide; pictures of the product
Section 5	white	product information section; gives detailed information: therapeutic indication, side effects, contraindications, dosages, etc. alphabetically by manufacturers
Section 6	green	diagnostic products information section (dyes used in procedures)

Poison control centers

Discontinued products

FDA telephone directory

Key to controlled substances categories

Key to FDA use-in-pregnancy ratings

Drug information centers

Adverse event report forms

There are separate PDRs for ophthalmology, nonprescription drugs, and drug interactions/side effects. There are also other references for drugs to be found in the public libraries and (perhaps) in doctors' offices.

Every drug has several different names; this can be confusing to the uninitiated. Here are a few examples of generic names with corresponding trade names:

*See Appendix G for list of drugs.

Generic	Trade
tetracycline (tĕ-tră-**sī**-klēn)	Achro **my** cin, Topicycline
acetylsalicylic acid (ă-sē-tĭl-săl-ĭ-**sī**-lĭk)	Easprin, **Ec** otrin, Healthprin aspirin
acetaminophen (ă-sē-tă-**mĭn**-ō-fĕn)	**Ty** lenol, Aspirin Free Excedrin, Fioricet
ibuprofen (ī-bū-**prō**-fĕn)	**Ad** vil, **Mo** trin

Drugs are classified by the type of action they produce. For example:

analgesic drugs (ăn-ăl-**jē**-sĭk)	relieve pain; including over-the-counter (OTC) pain relievers and narcotic drugs such as **Dem** erol or **mor** phine
diuretic drugs (dī-ū-**rĕt**-ĭk)	increase urinary output (**Di** uril)
antibiotic drugs (ăn-tī-bī-**ŏt**-ĭk)	inhibit or destroy bacterial life (peni **cill** ins)
tranquilizers (**trăn**-kwĭl-ī-zĕrs)	reduce anxiety (**Val** ium, **Com** pazine)
decongestants (dē-kŏn-**jĕs**-tănts)	relieve nasal congestion (Contac, **Su** dafed)
sedatives (**sĕd**-ă-tĭvs)	produce sleep (**Sec** onal, **Nem** butal)
immunosuppressants (ĭm-mū-nō-sūp-**prĕs**-sănts)	help to prevent rejection in organ transplantation (**Im** butal)

If a physician specifies a particular trade name in a drug prescription, in most states the pharmacist must supply the trade-name drug. However, the prescription may state "may substitute generic" when a trade-name drug is prescribed. If the prescription is written for a generic drug, the pharmacist chooses which brand to dispense. Generic drugs are generally less expensive than trade-name drugs.

Only the first letter of most brand-name drugs is a capital letter, with a few exceptions such as **phi** soHex, **Rho** GAM, Hydro **DI** URIL. Most hyphenated brand names also have a capital letter after the hyphen, as in **Ser-Ap-Es**. **A generic name is not capitalized.** In some cases the brand name and the generic name are the same, or almost the same. *Melatone* is a brand name; *melatonin* is a generic name.

Here is a typical drug listing in the white information section (Section 5) of the PDR:

Gan trisin (listed under Roche)	(brand name, by manufacturer)
sulfi *sox* azole—tablets	(generic name and form)
acetyl sulfisoxazole—syrup	
Description	
Clinical pharmacology	(composition)
Indications and usage	
Contraindications	
Warnings and precautions	
Adverse reactions, overdosage	
Dosage and administration	
How supplied	

To identify an unfamiliar drug name, or to verify its spelling, refer first to the alphabetical index in Section 2. If it is underlined, it is a generic name and you should not capitalize it. To check for unusual capitalization in a brand name, find the page number in the pink index (Section 2) and check the long white section for product information (Section 5). This section is somewhat awkward to use because the listings in the white section are by manufacturer (alphabetically), so you must first find the page number in the index.

If you know the brand name and wish to find the generic term, find the page number in the pink index, then look in the white Product Information Section (Section 5). The generic name is generally listed in parentheses below the brand name.

Related Pharmacology Terms

pla ce bo   an inert substance substituted for a drug; used in double-blind studies to test drug effectiveness; there is documented evidence that a placebo can provide relief in some cases, especially if the patient has confidence in the physician

tolerance   capacity for ingesting an increased amount without effect (usually a narcotic-type drug)

interaction   chemical reaction when two or more drugs are taken simultaneously; may also apply to some foods or alcoholic substances in combination with drugs

■ **Note:** The dosage of a drug is usually based on the size of the patient (body weight). Age is also a factor, because old people usually have an increased vulnerability to side effects, and a decreased ability to handle the effects of drugs. Since they may be taking many prescription drugs, and may be under treatment by several physicians, the possibility of interaction is increased.

Rx   prescription symbol; means "recipe," or "Take:"

OTC   over-the-counter drugs

generic   a drug comparable to the "trade name" substance, after the original producer's exclusive rights have run out; nonproprietary name

detail rep   representative of pharmaceutical company who calls upon physicians and introduces new drugs, leaves samples and sometimes gifts (to sell the product)

chemical name   chemical formula (with which you need not be concered)

street drugs   a number of illegal drugs sold "on the street" to users and addicts, at high prices and in varying degrees of purity. Examples: cocaine, including crack; marijuana; heroin; tranquilizers; narcotic sedatives; amphetamines; speed

IND   investigational new drug

FDA   Food and Drug Administration, a federal regulatory agency that must approve new drugs

USP   United States Pharmacopeia

General Information About Drugs

Many drugs must be stored in the refrigerator, especially those used in injectables and suppositories. *Important:* **All drugs have an expiration date after which time they should be discarded.** In fact, all unused prescription drugs should be discarded when they are no longer in use; antibiotic drugs should never be leftover, as the patient should continue to take them until they are used up. It is not wise to save leftover pills for the next illness, nor should they be given to someone else.

Worksheet

Define:

1. PDR _____

2. OTC _____

3. Rx _____

4. What is the action generally produced by the following drugs?

   a. a diuretic drug _____

   b. an analgesic drug _____

   c. a decongestant _____

   d. an immunosuppressant drug _____

5. Explain generic and brand names of drugs: _____

   _____

   May the pharmacist substitute one for the other? Explain: _____

   _____

6. What is a "detail rep"? _____

True/False: Circle the number of the true statements only. Defend your answers. Explain why a statement is false.

7. Some drugs must be stored in a refrigerator.

8. Drugs never "expire." They should be used up when you get sick again.

9. To learn the proper spelling of any drug, the best place to look is in the dictionary.

10. Antibiotic drugs are used to treat bacterial infections.

11. Sedatives such as Seconal sodium are given to patients who have difficulty sleeping.

12. If you have access to the PDR, look up the *brand* names of drugs and see if you can pick out ten that you have heard of. Write them here: _____

    _____

    List five classifications (blue section of the PDR) not given in this text, with an example of each.

    _____

    _____

    _____

    _____

    _____

13. The next time you receive a prescription form from your doctor, try to read it and look up the drug. You should also be able to read the abbreviations that tell how often the drug should be taken (qid or tid, for example).

14. Find a drug advertisement in a medical journal (instructor may provide these or you may utilize your library medical journals, such as JAMA or, the New England Journal of Medicine). Read through all of the information about the drug. List new words and define them, noting especially their side effects.

_____

_____

_____

_____

_____

_____

_____

_____

ANSWER KEY **31** page 268

■ **Note:** Sometimes the trade name of a drug will give you a clue to its action. For example:

Ob etrol   obesity control

Di upres, **Di** uril   diuretic drugs

Tussafed, Robi **tus** sin   "tuss" means "cough"; any name with tuss is for a cough medication

-gesic   analgesic, a pain reliever

On the other hand, some drug names don't tell you anything.

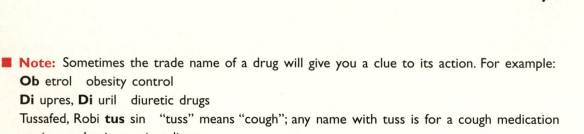

Worksheet

All of the following questions refer to the PDR.

1. Where would you look for the correct spelling of a trade-name drug? _Brand and Generic Name Index, pink section, section title, color_

2. Where would you look to find the names of some analgesics? _____

Name three analgesics: _____

3. What is indicated by the little black diamond shape shown before the names of some drugs in the pink section? _____

   Why are there two page numbers after these names? _____

4. Find the picture of Valium tablets. Who is the manufacturer? _____

   What is the generic name of this drug? _____

   Describe the tablets as to color and dosage: _____

5. These are generic names. What are some of their brand names?

   a. diazepam _____   b. meperidine _____

   c. norethindrone _____   d. allopurinol _____

6. These are brand names. Write their generic equivalents:

   a. Miltown _____

   b. Norinyl _____

   c. HydroDIURIL _____

   d. Sanorex _____

7. Correct spelling:

   a. Equanel _____

   b. Fasten _____

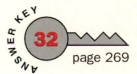

ANSWER KEY 32 page 269

Test p. 313

✔ Check Your Progress

Congratulations! You have made it to the end of Part I. By this point you should have a good basic foundation and framework in medical terminology. If you are still finding that certain words give you trouble, make and use flash cards for those terms. Review some of the worksheets from Part 1 that contain those terms. Be sure to discuss your problem with the instructor.

You may now be given a review test for Chapters 10–14, which can be found on page 315 in Appendix F. In this section, the end of Part 1, you have learned how to construct words that describe directional, positional, and numerical terms, general abbreviations and abbreviations for diagnostic and laboratory use, and basic pharmacology.

You will now move on to Part II, body system terminology. Remember to continue to review the completed Part I chapters as the foundation for the system terminology that you are learning and so that you do not forget what you have learned.

Body Systems Terminology

OVERVIEW

Beginning with basic body structures, this section focuses on each system's anatomy, physiology, and pathophysiology. Individual and group practice exercises, case histories, and health promotion tips conclude each system focus. Only the most frequently encountered medical terms are highlighted due to the nature and brevity of this course.

OBJECTIVES

1. To correctly locate and identify anatomical landmarks germane to each chapter.
2. To appropriately spell, define, and pronounce all medical terminology presented.
3. To apply medical terminology properly in context.

CHAPTER 15

Structure of
the Body

Anatomy and Physiology of Body Structure

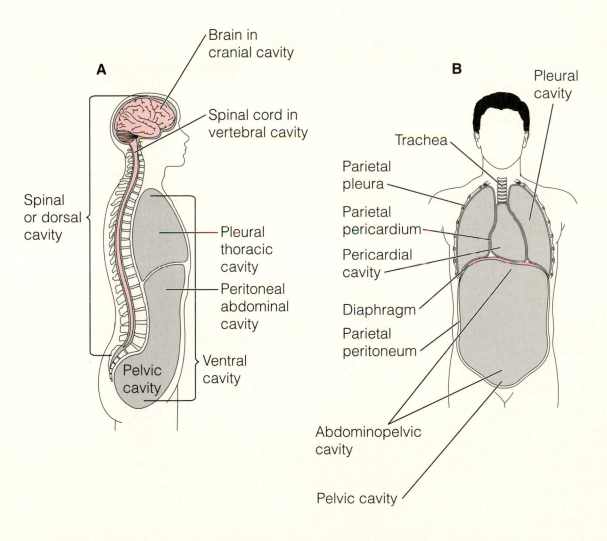

Figure 15.1 Body cavities. (**A**) Median section showing component parts of dorsal and ventral cavities. (**B**) Frontal section showing subdivisions of ventral cavity.

Body Cavities

pleural cavity (**plŭr**-ăl **kăv**-ĭ-tē) (tho **rac** ic cavity)   contains lungs, **tra** chea, e **soph** agus, **thy** mus.
  mediastinum (mē-dē-ă-**stī**-nŭm)   (in the middle) heart lies here.
peritoneal cavity (pĕr-ĭ-tō-**nĕ**-ăl)   (abdomino **pel** vic cavity) contains stomach, intestines, liver, gallbladder, pancreas, spleen, reproductive organs, and urinary bladder.

The pleural and peritoneal cavities derive their names from the membranes that line them—the pleura and the perito **ne** um. Related words: **pleur** isy, perito **ni** tis.

cranial cavity (**krā**-nē-ăl)   (skull) contains brain.
spinal cavity (**spī**-năl)   contains spinal cord.

The **di** aphragm is a dome-shaped muscle that separates the pleural and peritoneal cavities.

Structural Units of the Body

cells   the basic unit of all living things. They are microscopic in size and vary in shape, and each cell performs functions necessary for its own life. Cells multiply by dividing. This is called mi **to** sis. The following are the *main parts of a cell:*
  nucleus (**nū**-klē-ŭs)   contains **chro** mosomes; genes (hereditary units) are in the chromosomes.
  cytoplasm (**sī**-tō-plăzm)   protoplasm of the cell (the part outside of the nucleus).
  cell membrane (**sĕl mĕm**-brān)   holds the cell together (cell wall).
tissues   groups of cells that are alike.
  epithelial tissue (ĕp-ĭ-**thē**-lē-ăl)   protects, absorbs, and secretes (the skin and lining surfaces).
  connective tissue (fibrous)   connects and supports and also forms blood cells (bone, tendons, and so on).
  muscle tissue   contracts. Three types: (1) **stri** ated or striped (also called skeletal or voluntary); (2) cardiac; (3) smooth or involuntary.
  nerve tissue   conducts impulses (brain, spinal cord, and nerves).
  stroma (**strō**-mă)   type of connective tissue that supports an organ.
  parenchyma (păr-**ĕn**-kĭ-mă)   the essential parts of an organ concerned with its function, not framework.
organs   made up of more than one kind of tissue—heart, lungs, and liver, for example.
systems   groups of organs that work together. (Each system depends on the other systems of the body.)
  integumentary system (ĭn-tĕg-ū-**mĕn**-tăr-ē)   skin.
  musculoskeletal system (mŭs-kŭ-lō-**skĕl**-ĕ-tăl)   muscles, bones, and connective tissues: ligaments, tendons, and fasciae.
  cardiovascular system (kăr-dē-ō-**văs**-kū-lăr)   circulatory—heart and vessels.
  gastrointestinal system (găs-trō-ĭn-**tĕs**-tĭn-ăl)   (GI) digestive organs.
  respiratory system (**rĕs**-pĭr-ă-tŏr-ē)   lungs and airways.
  genitourinary system (jĕn-ĭ-tō-**ūr**-ĭ-nār-ē)   (GU) reproductive and urinary organs (also called urogenital). Also referred to separately as urinary and reproductive systems.
  endocrine system (**ĕn**-dō-krĭn)   ductless glands (for example: pituitary, thyroid).
  nervous system (**nĕr**-vŭs)   includes brain, spinal cord, and special senses.

Physiology Terms

Metabolism (mĕ-**tăb**-ō-lĭzm)   the process by which foods are changed into elements the body can use for growth, energy, and repair. Metabolism includes absorption, storage, and use of foods for the maintenance of the body; combining of foods and oxygen to produce energy; and elimination of waste materials.

Homeostasis (hō-mē-ō-**stā**-sĭs)   the state of equilibrium or relative constancy (sameness) that the body strives to maintain—for example, body temperature and cell division rate.

Body Openings

The following words refer to a body opening or entrance. Some are used interchangeably. You need not try to differentiate between them concerning usage. Merely become familiar with these terms so that if you hear them you will be able to recognize them. Watch the pronunciation of these terms.

meatus (mē-**ā**-tŭs)   passage or opening, such as urinary meatus.

orifice (**ŏr**-ĭ-fĭs)   entrance of any body cavity, such as anal orifice.

introitus (ĭn-**trō**-ĭ-tŭs)   vaginal cavity.

os (ōs)   mouth, opening; os uteri: mouth of the uterus, or cervix.

stoma (**stō**-mă)   artificial opening established by colostomy, ileostomy, and tracheostomy.

lumen (**lū**-měn)   opening within a hollow tube or organ.

patent (**pā**-těnt)   adjective, meaning open or not plugged, as in "The tube is patent."

perforation (pĕr-fō-**rā**-shŭn)   a hole in something; for example, a gastric ulcer can cause perforation of the stomach wall.

Related words:

dilatation or **dilation** (dĭl-ă-**tā**-shŭn), (dī-**lā**-shŭn)   making something wider or opened up.

constriction (kŏn-**strĭk**-shŭn)   making something smaller or narrower.

vasoconstriction (văs-ō-kŏn-**strĭk**-shŭn)   narrowing of vessels.

Define these other terms for kinds of body openings (use a dictionary).

aperture (**ăp**-ĕr-chŭr) _____

foramen (fō-**rā**-měn) _____

cavity (oral) _____

Pathophysiology

pathophysiology (păth-ō-fĭz-ē-**ŏl**-ō-jē)   the study of the nature and cause of physical disease.

pathology (pă-**thŏl**-ō-jē)   the study of the nature and cause of disease.

    etiology (ē-tē-**ŏl**-ō-jē)   cause

    epidemiology (ĕp-ĭ-dē-mē-**ŏl**-ō-jē)   frequency, distribution, occurrence, prevalence

Disease Origins

tumors or **neoplasms** (**tū**-mŏrs, **nē**-ō-plăzms)   malignancies; abnormal tissue formation.

traumatic (trăw-**mat**-ĭk)   accidental injuries; any physical or emotional injury.

metabolic (mět-ă-**bŏl**-ĭk)   hypoactive or hyperactive endocrine gland disorders, such as growth disorders, thyroid disorders, PKU.

infection (ĭn-**fĕk**-shŭn)   caused by any pathogenic agent, such as bacteria, viruses, fungi; all communicable diseases.

hereditary (hĕ-**rĕd**-ĭ-tăr-ē)   transmitted genetically from parent (such as Huntington's chorea).

congenital (kŏn-**jĕn**-ĭ-tăl)   present at birth; may be hereditary or acquired in the uterus (syphilis) or in the birth canal (gonorrhea).

vascular (**văs**-kū-lăr) occlusion or rupture of vessels, such as coronary occlusion, cerebrovascular accident, aneurysm.

degenerative (dē-**jĕn**-ĕr-ă-tĭv) result of wear and tear, especially on joints (as in osteoarthritis); includes eye conditions, some dementias.

immunologic (ĭm-ū-nō-**lŏj**-ĭk) immune-related diseases fall into three main groups: Those caused by action of antibodies, as in allergic hypersensitivity, autoimmune conditions in which the body produces antibodies against its own tissues, and immune deficiency disorders in which a weakened immune system is unable to fight off infection.

iatrogenic (ī-ăt-rō-**jĕn**-ĭk) caused by treatment by a physician.

nosocomial (nŏ-sō-**kō**-mē-ăl) caused by being in a hospital or treatment facility.

idiopathic (ĭd-ē-ō-**păth**-ĭk) disease for which no cause can be determined; peculiar to one person.

Worksheet

Fill in the blank:

1. Another name for the abdominopelvic cavity is _____

   Two other names for the chest cavity are _____ and _____

2. The cavity that contains the brain is _____

3. The smallest unit of living matter is _____

4. Name the main parts of a cell (3): _____

   _____

   What part contains the genes? _____

5. A catheter can be said to be _____ if its opening (_____) is not

   plugged up.

6. A gastric ulcer can eat through the stomach lining. This is called a _____ ulcer.

7. Three words that mean natural body openings are _____, _____,

   and _____

8. The narrowing of blood vessels is called _____

9. A patient who has a colostomy wears a pouch or appliance over the _____

   (opening in abdominal wall).

10. _____ (medications) cause blood vessels to

    become wider.

11. The os uteri is the _____

Name the systems that include the following organs:

12. heart   *cardiovascular*

13. vertebra (bone)

14. lungs

15. stomach

16. skeletal muscle

17. adrenal glands

18. spinal cord

19. kidneys

20. ovaries

21. skin

22. testes

23. Name four kinds of tissues:

24. A system is a _____ of _____ that work together to perform a certain function.

25. What are some of the processes included in metabolism?

26. Organs are made up of several kinds of

27. The diaphragm is a _____ that separates chest and abdominopelvic cavities.

Define or describe:

28. mitosis   *cell division (means of multiplying)*

29. lower extremities

30. striated (muscle)

31. secretion

32. absorption

33. elimination

34. pathology

35. homeostasis

True/False: Circle the number of the true statements only. Explain why the other statements are false.

36. A nosocomial infection is one you catch from your brother in your home.

37. The elderly often develop degenerative disorders.

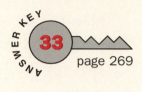
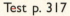

page 269

Test p. 317

▲ **Health Promotion Tip**

The following habits benefit the entire body structure:

- Adequate rest
- Proper nutrition
- Regular daily exercise
- Stress management
- Preventive medical care

CHAPTER 16

Integumentary System

Anatomy and Physiology of the Integumentary System

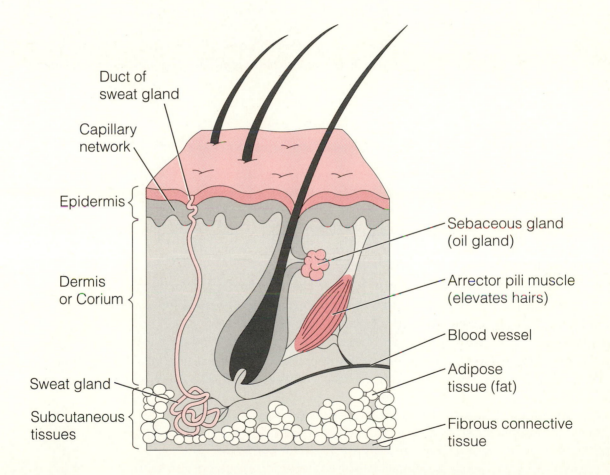

Duct of sweat gland

Capillary network

Epidermis

Dermis or Corium

Sweat gland

Subcutaneous tissues

Sebaceous gland (oil gland)

Arrector pili muscle (elevates hairs)

Blood vessel

Adipose tissue (fat)

Fibrous connective tissue

Figure 16.1 Cross section of normal skin showing epidermis, dermis (corium), and subcutaneous tissues. Note important structures in dermis: blood vessels, sweat glands, and sebaceous glands.

Function

The integumentary system is made up of skin and accessory structures; skin forms the external covering of the body. It plays the following roles:

- *Protection:* a waterproof overcoat that keeps body fluids in and harmful elements out (bacteria and sun, for example).
- *Sensory organ (receptor):* for sensations of touch, pain, and temperature.
- *Temperature regulator:* for cooling and heating (perspiration and "goose flesh").
- *Waste elimination:* disposal of wastes via perspiration.

Anatomy and Accessory Structures

skin   integument (from Latin, meaning "a covering"), or external covering.

epi der mis (cuticle)   nonvascular outer layer of skin; consists of four layers; epi **the** lial tissue. (See Figure 16.1 for cross section of normal skin.) Cells on the surface are dead cells. (*Epi* means "on top of.")

dermis or **corium**   deeper layer connective tissue containing nerves, nerve endings, blood vessels, sebaceous glands (sebum = oil), and sweat glands (sudo **rif** erous).

hair and **nails**   appendages of skin.

subcutaneous   "under the skin"; contains adipose tissue, connective tissue, vessels, and nerves.

breasts   mammary glands. Lactation is controlled by endocrine system. The a **re** ola mamma (plural = mammae) is the halo around nipple.

Pathophysiology of the Integumentary System

Descriptive Terms

See Figure 16.2.

bulla (plural, **-ae**) (**bŭl**-lă) (ā)   large blister, as in burns.

cyst (sĭst)   a type of nodule that is usually somewhat movable; contains fluid.

erosion (ē-**rō**-zhŭn)   "eating away," an early ulcer.

fissure (**fĭsh**-ŭr)   crack in skin surface (anal fissure or athlete's foot lesion, for example).

macule (**măk**-ūl)   spots, not elevated (freckle, flat mole, or rash of measles, for example).

nodule (**nŏd**-ūl)   larger raised lesion (cyst); can be felt more than seen.

papule (**păp**-ūl)   small, raised spots (wart, acne, mole, or psoriasis (sō-**rī**-ă-sĭs) for example).

plaque (plăk)   used to describe the silvery scales of psoriasis. (Other meanings refer to teeth and arteries.)

pustule (**pŭs**-tūl)   lesion containing pus (some acne, impetigo, pimple, for example); a large pustule is an **ab** scess.

scales or **crusts** (skāls, krŭsts)   flaking type of lesions (psoriasis, fungus, for example).

scar (skăr)   mark left by healing of a wound. *Cicatrix* (**sĭk**-ă-trĭks) is another word for scar. A **ke** loid is an overgrowth of scar tissue. Gelatin implants are used for scar correction.

tumor (**tū**-mŏr)   a swelling or large nodule (may be benign or malignant); also called a neoplasm.

ulcer (**ŭl**-sĕr)   tissue destruction, a deep lesion extending into subcutaneous tissue (**var** icose ulcer, de **cub** itus ulcer, for example).

vesicle (**vĕs**-ĭk-l)   lesion containing fluid (blister). (as in impetigo or varicella/chickenpox).

wheal (hwēl)   elevation (individual hive) or "bleb" produced by injection of a skin test.

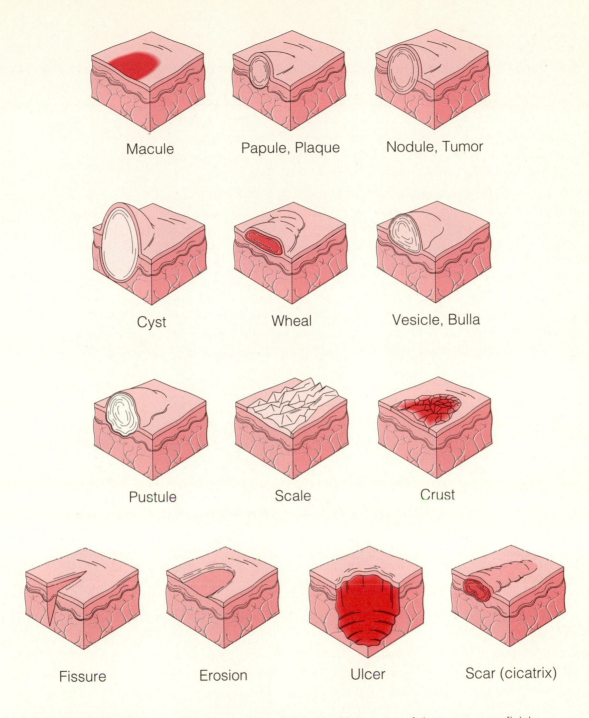

Macule

Papule, Plaque

Nodule, Tumor

Cyst

Wheal

Vesicle, Bulla

Pustule

Scale

Crust

Fissure

Erosion

Ulcer

Scar (cicatrix)

Figure 16.2 Primary and secondary lesions of the skin. Note some of these are superficial and some involve deeper tissues. (Adapted from Sims, L.K., D'Amico, D., et al., 1995. *Health Assessment in Nursing,* Redwood City, CA: Addison-Wesley Nursing.)

Surgical Terms

biopsy (**bī**-ŏp-sē)   excision of living tissue for examination.

cautery (**kăw**-tĕr-ē)   machine or methods used to destroy tissue by electricity, freezing, or chemicals (cauterization).

debridement (dĕ-**brēd**-mĕnt)   removal of dead tissue around a wound.

dermabrasion (**dĕrm**-ă-brā-zhŭn)   scraping off surface layers to remove scars or wrinkles.

dermatome (**dĕr**-mă-tōm)   instrument for cutting thin sections of skin for grafts.

electrodesiccation (ē-lĕk-trō-dĕs-ĭk-**kā**-shŭn)   destruction and drying out with electricity.

escharotomy (ĕs-kăr-**ŏt**-ō-mē)   removal of burn scar tissue.

fulguration (fŭl-gŭ-**rā**-shŭn)   destruction of tissue with electric sparks.

grafts (skin) (grăfts)   tissue taken from one place to replace a defect elsewhere: autogenous (ăw-**tŏj**-ĕ-nŭs; from self); homograft (from another person); pig skin may be used as a temporary graft. A new type of synthetic collagen is now being used for permanent skin grafts. A skin graft may be full-thickness, split-thickness, or pedicle graft.

Hyfrecator (**hī**-frĕk-ā-tŏr)   a type of machine for destroying tissue (high-frequency eradicator).

laser (**lā**-zĕr)   acronym for Light Amplification by Stimulated Emission of Radiation; intense heat to small areas in surgical procedures, such as some foot surgical procedures, especially toenails.

mammoplasty (**măm**-ō-plăs-tē)   surgery to reconstruct breasts after radical mastectomy.

theleplasty or **mammilliplasty** (**thē**-lĕ-plăs-tē, mă-**mĭl**-ĭ-plăs-tē)   plastic surgery of the nipple.

Common Growths

carcinoma (kăr-sĭ-**nō**-mă)   skin cancer; a malignant tumor. Examples include basal cell and squamous cell carcinomas; malignant mela **no** ma or "black tumor" is the only skin cancer that me **tas** tasizes (spreads to underlying tissues or through lymphatics).

keloid (**kē**-lŏyd)   abnormal scar formation, more common in dark skin (raised red scar).

keratosis (kĕr-ă-**tō**-sĭs)   thickened, horny skin; ac **tin** ic keratosis is due to exposure to sun and X rays.

nevus(i) (**nē**-vŭs)(ī)   mole; a discolored, flat or fleshy growth. A birthmark is a type of mole. See a medical dictionary for other types.

steatoma (stē-ă-**tō**-mă)   se **ba** ceous cyst, also called a wen; or a fatty tumor.

verruca(ae) (vĕr-**ū**-kă)   wart or epi **the** lial tumor. A plantar wart is one on the sole or plantar surface of the foot. (Warts are caused by viruses.) Venereal warts occur in genital area.

Bacterial Skin Diseases

Usually staphylo **coc** cal or strepto **coc** cal.

acne vulgaris (**ăk**-nē vŭl-**gā**-rĭs)   inflammation of the pilose **ba** ceous glands (pilo = hair, sebum = oil).

carbuncles and **furuncles** (**kăr**-bŭnk-ls, **fū**-rŭnk-ls)   pustular lesions, boils, abscesses.

cellulitis (sĕl-ū-**lī**-tĭs)   inflammation of skin and subcutaneous tissue. Ery **sip** elas is one type.

impetigo (ĭm-pĕ-**tī**-gō)   **pus** tular lesions, crusted vesicles or bullae, especially around mouth and nose. Com **mun** icable. (Often caused by staphylococci and/or streptococci.) Treated with antibiotics.

mastitis (măs-**tī**-tĭs)   breast inflammation.

Viral Skin Diseases

herpes genitalis (**hĕr**-pēz jĕn-ĭ-**tăl**-ĭs)   blister-type lesions in genital area; may endanger infant if mother is infected at time of delivery; causes damage to child's nervous system.

herpes ophthalmicus (ŏf-**thăl**-mĭ-kŭs)   severe type of herpes zoster, affecting the fifth cranial nerve (eye).

herpes simplex (sĭm-plĕks) "cold sores" or fever blisters.

herpes zoster (zŏs-tĕr) "shingles"—lesions follow the course of a nerve, usually only on one side of the trunk, pelvis, or eye.

verruca (vĕr-ū-kă) wart.

Parasitic Skin Diseases

Cause severe itching; communicable.

pediculosis capitis (pĕ-dĭk-ū-lō-sĭs kăp-ĭt-ĭs) head lice; sometimes epidemic in groups (school or child care populations, for example).

pediculosis corporis (kŏr-pŏr-ĭs) body lice.

pediculosis pubis (pū-bĭs) pubic lice or crabs.

scabies (skā-bēz) a small parasite called a mite, which burrows under the skin.

Fungal Skin Disorders

Communicable.

tinea (tĭn-ē-ă) ringworm—term used depends on body part involved.

    tinea barbae: (băr-bā) beard.

    tinea capitis: (kăp-ĭ-tĭs) scalp.

    tinea corporis: (kŏr-pŏr-ĭs) body.

    tinea cruris: (krū-rĭs) groin ("jock itch").

    tinea pedis: (pē-dĭs) foot (athlete's foot).

    tinea unguium: (ŭn-gwī-ŭm) nails.

Allergic Reactions

Due to sensitivity.

contact dermatitis (kŏn-tăkt dĕr-mă-tī-tĭs) caused by contact with some substance.

drug reactions usually rash-type lesions, caused by medication and/or photosensitivity reactions when exposed to sunlight.

eczema (ĕk-zĕ-mă) redness of skin, usually with itching, due to some substance or, possibly, food item.

insect bites local reaction usually due to bite or sting; may become life threatening if systemic reaction follows. (Examples: tick, spider, red ant, or chigger bites; bee, hornet, scorpion stings.)

Systemic Diseases

Those listed here may cause skin eruptions.

diabetes mellitus (dī-ă-bē-tēz mĕl-lī-tŭs) low insulin production affects metabolism; skin involvement includes various lesions and inability to heal.

erysipelas (ĕr-ĭ-sĭp-ĕ-lăs) acute febrile disease caused by "strep" infection; characterized by fiery red skin.

Hodgkin's disease (hŏdj-kĭnz) a type of cancer in which itching of the skin may occur.

Kaposi's (kă-pō-sēz) varicelliform eruption (named after an Austrian dermatologist); Kaposi's sarcoma is common in AIDS patients.

lupus erythematosus (lū-pŭs ĕr-ĭ-thē-mă-tō-sŭs) inflammatory dermatitis that may precede systemic lupus; characterized by "butterfly" lesions over nose and cheeks.

rubella (rū-bĕl-lă) three-day or German measles; characterized by rash.

rubeola (rū-bē-ō-lă) regular or hard measles; characterized by macular rash.

syphilis (sĭf-ĭl-ĭs)   chronic venereal disease with cu **tan** eous lesions in primary and secondary stages.
varicella (văr-ĭ-**sĕl**-lă)   chickenpox; vesicles that itch and later become scabs.

Skin Injuries

burns   first degree: red, tender, not blistered; second degree: blistered, dermal layer involved; third degree: subcutaneous tissue; white, charred; fat exposed; blisters often absent. Severe dehydration occurs in third degree burns.

■ **Note:** Important factors in burn injuries are parts of body involved (hands, feet, face, genitals, and joints are usually most serious); percentage of body burned and depth of burn; burns complicated by fractures with extensive soft tissue damage and respiratory involvement (most critical).

lacerations (lăs-ĕr-**ā**-shŭns)   cuts; deep lacerations involve meticulous care when large nerves and blood vessels are damaged.

Miscellaneous Terms

actinic (ăk-**tĭn**-ĭk)   pertaining to ultraviolet rays (sun).

albinism (**ăl**-bĭn-ĭzm)   lack of pigment; white skin and hair.

antibody (**ăn**-tĭ-bŏd-ē)   protein produced after foreign body invasion to react to the invading antigen.

antigen (**ăn**-tĭ-jĕn)   any foreign substance that stimulates antibody production.

alopecia (ăl-ō-**pē**-shē-ă)   baldness, hereditary or due to chemotherapy.

callus (**kăl**-lŭs)   localized hyper **pla** sia caused by friction.

cellulitis (sĕl-ŭ-**lī**-tĭs)   inflammation of connective tissue; skin infection that spreads through tissues (as in erysipelas).

cicatrix (**sĭk**-ă-trĭks)   (cicatricial) scar, scarred.

contusion (kŏn-**tū**-zhŭn)   bruise, black-and-blue mark, no break in skin.

decubitus (dē-**kū**-bĭ-tŭs)   ulcers on bony prominences due to prolonged lying down; bedsores.

dermatosis (dĕr-mă-**tō**-sĭs)   any skin condition without inflammation.

desensitization (dē-sĕn-sĭ-tī-**zā**-shŭn)   building tolerance to an antigen by giving small, increasingly pure doses of the specific allergic substance over 6–12 months; may or may not alleviate allergic symptoms.

ecchymosis (ĕk-ĭ-**mō**-sĭs)   bruise, black-and-blue mark due to bleeding under the skin.

eruption (ē-**rŭp**-shŭn)   any rash or "breaking out."

erythema (ĕr-ĭ-**thē**-mă)   redness.

eschar (**ĕs**-kăr)   hard crust over a burn.

exanthem (ĕks-**ăn**-thĕm)   rose-colored eruption.

excoriation (ĕks-kō-rē-**ā**-shŭn)   severe abrasion.

exfoliation (ĕks-fō-lē-**ā**-shŭn)   scaling, flaking.

fibrocystic disease (fī-brō-**sĭst**-ĭk)   of the breast; tumors in breast, nonmalignant (benign).

fungicide (**fŭn**-gĭ-sīd)   medication that destroys fungi; ointment.

gangrene (**găng**-grēn)   necrotic tissue (dead tissue).

hirsutism (**hŭr**-sūt-ĭzm)   excessive body hair, especially in women.

lesion (**lē**-zhŭn)   any kind of a "sore" is a lesion; a change in tissue structure.

neurodermatitis (nū-rō-dĕrm-ă-**tī**-tĭs)   usually severe itching and excoriation with unknown cause, presumed due to emotional or psychologic factors.

nummular (**nŭm**-ū-lăr)   having the shape of a coin; "size of a dime."

paronychia (păr-ō-**nĭk**-ē-ă)   inflammation around a nail.

pruritus (prŭ-**rī**-tŭs) itching.

psoriasis (sō-**rī**-ă-sĭs) chronic, hereditary derma **to** sis often associated with arthritis. Characterized by silvery flaking patches, especially on elbows and knees. Remissions and exacerbations are common, with periods of inflammation also common.

rhytidectomy (rĭt-ĭ-**dĕk**-tō-mē) face lift (wrinkles removed surgically).

superfluous hair (sū-**pĕr**-flū-ŭs) excessive hair on face of women.

urticaria (ŭr-tĭ-**kā**-rē-ă) hives; raised, itchy welts.

vitiligo (vĭt-ĭl-**ī**-gō) loss of pigment; white, patchy areas.

Skin Tests

The following tests are not related to skin disease, but skin reaction determines the outcome of the test.

coccidioidin (cocci) (kŏk-sĭd-ē-**ŏy**-dĭn) test for valley fever (respiratory fungal disease).

histoplasmosis (hĭs-tō-plăz-**mō**-sĭs) another fungal disease.

Mantoux or **PPD** (măn-**tū**) test for TB (bacterial disease).

If result is positive (red, raised area of certain size where injection was made), the person has been exposed, may now have the disease, or has had it previously.

Other skin tests include:

Dick test for susceptibility to scarlet fever.

Schick test for susceptibility to diphtheria.

sweat test for presence of cystic fibrosis.

Specialists

Dermatology is the study of skin disorders. The dermatologist is the specialist who usually treats these, although internists often prescribe for the less complicated cases. Plastic surgeons may become involved when extensive skin damage has occurred, or for cosmetic surgery.

Treatment

When medications are used for treatment, topical (local, to surface) treatment is the most usual; various antibiotic and cortisone ointments are used. Systemic antibiotics may also be given.

Abbreviations

decub decubitus

FB foreign body

PPD tuberculin skin test

RPR rapid plasma reagent test for syphilis; may be done to diagnose source of lesions

STD skin test dose; or sexually transmitted disease

subcu or **subq (SQ)** subcutaneous

Worksheet

Fill in the blank:

1. The specialist who treats skin disorders is a _dermatologist_____

2. Two functions of the skin are _____

3. The outer (top) layer of the skin is the _____

4. Sweat glands are also called _____ glands.

5. Oil glands are also called _____ glands.

6. Three skin diseases are _____

7. The dermis is the deeper layer of skin and is also called the _____ . In this

   layer are found the _____ .

8. Cold sores are called _____

9. Three skin conditions related to allergy or sensitivity are _____

   _____

10. Inflammation around the fingernail is _____

11. Name two skin tests and their purposes: _____

    _____

    _____

True/False: Circle the number of the *true* statements only. Defend your answers. Explain why the other statements are false.

12. *Nummular* means "coin shaped."

13. A biopsy is an examination of living tissue to determine malignancy.

14. A wart is a verruca.

15. The halo around the nipple of the breast is the areola mamma.

16. A vesicle is a lesion full of pus.

17. *Pruritus* means "itching."

18. Vitiligo is an infectious disease.

Fill in the blank:

19. An instrument for cutting a thin section of skin is a _____

20. Hives are called _____

21. The plural of nevus is _____ . Nevus means _____

22. A term that means "redness of the skin" is _____

23. Three systemic diseases that have skin symptoms are _____

_____

24. Pediculosis is caused by a _____ (parasite).

25. The disease common in teenagers that produces skin lesions is called _____

26. Name some other terms not mentioned in this worksheet that describe skin lesions: _____

_____

27. The malignant skin condition that frequently occurs in AIDS victims is _____

28. Plastic surgery following mastectomy to restore the breast is called _____

29. Another word for ecchymosis is _____

30. Scar tissue grossly overgrown is called _____

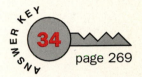

34 page 269

Test p. 319
Alternate Test p. 321

■ Case History ■

CASE HISTORY 1

DISCHARGE SUMMARY: Cellulitis of penis

Admitting Diagnosis   cellu li tis of penis

Discharge Diagnosis   same

This 40-year-old male reports an industrial injury to the *pubic area* by a piece of scaffolding 24 hours prior to admission. Penis was grossly *edematous* with moderate *erythema*. Admission diagnosis was *cellulitis*. Patient was treated with *intravenous* Kefzol. *Urethral* discharge cultured positive for *Staphylococcus aureus*. WBC was 26,100 with 32 *stabs*, 65 *neutrophils*; UA 2+ blood, 0–2 white cells. *RPR nonreactive*.

Over the next 6 days cellulitis persisted, and he began to show signs of *gangrene*. *Antibiotics* were changed to include clindamycin and minocycline during his hospital stay.

History and Physical Record

CC   Swelling of the penis.

PI   This 40-year-old male apparently was struck in the mid-lower abdominal area while working on the job. He noticed considerable discomfort and pain and some swelling, which increased over a 24-hour period, and he came to the Medical Center where he was admitted.

PH   Includes episode of a kidney stone, apparently was never hospitalized for it, and it seemed to pass rather quickly. He denies any other health problems, has had no surgery or fractures.

FH   Parents *L&W*. He is married, has three children all in good health. Denies any abnormal family health history.

SH   Construction worker. Denies use of medications or excessive use of alcohol or tobacco.

ROS   Generally has been in good health. Skin normal.

skin   Dry and warm. Some *ecchymosis* and gross swelling of penis.

HEENT   *Normocephalic* male. *TMs* clear. Eyes: *EOMS* intact, good *light reflex. Funduscopic* normal. Nose and throat normal.

neck   Good *ROM*. Negative for *palpable thyroid. Carotid* pulsations normal.

chest   Clear to *A and P* without *rales, rhonchi,* or *wheezes.* No history of *asthma, bronchitis,* or *pneumonia.*

cardiovascular   Regular *sinus rhythm* without *murmurs, rubs,* or *gallops.* Lymphatic negative.

abdomen   *Scaphoid. Negative organomegaly, masses,* or *tenderness.*

genitalia   Gross swelling of penis, patient in acute distress.

rectal, locomotor, extremities   *Unremarkable.*

neurologic   *DTRs* 2+ *bilaterally.* Cranial nerves grossly intact.

Impression   Cellulitis

■ **Assignment:** Write all of the italicized words and define them. Notice the use of the words *denies* and *unremarkable.* These are commonly used terms. With regard to the laboratory terms, are the results within normal limits? (Refer to laboratory forms in Chapter 13 for "normals.")

▲ **Health Promotion Tip**

For optimal health of the integumentary system:

- Avoid exposure to harmful substances.
- Maintain adequate hydration.
- Avoid sudden, extreme temperature shifts to aid temperature regulation.
- Maintain good hygiene
- Promote waste disposal (for example, wearing cotton clothing allows skin to perspire).

Safety tips regarding exposure of skin to harmful substances:

1.   Avoid harmful substances.

2.   If unavoidable, take measures to protect yourself.
    - Thoroughly apply SPF15 (or greater) sun lotion to exposed skin surfaces at least half an hour before going outside; reapply according to label directions.
    - Wear gloves to avoid contact with potentially harmful cleaning substances or chemicals.
    - Thoroughly rinse skin (for at least 15 minutes) in water as soon as possible if harmful substances come in contact with skin. Follow up with physician if necessary.

CHAPTER 17

Musculoskeletal System

Anatomy and Physiology of the Musculoskeletal System

Function

The musculoskeletal system supports and gives shape to the body; protects internal organs; makes movement possible; and forms blood cells.

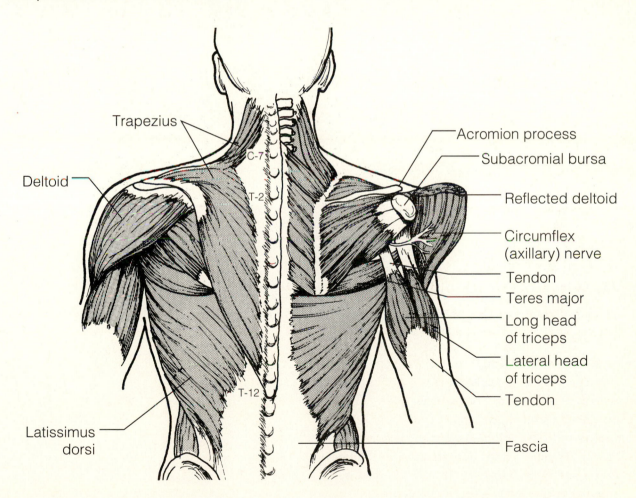

Figure 17.1 Shoulder dissection from rear (muscles, tendons, fascia, and bursa).
(© Copyright 1996. CIBA-GEIGY Corporation. Reprinted with permission from the Clinical Symposia, illustrated by Frank Netter, M.D. All rights reserved.)

1. Femur
2. Tibia
3. Fibula
4. Patella
5. Quadriceps tendon
6. Patellar tendon
7. Suprapatellar bursa
8. Lateral gastrocnemius bursa
9. Prepatellar bursa
10. Popliteus bursa
11. Bursa of biceps tendon
12. Deep infrapatellar bursa
13. Superficial infrapatellar bursa
14. Lateral collateral ligament

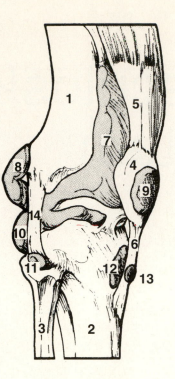

Figure 17.2 Knee, anterolateral aspect, with synovial sac and adjacent bursae. Shows large bones of the leg and some tendons and ligaments.

Anatomy of the Muscle

The three kinds of muscle are:
striated striped, voluntary, skeletal
nonstriated smooth, involuntary
cardiac heart muscle

Anatomy of the Skeleton

1. **Axial** (ăk-sē-ăl) skull, thorax (ribs and sternum), vertebral column.

2. **Appendicular** (ăp-ĕn-**dĭk**-ū-lăr) the appendages that hang from the axial skeleton; upper and lower extremities (includes shoulder and pelvic girdle).

Large Bones of the Body

  clavicle (**klăv**-ĭk-l) collarbone.
  sternum (**stĕr**-nŭm) breastbone.
  humerus (**hū**-mĕr-ŭs) upper arm.
  radius and **ulna** (**rā**-dē-ŭs, **ŭl**-nă) forearm.
  femur (**fē**-mŭr) thigh (longest bone in the body).
  fibula and **tibia** (**fĭb**-ū-lă, **tĭb**-ē-ă) lower leg.
  scapula (**skăp**-ū-lă) shoulder blade.
  vertebral column (**vĕr**-tĕ-brăl) starting at the neck: cervical vertebrae (there are 7), thoracic or dorsal (12), lumbar (5), sacral (5, fused), coccyx or tailbone (4) (see Figure 17.4 on p. 140).

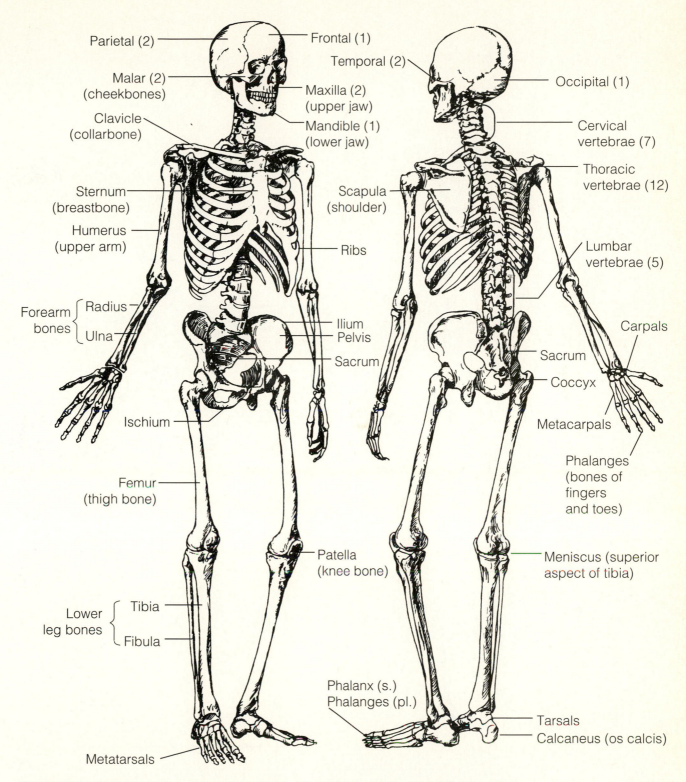

Parietal (2)

Frontal (1)

Temporal (2)

Malar (2)
(cheekbones)

Occipital (1)

Maxilla (2)
(upper jaw)

Mandible (1)
(lower jaw)

Clavicle
(collarbone)

Cervical
vertebrae (7)

Thoracic
vertebrae (12)

Sternum
(breastbone)

Scapula
(shoulder)

Humerus
(upper arm)

Lumbar
vertebrae (5)

Ribs

Forearm
bones

Radius

Carpals

Ilium
Pelvis

Ulna

Sacrum

Sacrum

Coccyx

Ischium

Metacarpals

Phalanges
(bones of
fingers
and toes)

Femur
(thigh bone)

Patella
(knee bone)

Meniscus (superior
aspect of tibia)

Lower
leg bones

Tibia

Fibula

Phalanx (s.)
Phalanges (pl.)

Tarsals
Calcaneus (os calcis)

Metatarsals

Figure 17.3 Skeleton. Left, anterior view, showing large bones of the body. Right, posterior view, showing large bones and sections of vertebral column. *Note:* (1) For cranial bones and vertebrae, the number of bones of that type are shown in parentheses. (2) There are several gender and age differences in skeletons. Females have a wider pelvis. Infants have a larger head in proportion to the body, more cartilage, and soft spaces in the skull called *fontanels*.

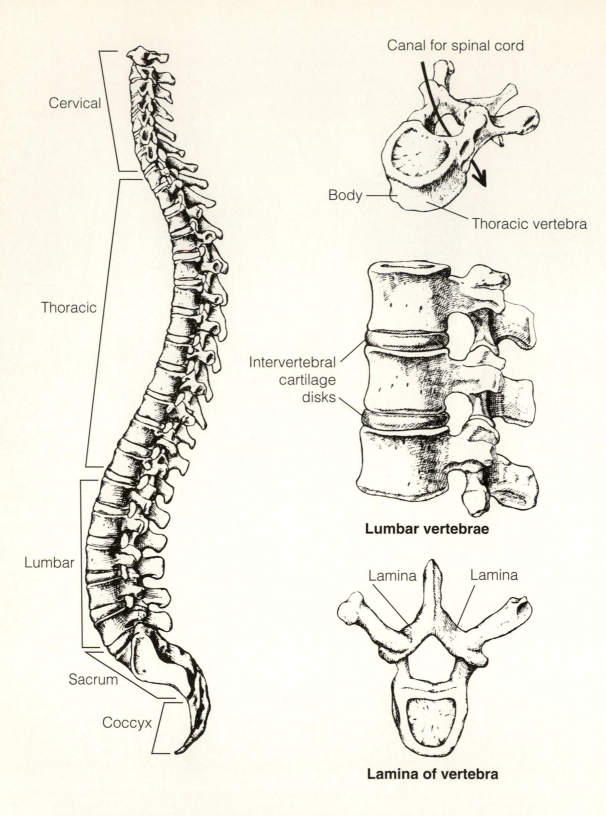

Lumbar vertebrae

Lamina of vertebra

Figure 17.4 On the left, spinal column showing cervical, thoracic, lumbar, sacral, and coccygeal sections. On the right, individual vertebra showing spinal canal and laminae.

Cranial Bones (also called *skull* or *calvarium*)

frontal (**frŏn**-tăl) forehead (1).

parietal (pă-**rī**-ĕ-tăl) top of head (2).

temporal (**tĕm**-pō-răl) temples (2).

occipital (ŏk-**sĭp**-ĭ-tăl) back of head (1).

ethmoid (**ĕth**-mŏyd) upper nasal, between eyes (1).

sphenoid (sfē-**nŏyd**) behind eyes (base of skull), and laterally between parietal and temporal bones (1).

mandible (**măn**-dĭ-bl) lower jaw (1).

maxilla (măk-**sĭl**-ă) upper jaw (2).

turbinates (**tŭr**-bĭ-nāts) cone-shaped nasal bones (2).

malar (**mā**-lăr) cheekbone (2); also called zygomatic.

Joints and Related Structures

aponeurosis (ăp-ō-nū-**rō**-sĭs) flattened tendon; resembles a membrane that attaches muscle to bones or tissue.

ball and socket joint hip and shoulder joints.

bursa (plural, **-ae**) (**bŭr**-să) (ā) small sacs that cushion joints between tendons and bones.

fascia (ae) (făs-sē-ă) (ā) connective tissue sheath; covers, supports, and separates muscles; holds muscle fibers.

hinge joint elbows, knees, fingers.

interphalangeal joints (ĭn-tĕr-fă-**lăn**-jē-ăl) fingers and toes; DIP is distal interphalangeal and PIP is proximal interphalangeal.

intervertebral disks (ĭn-tĕr-**vĕr**-tĕ-brăl) cartilaginous material between vertebrae.

lamina (ae) (**lăm**-ĭ-nă) (ā) flattened part of the vertebral arch (thinnest part of vertebrae).

ligament (**lĭg**-ă-mĕnt) strong fibrous tissue that connects bone to bone.

meniscus (plural, **-ci**) (mĕ-**nĭs**-kŭs) (kī) lateral and medial knee cartilage.

sutures (**sū**-chŭrs) articulations in the cranial bones; immovable joints.

synovial fluid (sĭn-**ō**-vē-ăl) clear joint fluid that acts as lubricant.

temporomandibular joint (TMJ) (tĕm-pō-rō-măn-**dĭb**-ū-lăr) connecting point of lower jawbone and temporal bone.

tendon (**tĕn**-dŏn) fibrous tissue attaching muscle to bone.

theca (**thē**-kă) covering or sheath of a tendon.

Projections, Openings, and Indentations in Bones

acetabulum (ăs-ĕ-**tăb**-ū-lŭm) large socket for head of femur (hip).

foramen (plural, **foramina**) (fōr-**ā**-mĕn, fōr-**ăm**-ĭ-nă) holes in a bone for large vessels and nerves to pass through; for example, for **a** men **mag** num.

fossa (ae) (fŏs-ă) (ā) depressions or hollows.

grooves shallow linear depressions in bone (or tooth).

malleolus (măl-**ē**-ō-lŭs) hammerlike protuberance (either side of ankle).

olecranon (ō-**lĕk**-răn-ŏn) a process on the ulnar bone (elbow).

prominences, processes, tuberosities (**prŏm**-ĭ-nĕn-sĕz, **prŏ**-sĕs-ĕz, tū-bĕr-**ŏs**-ĭ-tēz) projections.

sinuses (**sī**-nŭs-ĕz) air spaces in cranium that lighten the skull and serve as voice resonating chambers.

Names of the small bones of the ankle, foot, and wrist are not given in this text. Should you need these, most medical dictionaries list bones in the appendix. Taber's dictionary lists them under *skeleton*. Similar lists of muscles, joints, ligaments, and so on are also usually given in the appendices of medical dictionaries.

Pathophysiology of the Musculoskeletal System

fractures   Figure 17.5 describes kinds of fractures.

skull fractures   possible damage to brain.

spondylolisthesis (spŏn-dĭl-ō-lĭs-**thē**-sĭs)   forward displacement of a vertebra (type of dislocation).

subluxation (sŭb-lŭks-**ā**-shŭn)   partial dislocation (luxation = dislocation).

"torn" ligaments, tendons, cartilage   common sports injuries.

contracture (kŏn-**trăk**-chŭr)   permanent contraction of a muscle.

muscle atrophy (**ăt**-rō-fē)   wasting away, shrinkage; from disuse.

muscle hypertrophy (hī-**pĕr**-trō-fē)   increase in muscle size; from overuse.

muscle tone   muscles partially contracted, enough to make them feel firm.

paralysis (pă-**răl**-ĭ-sĭs)   inability to contract muscle, due to nerve damage.

paresis (pă-**rē**-sĭs)   marked weakness, incomplete paralysis.

Musculoskeletal and Neuromuscular Disorders

ALS, amyotrophic lateral sclerosis (ă-mī-ō-**trŏf**-ĭk lăt-ĕr-ăl sklĕ-**rō**-sĭs)   a syndrome marked by muscular weakness and atrophy with spasticity and hyperreflexia (neurologic disorder with poor prognosis) also called **Lou Gehrig's disease.**

ankylosing spondylitis (**ăng**-kĭ-lō-sĭng spŏn-dĭ-**lī**-tĭs)   chronic, progressive inflammation of the vertebrae with spontaneous fusion causing deformity; also called **Marie-Strümpell disease** and "poker spine."

arthritis (ăr-**thrī**-tĭs)   inflammation of a joint; a group of diseases including: **rheumatoid arthritis,** which starts at any age and causes severe deformity; **osteoarthritis** or **DJD** (degenerative joint disease), which begins at older ages (painful but less deformity).

ataxia (ā-**tăk**-sē-ă)   without muscle coordination.

atonic (ā-**tŏn**-ĭk)   lack of muscle tone.

"backache" or back pain   the most common medical complaint. 85% of all adults have episodes of back pain. According to the National Center of Health Statistics, money spent on back problems surpasses all funds spent on AIDS patients. Back problems often are the result of improper body mechanics or weak abdominal muscles from inadequate exercise and are usually not serious, although they are often incapacitating.

bursitis (bŭr-**sī**-tĭs)   inflammation of a bursa; very painful, acute condition often treated with injection of hydrocortisone into joint area.

carpal tunnel syndrome (**kăr**-păl **tŭn**-nĕl **sĭn**-drōm)   pain, edema, and atrophy usually on thumb side of hand, due to pressure on median nerve in the wrist; often associated with repetitive hand motions.

clonic (**klŏn**-ĭk)   muscular relaxation and contraction.

collagen disease (**kŏl**-ă-jĕn)   any of several diseases of the connective tissue, including **SLE (systemic lupus erythematosus), rheumatoid arthritis, polyarteritis.**

de Quervain's disease (dĕ-**kār**-vănz)   tenosyno **vit** is caused by narrowing of tendon sheath (wrist area).

genu (**jē**-nū)   means "knee"; *genu valgum* means "knock knees"; *genu varum,* "bow legs."

gout (gŏwt)   a type of acute arthritis, due to accumulation of uric acid crystals, especially in the great toe.

herniated nucleus pulposus (HNP) (**hĕr**-nē-ā-tĕd **nū**-klē-ŭs pŭl-**pō**-sŭs)   ruptured intervertebral disk (see Case History 3, p. 150, and Figure 17.6 on p. 144).

kyphosis (kī-**fō**-sĭs)   hunchback deformity of spine (see *lordosis* and *scoliosis*).

Legg-Calve-Perthes disease (**lĕg**-kăl-**vā**-**pĕr**-tĕz)   osteochondritis of head of femur.

lordosis (lŏr-**dō**-sĭs)   convex curvature of spine (swayback).

lupus erythematosus (systemic) **SLE** (**lū**-pŭs ĕ-rĭ-thē-mă-**tō**-sŭs)   collagen disease affecting connective tissues, thought to be due to abnormal immuno **log** ic response.

Simple (closed)

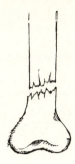

Greenstick
(also simple fx)

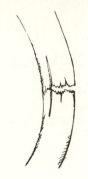

Comminuted (fragmented)

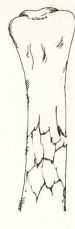

Compound
(protrudes through the skin)

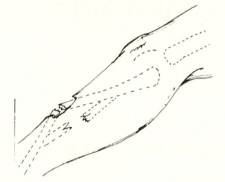

Transcervical
(neck of femur)

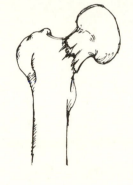

Intercondylar
(T shaped)

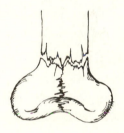

Impacted

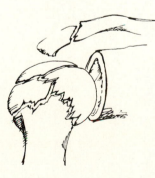

Pott's
(fracture of lower fibula,
usually with a chipped tibia)

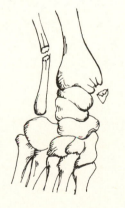

Colles'
(fx of lower end of radius)

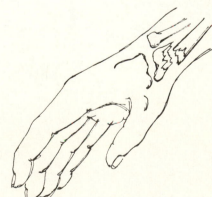

Figure 17.5 Examples of some types of fractures (fx).

Lyme disease (LD) (līm)   symptoms resemble arthritis. Caused by a spirochete transmitted by a tick. First seen in Lyme, Connecticut, it is now found in many other states. First presents as a skin lesion (history of tick bite); skin lesion is called *ECM,* which stands for *erythema chronicum migrans.* Neurologic, cardiac, and joint abnormalities may follow. Treated with antibiotics.

muscular dystrophies (MD) (**mŭs**-kū-lăr **dĭs**-trō-fēz) and related disorders   motor dysfunction and weakness; inherited diseases with progressive weakness and degeneration of muscle fibers without neural degeneration. Pseudohyper **tro** phic muscular dystrophy (also called Duchenne disease) is most common, occurring in boys ages 3–7 and progressing to wheelchair status by ages 10–12. Muscle biopsy helpful in making diagnosis, especially to differentiate from treatable polymyo **si** tis.

myasthenia gravis (mī-ăs-**thē**-nē-ă **grăv**-ĭs)   severe fatigability and weakness of muscles; more common in females, ages 20–50. May be mild or severe (fatal) and may have prolonged remissions.

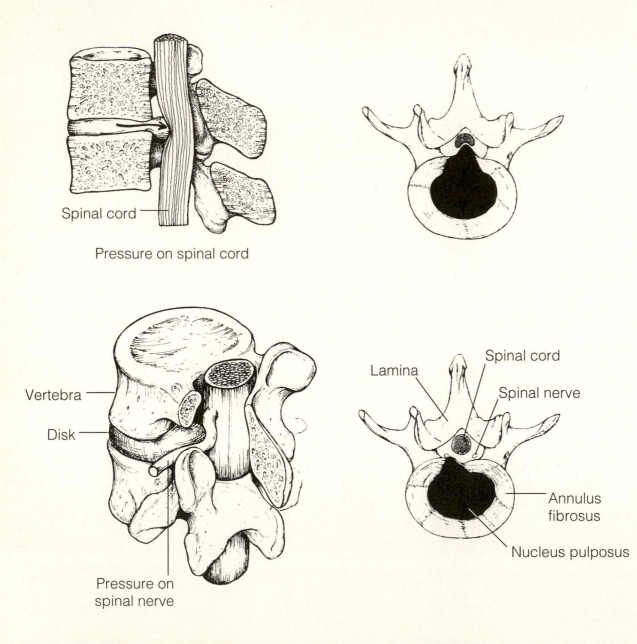

Spinal cord

Pressure on spinal cord

Vertebra

Disk

Pressure on spinal nerve

Lamina

Spinal cord

Spinal nerve

Annulus fibrosus

Nucleus pulposus

Figure 17.6   Sections of spinal column showing hernia of intervertebral disk (HNP). (Adapted from Medical Times Patient Education Chart. Romaine Pierson Publishers, Inc., New York.)

myositis (or **myitis**) (mī-ō-**sī**-tĭs, mī-**ī**-tĭs)   inflammation of muscles (especially skeletal).

Osgood-Schlatter disease (**ŏz**-good **shlăt**-ĕr)   osteochondrosis of end of tibia (knee); occurs in adolescent boys especially.

osteochondrosis and **osteochondritis** (ŏs-tē-ō-kŏn-**drō**-sĭs, ŏs-tē-ō-kŏn-**drī**-tĭs)   degenerative changes and chronic inflammation of bone and cartilage; Scheuermann's disease, osteochondrosis of vertebrae (swimmer's back) from butterfly stroke.

osteogenesis imperfecta (ŏs-tē-ō-**jĕn**-ĕs-ĭs ĭm-pĕr-**fĕk**-tă)   congenital, cause unknown; brittle bones, and many fractures occur in those afflicted.

osteomalacia (ŏs-tē-ō-mă-**lā**-shē-ă)   softening of bone, caused by vitamin D deficiency.

osteomyelitis (ŏs-tē-ō-mī-ĕ-**lī**-tĭs)   inflammation of bone and marrow caused by bacterial invasion; often occurs with fracture injuries and bone surgery.

osteoporosis (ŏs-tē-ō-pŏr-**ō**-sĭs)   porous condition of bones, especially in elderly women (postmenopausal), causing fractures, severe pain. Some factors thought to be involved: exercise or lack of it, estrogen deficiency, calcium deficiency, and genetic factors (spine often affected, leading to severe kyphosis). Medicines that increase calcium excretions, such as corticosteroids, antacids, tetracycline, and some diuretics, also contribute to osteoporosis.

Pott's disease (pŏts)   oste **it** is of the vertebrae, usually of tuberculous origin. (Percival Pott, British surgeon)

Pott's fracture   fracture of the lower end of the fibula and medial mal **le** olus of the tibia with dislocation of foot outwards and backwards; treated with walking cast.

rachitis (ră-**kī**-tĭs)   inflammation of the spine.

rheumatism (**rū**-mă-tĭzm)   general term for soreness and stiffness of joints, tendons, muscles, bones.

rickets (**rĭk**-ĕts)   juvenile osteomalacia.

sarcoma (osteogenic) (săr-**kō**-mă, ŏs-tē-ō-**jĕn**-ĭk)   malignant bone tumor (primary tumor); secondary (meta **stat** ic) tumors of the bone are more common.

scoliosis (skō-lē-**ō**-sĭs)   lateral curve of the spine; should be detected early in childhood to avoid deformity (school screening programs).

Sjögren's syndrome (**shō**-grĕns)   an autoimmune disorder; a progressive type of collagen disease that occurs postmenopause; cause unknown.

SLE (see *lupus erythematosus, systemic*)

spina bifida (**spī**-nă **bĭf**-ĭd-ă)   a congenital defect of the spine; may be occult, causing no symptoms, or can be severe, as in **myelomeningocele** (mī-ĕ-lō-mĕ-**nĭn**-gō-sēl)   allowing the spinal cord and meninges to protrude on the surface of the back, requiring surgery and leaving residual paralysis in most cases.

spondylitis   (see *ankylosing*)

talipes (ankle, foot) (**tăl**-ĭ-pēz)   any of a number of deformities of the foot, especially congenital clubfoot; talipes valgus, heel turned outward; talipes varus, heel turned inward.

tendinitis (tendonitis) (tĕn-dĭn-**ī**-tĭs)   inflammation of a tendon.

thoracic outlet syndrome (thō-**răs**-ĭk ŏwt-lĕt)   brachial neuritis with or without vasomotor disturbance in the upper extremities; pain, tingling, numbness anywhere from shoulder to fingers with atrophy of small muscles of the hand or other muscles of arm. Also called *scalenus syndrome*.

tonic (**tŏn**-ĭk)   muscular tension (state of).

Surgical, Diagnostic, and Treatment Terms

amputation (ăm-pū-**tā**-shŭn)   removal of a limb, partial or whole; AK = above knee, BK = below knee.

arthrocentesis (ăr-thrō-sĕn-**tē**-sĭs)   puncture into joint to remove liquid.

arthroscopy (ăr-**thrŏs**-kŏ-pē)   procedure of looking into joint with scope.

arthrotomy (ăr-**thrŏt**-ō-mē)   incision into a joint.

chemonucleolysis (kē-mō-nū-klē-**ōl**-ĭ-sĭs)   dissolving herniated nucleus pulposus by injecting an enzyme.

electrical stimulation (or electric "stim")   used to quickly heal fractures or traumatic injuries to cartilage or tendons.

electrodynogram (ē-lĕk-trō-**dī**-nō-grăm)   computer measurement of foot movement (force, range, timing).

electromyography (EMG) (ē-lĕk-trō-mī-**ŏg**-ră-fē)   recording of a muscular contraction for diagnostic purposes or treatment, such as biofeedback.

external fixation   fracture reduction devices (without casting).

fracture reductions   restoring bone to normal position, done without surgery as a **closed reduction,** as in a cast, or in surgery as an **ORIF,** open reduction with internal fixation.

laminectomy with diskectomy (lăm-ĭ-**nĕk**-tō-mē, dĭs-**kĕk**-tō-mē)   surgical excision of part or whole of intervertebral disk by incising the lamina.

meniscectomy (mĕn-ĭ-**sĕk**-tō-mē)   excision of part or whole of meniscus of the knee (see Figure 17.3 on p. 139), often to treat "torn cartilage in knee."

myelogram (mī-ĕl-ō-grăm)   diagnostic X-ray exam of the spinal cord after dye has been introduced into the spinal cavity (to diagnose a herniated disk for example).

myogram (mī-ō-grăm)   an electromyogram; *not* the same as myelogram.

reconstructive knee surgery   arthroscopic surgery to replace torn ligaments.

replantation   reattaching a severed body part (often with microsurgery).

spondylosyndesis (spŏn-dĭ-lō-**sĭn**-dē-sĭs)   spinal fusion via surgical formation of ankylosis.

synovectomy (sĭn-ō-**vĕk**-tō-mē)   excision of synovial membrane.

total hip replacement   hip joint replaced using prosthetic devices for the head of the femur and the bone cavity above that it rotates in, the acetabulum.

traction (**trăk**-shŭn)   process of drawing or pulling.

Laboratory Arthritis Profile

Several laboratory tests are often ordered together to help the physician establish the presence of a disease, to determine its severity, and to help in determining which of several possible diseases with similar symptoms is present. Such an *arthritis profile* includes these tests:

sedimen **ta** tion rate (SR or ESR)

antinuclear antibodies (ANA)

C-reactive protein (CRP)

rheumatoid (RA) factor

LE (lupus erythema **to** sus) cell prep

latex floccu **la** tion or bentonite aggluti **na** tion

ASO (antistreptolysin O) titer

■ **Note:** Autoimmune antibodies are associated with many diseases, and their identification may provide diagnostic and prognostic information for management of the disease. Collagen or rheumatic diseases overlap in their clinical picture; the ANA findings support the diagnosis. Autoimmune diseases, a group of diseases in which the immune system apparently mistakes "self" cells for invaders, cause the body to produce antibodies against its own tissues. Normally, the immune system protects the body by producing antibodies against invaders and harmful substances.

Specialists

A great variety of practitioners treat musculoskeletal and neuromuscular disorders: rheuma **tol** ogist, ortho **ped** ist, ortho **ped** ic surgeon, hand surgeon, head and neck surgeon; in some cases plastic surgeon, neurosurgeon and vascular surgeon; general practitioners, both MD and DO; **chi** ropractors, physi **at** rists, physical therapists, and occupational therapists. In **tern** ists and family practice specialists often treat patients with arthritis, gout, lupus, and so on.

Treatment

A great many methods are used in treating musculoskeletal disorders and injuries. Among these are the various analgesics, anti-inflammatory drugs, and cortisone drugs, immobilization and fixation for fractures, joint replacement surgical procedures, and reattaching body parts, as well as "adjustment" procedures and physical therapy treatment of several kinds, prosthetic devices, and equipment to aid ambulation.

Bonus: When you have learned the names of bones, you have also learned names of some blood vessels and nerves (for example: femur, femoral artery and nerve; tibia, tibial artery and nerve). The lobes of the brain are named the same as the cranial bones (for example, frontal, parietal, and so on).

Abbreviations

AE or BE   above elbow or below elbow
AK or BK   above knee or below knee
ALS   amyotrophic lateral sclerosis
ANA   antinuclear antibodies
DIP or PIP   distal or proximal interphalangeal (joint of digit)
DJD   degenerative joint disease
EDG   electrodynogram
EMG   electromyography

HNP   herniated nucleus pulposus
LD   Lyme disease
LE   lupus erythematosus
MD   muscular dystrophy
NSAID   nonsteroidal anti-inflammatory drugs
ORIF   open reduction internal fixation
PIP   proximal interphalangeal (joint of digit)
RA   rheumatoid arthritis: RA lab test
SLE   see *LE* (systemic)

Worksheet

Fill in the blank:

1. Another word for skull is _____

2. Air spaces in the skull are called _____

3. "Cracks" in the skull are called _____

4. Soft spots normally found in an infant's skull are called _____

5. Name five sections of the vertebral column (spine), in order, starting at the neck:

   _____   _____

   _____   _____

   _____

Define:

6. adduction   *movement toward the midline* _____

7. ligament _____

8. tendon _____

9. bursa _____

10. Name and describe three kinds of fractures:

_____

_____

_____

11. Name three types of practitioners for bone disorders:

_____

_____

_____

12. What does "ortho" mean? _____

Define orthopedic: _____

13. Define osteopath: _____

_____

14. Name the common words for flexion: _____

extension: _____

15. Fixed ribs are attached anteriorly to the _____ and

posteriorly to the _____

Define:

16. paralysis _____

17. atrophy (muscle) _____

18. hypertrophy _____

19. meniscus _____

20. Name three cranial bones: _____

21. Intercostal muscles are between the _____

22. Skeletal muscle is attached to _____

23. The dome-shaped muscle that aids breathing is called the _____

24. Name three kinds of muscle tissue: _____

_____

25. Name three diseases of the musculoskeletal system: _____

_____

26. "Foramina," "grooves," and "processes" are all terms used in relation to _____

27. The two main divisions of the skeleton are _____ and _____

28. How does the infant skeleton differ from that of the adult? _____

_____

29. Spell out:

SLE _____

RA _____

NSAID _____

30. Diagram the skeleton and label all of the large bones.

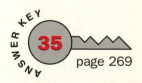

ANSWER KEY
35
page 269

Test p. 323
Alternate Test p. 325

■ Case Histories ■

CASE HISTORY 2

DISCHARGE SUMMARY: Torn medial meniscus

Admission Diagnosis   Torn medial me **nis** cus, left knee.

Discharge Diagnoses   Torn medial me **nis** cus, left knee; chondroma **la** cia of the medial **fem** oral **con** dyle.

History of Present Illness   The patient injured her left knee on June 10, 1996, while playing tennis. She subsequently had difficulty with persistent ef **fu** sion and pain in the left knee. An **ar** throgram prior to admission revealed a tear of the medial meniscus.

Physical Examination   Absence of tenderness to pal **pa** tion of any of the joint structures. There was approximately 30–55 mL* of fluid within the joint. Range of motion was full (FROM).

Laboratory Data   Admission hemoglobin was 15.9, hematocrit 47%, white count 7400, with normal differential. Urinalysis was WNL (within normal limits). Chemistry profile showed an elevated cho **les** terol of 379 mg/dL. Chest X-ray examination was negative.

Treatment and Hospital Course   The patient had surgery on the day of admission, at which time she underwent ar **thros** copy. This revealed a tear of the medial me **nis** cus. Ar **throt** omy was performed, with medial menis **cec** tomy. A **chon** dral fracture was noted in the medial femoral **con** dyle, measuring approximately 5 mm in greatest diameter. The edges of this were sheathed. Postoperatively, the patient's course was benign. There was no significant temperature elevation. She was ambulatory with crutches on the first postoperative day with no difficulty with straight leg raising.

Disposition   Discharged to home with crutches and exercise program. To return in 1 week for suture removal.

CASE HISTORY 3

REPORT OF OPERATION: Herniated nucleus pulposus

Preoperative Diagnosis   Her niated **nu** cleus pul **po** sus, L5, S1 on the left (herniated disk).

Operation Performed   Lamin **ec** tomy and excision of disk.

Pathologic Operative Findings   The disk had completely ruptured through the ligament, and the nerve root was compressed against the liga **men** tum **fla** vum.

Operative Procedure   Under general endo **tra** cheal anes **the** sia, with the patient in the prone position, the patient was prepped and draped in the usual manner. A linear incision extending from approximately L3 down to the sacrum was made over the spinous process through the skin and subcutaneous tissue. By means of subperi **os** teal dissection the posterior bony elements were exposed. The interspace was identified and the superior aspect of S1 and inferior aspect of L5 from the spinous processes were ron **guered.** By means of a cu **rette** the borders of the **lam** inae were identified and a Kerrison ronguer used to remove the superior aspect of S1 and the inferior aspect of L5.

The ligamentum flavum was cut in the midline and retracted lateralwards and removed. The nerve root was then identified, and it was markedly tight in this area. This required dissection starting superiorly to get the nerve root off the disk. After it was off the disk, the disk ruptured right into the wound, and the major fragment was removed. At this time the nerve root was held medialwards, and the remaining disk was removed from the intervertebral space.

A **cru** ciate incision was made into the **an** nulus so the pituitary ronguer could get into the interspace. After removal of the disk, the disk space was curetted, and the pituitary ronguer was used again to remove the further disk material. At this time the bleeding was controlled with Gelfoam packing. The

---

*Other common abbreviations for milliliter are ml and cc (I cc = I mL). However, the preferred form is mL.

wound was copiously irrigated and closed with interrupted nylon suture for the inner spinous ligament and posterior fascia, interrupted plain suture for the subcutaneous tissue, and a continuous subcuticular nylon suture for the skin. Steristrips were applied. Estimated blood loss was 200 mL. Blood replaced, none. All bleeders were clamped as encountered.

The patient tolerated the procedure well and returned to the recovery room in satisfactory condition.

■ **Assignment:** You have just read Case Histories 2 and 3: Discharge Summary and Report of Operation. It is helpful to read them aloud, your instructor may ask you to do this in class. Look up all of the root words that you do not know. Write them and write the definitions.

Health Promotion Tip

Exercise, adequate nutrition, and appropriate posture are essential to promote a healthy musculoskeletal system throughout your life. When indicated, some women may consider ERT (estrogen replacement therapy) under their physician's care.

Good nutrition:

- Molasses, turnip greens, cheese, yogurt, and milk are rich sources of calcium.
- Calcium is important in helping the heart beat, the blood clot, and the musculoskeletal system function.
- Skim milk taken daily in appropriate amounts is especially important to children and to women over 35 years old.

Appropriate posture and lifting techniques:

- Practice healthy body mechanics—especially important for allied health professionals who often support patients, or anyone who does lifting.
- Do not use your back when lifting. Make sure to bend your knees and lift with the thigh muscles.
- Employ good posture, such as sitting up straight in a chair. This helps prevent back discomfort and abnormalities later.
- Excercise to strengthen abdominal and lower back muscles and skeletal bones.

CHAPTER 18

Cardiovascular System

Anatomy and Physiology of the Cardiovascular System

Function

The cardiovascular system provides oxygen and food to the cells of the body and carries carbon dioxide and wastes to lungs for expulsion (elimination); includes the heart, blood vessels, and blood.

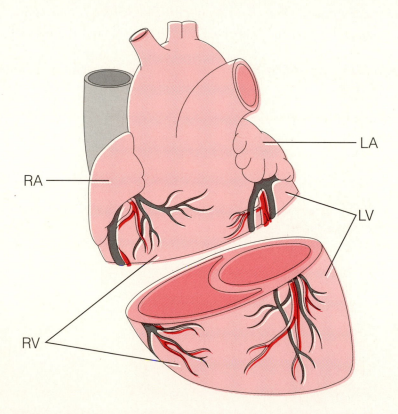

Figure 18.1   Cross section of the heart showing globular shape of left ventricle (LV) and half-moon shape of right ventricle (RV) as it drapes around LV. Above them are the right atrium (RA) and left atrium (LA). The coronary arteries are also shown. Adapted from Guyton, A.C., *Medical Physiology* (Philadelphia: W.B. Saunders Company, 1956)

Heart

The heart lies in the **media** *sti* **num,** between the lungs. It has *four chambers:* the **right** and **left atria** (singular, **atrium**) are receiving chambers (also called *auricles*); the **right** and **left ventricles** are pumping chambers. See Figure 18.1. The **apex** is the pointed part (bottom of the heart). The function of the heart is to pump blood, thereby maintaining circulation.

valves (vălvs)   keep blood from backflowing.

> **tricuspid** (trī-**kŭs**-pĭd)   between right atrium and right ventricle.
>
> **pulmonary semilunar** (pŭl-mō-nĕ-rē sĕm-ē-**lū**-năr)   between right ventricle and pulmonary artery.
>
> **mitral** (**mī**-trăl)   between left atrium and left ventricle (also called bi **cus** pid valve).
>
> **aortic** (ā-**ŏr**-tĭk)   between left ventricle and aorta.

septum (**sĕp**-tŭm)   wall that divides the right and left *sides* of the heart.

muscle   myo **card** ium is the heart muscle.

membranes   endo **car** dium lines inside of heart chambers; peri **car** dium is the outer double membranous sac consisting of the epi **car** dium (visceral layer); and outer pa **ri** etal layer.

Electrical Conduction System

sinoatrial node or **SA node** (sī-nō-**ā**-trē-ăl nōd)   this is the pacemaker (right atrium).

atrioventricular node (ā-trē-ō-vĕn-**trĭk**-ū-lăr nōd)   in septum.

bundle of His   conducting fibers.

Blood Vessels

The blood vessels consist of arteries, veins, and **cap** illaries (see Figure 18.2).

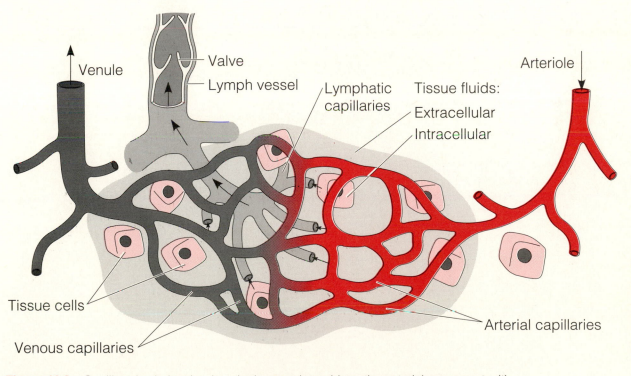

Figure 18.2   Capillary bed showing lymphatic vessels and how tiny arterioles connect with tiny venules. Gas, nutrient, and waste exchanges between blood and tissue take place in capillary beds. Adapted from Sloane, S.B., *The Medical Word Book* (Philadelphia: W.B. Saunders Company, 1991)

arteries (ăr-tĕr-ēz) always carry blood *away* from the heart (oxygenated blood except in pulmonary arteries).

veins (vānz) always carry blood *toward* the heart (deoxygenated blood except in pulmonary veins).

aorta (ā-ŏr-tă) largest artery (sections are ascending, aortic arch, tho **rac** ic, and ab **dom** inal).

vena cava (vē-nă **kā**-vă) largest vein (there are two: the superior and inferior venae cavae).

capillaries (kăp-ĭ-lăr-ēz) tiny blood vessels that connect arteries and veins; sites in which substances are exchanged between blood and tissues.

coronary arteries (kŏr-ō-nă-rē) supply the heart muscle with blood; arise from the base of the aorta. Oc **clu** sion of these causes heart attack (coronary oc **clu** sion). (See Figure 18.3.)

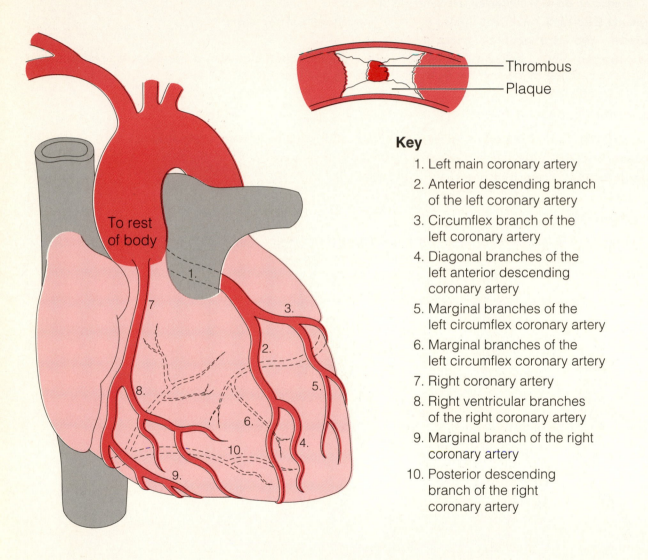

Thrombus
Plaque

Key

1. Left main coronary artery
2. Anterior descending branch of the left coronary artery
3. Circumflex branch of the left coronary artery
4. Diagonal branches of the left anterior descending coronary artery
5. Marginal branches of the left circumflex coronary artery
6. Marginal branches of the left circumflex coronary artery
7. Right coronary artery
8. Right ventricular branches of the right coronary artery
9. Marginal branch of the right coronary artery
10. Posterior descending branch of the right coronary artery

To rest of body

Figure 18.3 Coronary arteries and section of artery showing thrombus and plaque formation.

Circulation

The function of circulation is to carry oxygen and nutrients to cells and to carry carbon dioxide and wastes away from the cells (see Figure 18.4).

pulmonary circulation (pŭl-mō-nĕ-rē sĕr-kū-lā-shŭn)   starts in the right side of heart: blood returning from the body is received in the right atrium, goes to the right ventricle and through the pulmonary artery to the lungs. It returns to the left atrium by way of the pulmonary veins.

systemic circulation (sĭs-tĕm-ĭk)   from the left atrium, blood flows to the left ventricle and is pumped out through the aortic valve to the aorta and goes to the entire body.

portal circulation (pŏr-tăl)   circulation from the intestines, stomach, pancreas, and spleen to the liver.

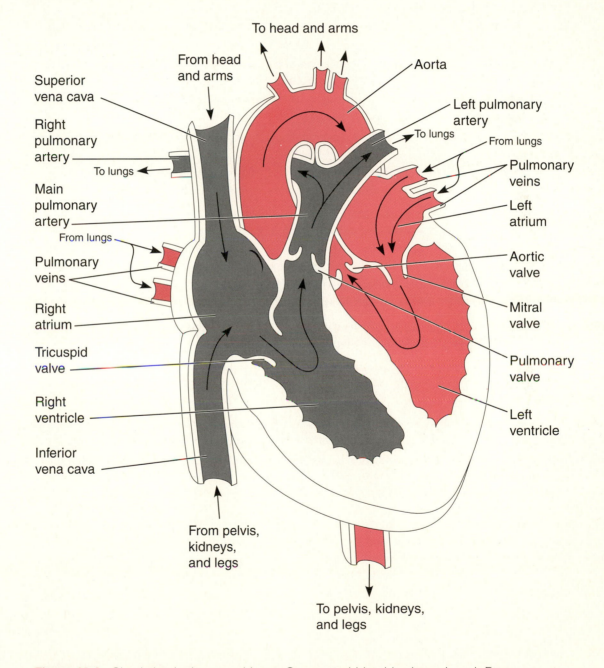

Figure 18.4   Circulation in the normal heart. Oxygenated blood is shown in red. Deoxygenated blood is shown in gray.

Lymphatic System

Lymph fluid comes from the blood; it filters out into the spaces between tissue cells, and returns to the blood via **lymphatic vessels. Lymph nodes** are numerous in certain parts of the body; nodes are palpable in the neck (cervical nodes), in the axilla (axillary nodes), and in the groin (inguinal nodes); they help filter out harmful substances such as bacteria and cancer cells. The **spleen** is the largest lymphatic organ of the body. In youth it helps build up blood cells; it also destroys old blood cells.

Blood

red blood cells (RBCs)   called **e ryth rocytes;** they contain hemoglobin, which carries oxygen to the cells and carries carbon dioxide away from the cells.

white blood cells (WBCs)   called *leu kocytes.* There are five basic kinds of white blood cells:

   Gran ulocytes (have granules in cytoplasm) are formed in bone marrow. There are three types:

      1.   *Neu trophils**: also called polymorpho **nu** clear leukocytes or PMNs because their nuclei have many shapes or forms. They defend the body by means of phagocy **to** sis (ingesting invaders).

      2.   **Eosinophils** (ē-ō-sĭn-ō-fĭls): are thought to be active and increased in allergic conditions.

      3.   **Basophils** (bā-sō-fĭls): function is unclear.

   Agranulocytes (ă-grăn-ū-lō-sīts)   (have no granules) are produced by spleen and lymph nodes. There are two types:

      4.   **Lymphocytes** (lĭmf-ō-sīts): produce antibodies and destroy foreign material.

      5.   **Monocytes** (mŏn-ō-sīts): perform phagocytosis and destruction of invaders.

plasma (plăz-mă)   the liquid part of the blood, minus the cells. It is amber colored. If whole blood is allowed to stand in a container, the cells will settle to the bottom (clot), and the clear plasma will rise to the top.

serum (sĭr-ŭm)   plasma minus the fi **brin** ogen that promotes clotting.

platelets (plāt-lĕts)   also called **throm** bocytes (clotting particles).

reticulocyte (rĕ-tĭk-ū-lō-sīt)   immature red blood cell, in bone marrow.

◼ **Note:** An order for *WBC and diff* means a white blood count and differential. A differential lab test determines the percentage of each kind of leukocyte. The hematology form in Figure 13.1 shows normal ranges on the right side.

Blood Types

Landsteiner types   based on type of red blood cells: A, B, AB, and O. (Type O is sometimes referred to as a universal donor, and type AB is sometimes referred to as a universal recipient.)

distribution   our population shows 3% AB, 10% B, 40–44% A, and 40–44% O. When incompatible bloods are mixed, clumping of cells occurs. Example: Type A red cells that are dropped into type B blood cause clumping or sticking together. These clumps could cause fatal injury as they pass through the heart or brain.

type and crossmatch (x-match)   done to determine compatibility before a transfusion is given. Cells from the donor and serum from the recipient are mixed to see if clumping occurs. A second test may also be done using the cells of the recipient and the serum of the donor. If no clumping occurs, it can be assumed that the two bloods are of the same type.

---

*Neutrophils are generally not called neutrophils on laboratory forms. They may be called *segs* because of their segmented nuclei, or they may be called *polys* or *PMNs*. Immature forms are often called *bands* or *stabs* or *juvs*. (See hematology laboratory form, Figure 13.1, p. 101.) *-phil* as in *neu-trophil* may also be spelled *-phile.*

Even the most carefully handled transfusions may have complications, so they are being done less frequently. Individuals who must receive transfused blood and are able to prepare for their operations may "bank" their own blood in advance.

Rh Factor

Rh factor is so named because it was first found in the blood of the rhesus monkey.

> 85% of population have this factor; they are **Rh-positive** (written **Rh+**).
>
> 15% do *not* have this factor; they are **Rh-negative** (**Rh−**).

The Rh factor acts like a foreign substance to anyone who is negative for it. If an Rh-negative person receives Rh-positive blood, that person's own blood will make an antibody that acts against the Rh-positive blood. If an Rh-negative woman mates with an Rh-positive man, their child may inherit the Rh factor from his father. The mother's blood may produce so many antibodies against it that the baby may die before or shortly after birth. This does not usually affect the first child of these parents because not enough antibodies are present, but it will affect subsequent pregnancies.

Antibody titers (tests) done during pregnancy aid the doctor in determining when intervention is necessary. If the titer rises rapidly, the pregnancy can be terminated early or preparation for exchange transfusion at time of delivery can be made. *RhoGAM* can be given to the Rh-negative mother following her first delivery to prevent Rh antibodies from forming.

Blood Pressure

Blood pressure (B/P) is the amount of pressure on the walls of blood vessels as blood passes through.

hypertension (hī-pĕr-**tĕn**-shŭn)   high blood pressure. *Essential hypertension* is high blood pressure with no apparent cause.

sphygmomanometer (sfĭg-mō-mă-**nŏm**-ĕt-ĕr)   B/P cuff (mercury and aneroid types).

systolic pressure (sĭs-**tŏl**-ĭk)   Top number in B/P reading. The greatest force exerted on the walls of the artery when the ventricles contract.

diastolic pressure (dī-ăs-**tŏl**-ĭk)   Bottom number in B/P reading. The least amount of force exerted on the walls of the artery when the ventricles relax.

normal B/P   Pressure up to about 140/90 in a healthy person is usually considered "within normal range." Anything above this bears watching.

- ■ **Note:** One B/P reading that is above normal does not constitute high blood pressure. Several readings, at intervals, are taken over a period of several weeks before a diagnosis of hypertension is made. Factors that affect blood pressure include:

  1. The volume or amount of blood

  2. The force or strength of the heart beat

  3. The condition of the arteries; if narrowed by disease, pressure will be higher

  4. Thickness or viscosity of the blood

Blood pressure may also vary with exercise or lack of it; eating, smoking, or fasting; taking stimulants or other drugs; strong emotions, fever, fatigue, hemorrhage, or shock.

Treatment of essential hypertension: lose weight if overweight, eliminate salt from diet, exercise. If these do not lower the B/P sufficiently, a diuretic medication is given. If further treatment is needed, antihypertensive drugs may be prescribed. These medications must be taken regularly and usually for a lifetime. The problem in treating hypertensives is that they do not feel ill and often do not take the medication as prescribed.

Pathophysiology of the Cardiovascular System

Cardiovascular Diseases and Disorders

AIDS   see Chapter 23 section on sexually transmitted diseases, page 214.

anemias (ă-**nē**-mē-ăz)   a group of diseases characterized by insufficient red blood cells; may be due to iron deficiency, some life-threatening condition (such as aplastic anemia, sickle cell anemia), a bone marrow defect, or heredity.

aneurysm (**ăn**-ū-rĭzm)   a weak, ballooned area in a vessel.

angina pectoris (ăn-**jī**-nă **pĕk**-tŏr-ĭs)   pains in the chest due to spasm of coronary arteries.

arrhythmia (ă-**rĭth**-mē-ă)   irregular heartbeat; often occurs after MI.

arteriosclerosis (ăr-tĕr-ē-ō-sklĕ-**rō**-sĭs)   thickening, hardening, and loss of elasticity of blood vessel walls, causing the lumen to become narrowed.

asystole (ă-**sĭs**-tō-lē)   cardiac standstill.

atherosclerosis (ăth-ĕr-ō-sklĕ-**rō**-sĭs)   a form of arteriosclerosis due to buildup of fatty material (plaque) in arteries.

cardiac arrest (**kăr**-dē-ăk ăr-**rĕst**)   cessation of heart action (CPR is indicated).

cardiomyopathy (kăr-dē-ō-mī-**ŏp**-ă-thē)   see *idiopathic cardiomyopathy*.

cerebrovascular accident (CVA) (sĕr-ĕ-brō-**văs**-kū-lăr)   change in blood supply of brain: either a vessel ruptures and bleeds into the skull, putting pressure on surrounding tissue that produces neurological symptoms, or a vessel blocked by an embolism or clot deprives the brain of oxygen and nutrients. (See *stroke*.)

cholesteremia, cholesterolemia, or **hypercholesterolemia** (kŏl-ĕs-tĕr-ē-mē-ă)   high cholesterol levels. The LDL (low-density lipoproteins) are a contributing factor in coronary artery disease. But high levels of HDL (high-density lipoproteins) are considered to be beneficial.

coarctation (kō-ărk-**tā**-shŭn)   compression or narrowing of the walls of a vessel, especially the aorta.

congenital defects (kŏn-**jĕn**-ĭ-tăl)   include septal defects (atrial, ASD; ventricular, VSD), **pa** tent **duc** tus arteri o sus, tet **ral** ogy of Fallot (făl-**ō**).

congestive heart failure (CHF) (kŏn-**jĕs**-tĭv)   inability to pump blood effectively throughout the body.

coronary occlusion (**kŏr**-ō-nă-rē ŏ-**klū**-zhŭn) and **coronary thrombosis**   see *heart attack*.

CVA   see *cerebrovascular accident*.

embolus, embolism (**ĕm**-bō-lŭs, **ĕm**-bō-lĭzm)   a thrombus that has broken loose and been carried along in the circulation until it blocks a vessel (air and fat globules may also cause this).

endocarditis (ĕn-dō-kăr-**dī**-tĭs)   inflammation of the endocardium.

fibrillation (fĭ-brĭ-**lā**-shŭn)   quivering or trembling type of contraction caused by injury to heart, as in MI, or by certain drugs; a heart in fibrillation cannot maintain circulation. Treatment is defibrillation.

heart attack   a clot in a coronary artery, cutting off circulation to the heart muscle; also called coronary oc **clu** sion, coronary throm **bo** sis, myo **car** dial in **farc** tion or **in** farct, MI (see Figure 18.5).

heart block   a type of ar **rhyth** mia; conduction of impulses from atrium to ventricle disturbed; pacemaker may be inserted.

heart murmur   a soft, blowing sound heard on auscul **ta** tion, indicating the valve may be incompetent and does not close properly.

hemophilia (hē-mō-**fĭl**-ē-ă)   congenital lack of clotting factor in blood.

hepatitis (hĕp-ă-**tī**-tĭs)   a liver disease; one type is spread by blood.

Hodgkin's disease   a type of malignant tumor of the lymph nodes and spleen.

hypertension (hī-pĕr-**tĕn**-shŭn)   *essential* hypertension (cause unknown) is high blood pressure.

idiopathic cardiomyopathy (ĭd-ē-ō-**păth**-ĭk kăr-dē-ō-mī-**ŏp**-ăth-ē)   and idiopathic hyper **troph** ic sub a **ort** ic sten **os** is—thickening of heart walls and septum that obstructs the flow of blood. Cause unknown. Occurs in young athletes, causing sudden death.

ischemia (ĭs-**kē**-mē-ă)   insufficient blood supply to a body part.

leukemias (lū-**kē**-mē-ăz) a group of diseases of the blood-forming organs and white blood cells; acute or chronic.

MI (myocardial infarct) (mī-ō-kăr-**dē**-ăl **ĭn**-fărkt) see *heart attack.*

myocarditis (mī-ō-kăr-**dī**-tĭs) inflammation of the heart muscle.

pericarditis (pĕr-ĭ-kăr-dī-tĭs) inflammation of the double membranes surrounding the heart.

rheumatic heart disease (rū-**măt**-ĭk) a form of myocarditis with mitral valve insufficiency; occurs as a sequela (sē-**kwē**-lă, aftereffect) to rheumatic fever. Beta strepto **coc** cus is the causative organism.

shock inadequate amount of circulating blood (cardiogenic); see index and dictionary.

stroke cerebrovascular accident (CVA); damage to the cerebrum due to ruptured vessel or clot occluding vessel.

thrombophlebitis (thrŏm-bō-flĕ-**bī**-tĭs) inflammation in a vein with clot formation.

thrombus (thrŏm-bŭs) blood clot in a vessel.

transient ischemic attack (TIA) (trăn-zē-ĕnt ĭs-**kē**-mĭk) brief period of inadequate blood supply to brain, sometimes referred to as "small strokes." Temporary occlusion resulting in impairment of blood flow to the brain (due to thrombus or embolism).

varicose veins (**văr**-ĭ-kōs) dilated veins caused by defective valves; also called **var** ices. Heredity is a factor. Surgical stripping removes varicosities.

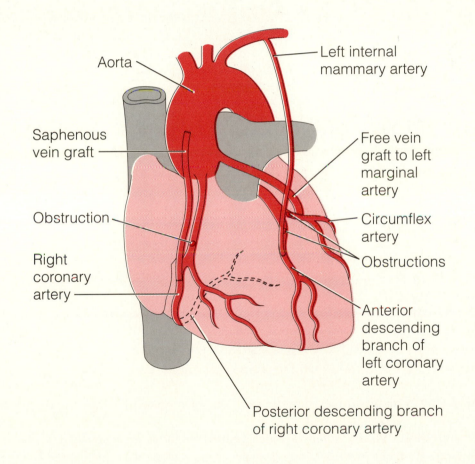

Figure 18.5 Triple coronary artery bypass graft.

Surgical, Diagnostic, and Treatment Terms

angiography (ăn-jē-**ŏg**-ră-fē)   X-ray examination of vessels.

angioplasty (**ăn**-jē-ō-plăs-tē)   see *percutaneous transluminal coronary angioplasty*. Tube inserted in the artery and inflated to open the artery.

anticoagulant (ăn-tē-kō-**ăg**-ū-lănt)   medication to delay clotting (blood thinner).

antihypertensive drugs (ăn-tē-hī-pĕr-**tĕn**-sĭv)   to relax artery walls or neutralize a hormone that causes arterial spasm.

atherectomy (ăth-ĕ-**rĕk**-tō-mē)   excision of plaque (same as *endarter **ec** tomy*).

bone marrow transplant   cells from marrow of a matched donor given to patients with leukemia.

bradycardia (brā-dē-**kăr**-dē-ă)   slow heart rate, less than 60 beats per minute.

bypass (**bī**-păs)   see *coronary artery bypass graft*.

cardiac catheterization (**kăr**-dē-ăk kăth-ĕ-tĕr-ī-**zā**-shŭn)   catheter passed into heart through a vein in the arm or leg to detect abnormal flow in coronary arteries.

cardiectomy (kăr-dē-**ĕk**-tō-mē)   the procedure of excising the donor's heart in transplant surgery.

cardioversion (**kăr**-dē-ō-vĕr-zhŭn)   treatment for tachycardia (rapid heart rate) using a dose of electrical energy or medication.

carotid endarterectomy (kă-**rŏt**-ĭd ĕnd-ăr-tĕr-**ĕk**-tō-mē)   surgically cleaning the carotid artery (especially successful with vessels that are blocked 70–99%).

claudication (clăw-dĭ-**kā**-shŭn)   cramplike pains in legs due to insufficient arterial blood supply to the muscles.

collateral circulation (kŏ-**lăt**-ĕr-ăl sĕr-kū-**lā**-shŭn)   "new" expanded small vessels that try to accommodate ischemic area when primary circulation has been blocked.

commissurotomy (kŏm-ĭ-shŭr-**ŏt**-ō-mē)   cutting defective heart valve (mitral stenosis) to improve flow of blood. (A commissure is any union of corresponding parts, such as the sides of the mitral valve.)

compression sclerotherapy (kŏm-**prĕ**-shŭn sklĕr-ō-**thĕr**-ă-pē)   injection along with compression for treatment of varicose veins and spider veins.

coronary artery bypass graft (**kŏr**-ō-nă-rē **ăr**-tĕr-ē **bī**-păs grăft)   substituting a vein from the leg to bypass the occluded artery in MI patients (see Figure 18.5); ileo **fem** oral bypass is similar, to supply blood to ischemic lower extremities.

digital subtraction angiogram (angi og raphy) (**dĭj**-ĭt-ăl sŭb-**trăk**-shŭn **ăn**-jē-ō-grăm)   uses computer; unwanted parts of X-ray picture are subtracted, giving a clear, precise image of vessels.

digitalized (**dĭj**-ĭ-tăl-īzĕd)   subjection of the patient to the drug digitalis (dĭj-ĭ-**tăl**-ĭs) in a quantity sufficient to maintain heart contraction force without side effects. (The process is called **digitalization.**)

diuretic (dī-ū-**rĕt**-ĭk)   a type of medication, often called a "water pill," that lowers blood pressure by reducing blood volume.

Doppler (**dŏp**-lĕr)   ultrasonic probe that checks blood flow in artery under it.

dyscrasia (blood) (dĭs-**krā**-zē-ă)   any abnormal condition.

echocardiogram   using ultrasound to visualize internal heart structures.

electrocardiogram (ECG, EKG) (ē-lĕk-trō-**kăr**-dē-ō-grăm)   picture of electical impulses of the heart (see Figure 18.6).

endarterectomy (ĕnd-ăr-tĕr-**ĕk**-tō-mē)   "boring out" the inner lining of artery to increase size of the lumen.

halocath laser (hăl-ō-**kăth lā**-zĕr)   used to widen vascular openings in lower limbs.

hemoglobin (**hē**-mō-glō-bĭn)   iron-containing pigment in red blood cells, essential for transport of oxygen.

heparin (**hĕp**-ă-rĭn)   an anticoagulant in the blood; also given as a medication.

Holter monitor (**hŏl**-tĕr **mŏn**-ĭt-ŏr)   portable ECG.

intra-aortic balloon pumping (ĭn-tră-ā-**ŏr**-tĭk)   to push more blood into coronary arteries following a severe MI or open-heart surgery.

ECG CHARACTERISTICS OF SELECTED
CARDIAC RHYTHMS AND DYSRHYTHMIAS

Rhythm/ECG Appearance	ECG Characteristic	Management

Superventricular Rhythms

Normal sinus rhythm (NSR)

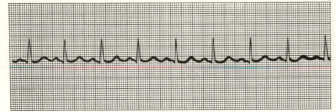

Rate: 60 to 100 BPM

Rhythm: Regular

P:QR5: 1:1

PR interval: 0.12 to 0.20 sec

QRS complex: 0.6 to 0.10 sec

None; normal heart rhythm.

Sinus arrhythmia

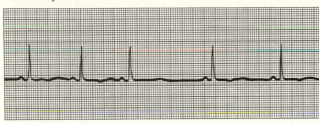

Rate: 60 to 100 BPM

Rhythm: Irregular, varying with respirations

P:QRS: 1:1

PR interval: 0.12 to 0.20 sec

QRS complex: 0.6 to 0.10 sec

Generally none; considered a normal rhythm in the very young and very old.

Sinus tachycardia

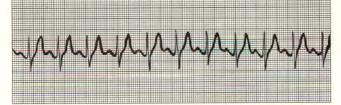

Rate: 101 to 150 BPM

Rhythm: Regular

P:QRS: 1:1 (With very fast rates, P wave may be hidden in preceding T wave)

PR interval: 0.12 to 0.20 sec

QRS complex: 0.6 to 0.10 sec

Treated only if the client is experiencing symptoms or is at risk for myocardial damage.

Treat underlying cause (e.g., hypovolemia, fever, pain).

Beta blockers or verapamil may be used.

Sinus bradycardia

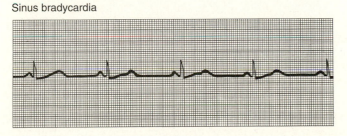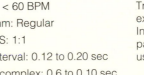

Rate: < 60 BPM

Rhythm: Regular

P:QRS: 1:1

PR interval: 0.12 to 0.20 sec

QRS complex: 0.6 to 0.10 sec

Treated only if the client is experiencing symptoms. Intravenous atropine and/or pacemaker therapy may be used.

Figure 18.6 Examples of ECGs. (Adapted from LeMone, P., Burke, K.M., 1996. *Medical-Surgical Nursing*, Redwood City, CA: Addison-Wesley Nursing.)

low-salt diet   lowers blood pressure by reducing blood volume; reduces edema.

lumen (lū-měn)   the opening within a tubal structure, such as a blood vessel.

open heart surgery   coronary artery bypass and other surgical procedures in which the heart is exposed.

pacemaker   a battery-powered device implanted under the skin to regulate heart rate.

percutaneous excimer laser angioplasty (PELA) (pěr-kū-tā-nē-ŭs ěk-sǐm-ěr lā-zěr ăn-jē-ō-plăs-tē) uses high-energy "cool" laser to open blocked arteries; procedure is similar to standard heart catheterization. Atherosclerotic material is removed by vaporization without damage to surrounding tissue. (See *percutaneous transluminal coronary angioplasty*.)

perfusion (pěr-fū-shŭn)   injecting fluid to thoroughly permeate (blood).

phlebotomy (flě-bŏt-ō-mē)   incision of a vein when venipuncture is unsuccessful, or for longer-term use than a simple IV.

percutaneous transluminal coronary angioplasty (PTCA) (pěr-kū-tā-nē-ŭs trăns-lŭm-ĭn-āl kŏr-ō-nă-rē ăn-jē-ō-plăs-tē)   an alternative to bypass surgery in selected cases; balloon-type catheter exerts pressure on area of plaque, thus opening the blocked area of vessel. (See *cardiac catheterization*.)

rotoblator (rŏ-tō-blă-tŏr)   burrowing instrument used for endarterectomy.

sinus rhythm (sī-nŭs rĭth-ŭm)   normal cardiac rhythm initiated by the SA node.

stent   a metallic support mounted on a balloon catheter and passed into artery; when balloon is removed, stent is left in place to hold artery open.

sternotomy (stěr-nŏt-ō-mē)   incision into sternum, for heart surgery.

stress ECG   electrocardiogram taken while patient is on the treadmill.

Swan-Ganz catheter (swăn gănz kăth-ě-těr)   pulmonary-artery balloon catheter; when inflated in pulmonary artery it blocks the flow of blood from the right heart to the lungs in order to measure pressures within the heart, central venous pressure.

tachycardia (tăk-ě-kăr-dē-ă)   rapid heart rate.

transplant (trăns-plănt)   implanting a donor heart (and lungs, sometimes) into a patient with life-threatening cardiac condition. Many other organs can also be transplanted.

valvulotomy, valvuloplasty (văl-vū-lŏt-ō-mē, văl-vū-lō-plăs-tē)   surgical procedures to repair or replace heart valves, especially the mitral valve.

vasodilator (văs-ō-dī-lā-tŏr)   agent that causes dilatation.

vasopressor (văs-ō-prěs-ŏr)   agent that causes constriction.

venipuncture (věn-ĭ-pŭnk-chūr)   puncturing a vein for any purpose, usually to draw blood or to introduce some medication.

Specialists

Medical doctors involved in treating cardiovascular disorders include: cardiologist, internist, cardiovascular surgeon, hematologist, oncologist; pediatric cardiologist and hematologist.

Treatment

Treatment for cardiovascular disorders varies from encouraging patients to change their lifestyle (lose weight, exercise, stop smoking, and so on) to prescribing a great variety of drugs and surgical correction of various heart and vessel disorders. Biofeedback may also be used.

Abbreviations

ABP   arterial blood pressure.

ACE   angiotensin-converting enzyme; ACE inhibitors are medications to lower blood pressure.

AIDS acquired immune deficiency syndrome.

ALL acute lympho **cyt** ic leukemia.

AML acute myelo **blas** tic (myelomonocytic) leukemia (**my** eloblast is a primitive bone marrow WBC).

ARC AIDS-related complex.

ASD atrial septal defect (often referred to as a "hole in the heart").

baso basophil (kind of WBC).

B/P blood pressure.

CABG coronary artery bypass graft.

CAC cardiac arrest case.

CBC complete blood count.

CCU coronary care unit.

CHF congestive heart failure.

CO₂ carbon dioxide (a colorless gas).

CPR cardiopulmonary resuscitation.

CVA cerebro **vas** cular accident (a stroke); *cva* (lowercase letters) means "costovertebral angle."

CVP central venous pressure, revealed by Swan-Ganz catheter.

ECG, EKG electro **car** diogram.

eos eo **sin** phil (type of WBC).

HDL high-density lipoprotein ("good" cholesterol).

HIV human immunodeficiency virus.

IHSS idiopathic hypertrophic subaortic stenosis.

ITP idiopathic thrombocytopenic purpura.

IVUS intravascular ultrasound for blood vessel imaging.

LDL low-density lipoprotein ("bad" cholesterol).

lymph **lymph** ocyte (type of WBC).

MI myo **car** dial **in** farct (heart attack).

mono **mon** ocyte (type of WBC); *mono* can also mean "mononucleosis."

O₂ oxygen (a colorless gas); essential for life.

PELA percu **ta** neous **ex** cimer **la** ser **an** gioplasty.

PICC peripherally inserted central catheter.

PMI point of maximal impulse (of heart on chest wall).

PMN polymorpho **nu** clear (leukocyte).

PTCA percu **ta** neous trans **lu** minal **cor** onary **an** gioplasty.

PVC premature ven **tric** ular contractions.

RBC red blood cell; red blood count.

segs white blood cells with segmented nuclei.

TEE transesophageal echocardiogram; ultrasound to view heart from the back.

TIA **tran** sient is **che** mic attack.

TPA tissue plasminogen activator (opens vessel occluded by clot).

VSD ven **tric** ular septal defect.

WBC white blood cell; white blood count.

Worksheet

Fill in the blank:

1. Define cardiovascular disease *disease of the heart and/or blood vessels* _____

   _____

2. What is CVA or stroke? _____

   _____

3. There are two phases to circulation of blood in the body. In one, deoxygenated blood is sent to the

   lungs; this is _____ circulation. In the other, the oxygenated blood is sent

   to the rest of the body; this is _____ circulation.

4. Blood from the right ventricle passes through the pulmonary valve and goes to the _____

   _____ (vessel) and _____ (organ); it returns to the

   (chamber) _____ of the heart, through the _____ (vessel).

5. Blood from the left ventricle goes to the entire body, leaving the left ventricle through the _____

   _____ valve to the _____ (artery).

6. The heart valves between the atria and ventricles are the _____ (right side)

   and the _____ (left side).

7. The largest veins in the body, which return blood to the heart from the upper and lower parts of the

   body, are the _____

   and the _____

8. The function of valves in the heart and in the veins is to _____

   _____

9. Arteries, veins, arterioles, venules, and capillaries are all _____

10. Circulation that takes over when regular circulation is cut off or blocked is called _____

    circulation.

11. The blood carries _____ (gas) and _____ to all tissues

    of the body and carries away _____ (gas) and _____

    for excretion.

Define:

12. septum (heart) *dividing wall between right and left sides of heart* _____

13. systole _____

14. diastole _____

15. myocardium _____

16. type and x-match _____

17. hematology _____

18. deoxygenated _____

19. varicose _____

20. coronary arteries _____

Fill in the blank:

21. The four main blood types (Landsteiner) are _____

22. a. Red blood cells (RBCs) are called _____

    b. White blood cells (WBCs) are called _____

    c. Cells that aid clotting are _____

    d. Name five kinds of white blood cells: _____

    _____

23. If a person does not have the Rh factor in his blood, he is said to be _____

24. The sinoatrial node is called the _____

25. Name the specialist who diagnoses and treats circulatory disorders: _____

    "blood" diseases (diseases of bone marrow) _____

26. Give three names for a heart attack: _____

    _____

27. The outer and inner membranes of the heart (in order) are _____

    and _____

28. Identify: ECG _____

    CCU _____

29. Factors that can affect B/P (give three): _____

    _____

    _____

30. Give root words for

    heart _____   (blood) vessels _____

    vein _____   blood clot _____

    artery _____   circulating clot _____

31. The universal donor is type _____

32. RhoGAM is given following delivery (of Rh-negative mother). What does it do? _____

    _____

    _____

33. Name three disorders of the heart, vessels, or blood not mentioned in this worksheet:

_____

_____

34. Identify:

a. MI _____

b. CHF _____

c. CVA _____

d. ASD _____ (congenital)

e. TIA _____

35. What is the usual treatment for essential hypertension?

a. _____

b. _____

c. _____

d. _____

36. What do these terms mean (in medicine)?

a. idiopathic _____

b. essential _____

c. transluminal _____

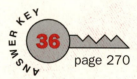

ANSWER KEY 36 page 270

Test p. 327
Alternate Test p. 329

■ Case History ■

CASE HISTORY 4

DISCHARGE SUMMARY: Chest pain

Final Diagnosis   1. Recurrent episode of chest pain, probably on an ischemic basis.

2. History of an inferior wall MI, August 1996, with cardiac arrest, which was apparently not due to atherosclerosis.

3. Hiatal hernia by history.

4. Type IV hyperlipoproteinemia

The patient is a 48-year old male admitted to this hospital for evaluation of an episode of chest pain on the morning of admission. He has a history of undergoing cardiac catheterization and coronary angiography in January 1995 because of persistent PVCs and atypical chest pain. This catheterization gave completely normal results with normal left ventricular function and completely normal coronary arteries. He subsequently sustained an acute transmural inferior wall myocardial infarction with secondary cardiac arrest in August 1996, for which he was hospitalized. Repeat cardiac catheterization and coronary angiography performed subsequent to his MI showed total occlusion of his right coronary artery but no other abnormalities aside from markedly abnormal left ventricular function secondary to his infarct.

He has been maintained on no cardiac medications. A stress test was apparently performed approximately one month prior to his admission and, according to the patient, gave normal results.

He was in his usual state of health until breakfast time on the morning of admission when he noted the gradual onset of crampy type discomfort between the shoulder blades and a substernal heaviness with radiation into his jaw, accompanied by chills and slight nausea. These symptoms lasted a total of approximately 20 minutes. He described the back and chest discomfort as being more severe than that which occurred with his prior MI. He denies any other accompanying symptoms. He came to the ER for evaluation where an ECG was obtained, which showed a normal sinus rhythm with changes consistent with an old inferior-wall MI without other definite acute changes except for some frequent unifocal PVCs. He was given a bolus of lidocaine and started on lidocaine drip. Because of his past and present history he was admitted for further evaluation and treatment.

Physical Examination   Well-nourished, well-developed, alert, cooperative, responsive white male resting comfortably in no apparent distress.

Pertinent diagnostic data: Admisstion CBC—hemoglobin 15.3g, hematocrit 45.8%, WBC 6900 with a normal differential; RPR nonreactive; prothrombin time and PTT WNL; Ua normal; electrolytes—sodium 143, potassium 4.2, chloride 102, CO_2 28; blood glucose 97; BUN 18; cholesterol 279; uric acid 7.6; phosphorus 2.8; calcium 9.8; total bilirubin 0.4; total protein 8.2; albumin 5.0; SGOT 18; LDH 109; alkaline phosphatase 79; CPK 60; serial cardiac isoenzymes completely WNL; lipid profile shows a pattern consistent with type IV abnormality; HDL level is not recorded; serial ECGs show a normal sinus rhythm with changes of an old transmural inferior-wall MI and some vacillating ST-T wave changes consistent with new inferolateral wall ischemia; chest X-ray examination WNL.

A recurrent acute MI was essentially ruled out with negative enzymes and ECGs. He was initally started on nitroglycerin ointment but did not tolerate this in any dose, developing severe headaches. His hospital course was totally uneventful except for the presence of some unifocal PVCs on admission, which responded to intravenous lidocaine and oral Norpace. He had no recurrent anginal symptoms whatsoever. At the time of discharge he was feeling well and was fully ambulatory. He will be followed as an outpatient.

Therapy on discharge: Low-saturated-fat diet and Norpace 150 mg po qid. Referral to a dietitian due to high cholesterol; follow up with cholesterol blood test in 3 and 6 months, then as needed.

■ **Assignment:** After reading the case history, write all new words and define them. Using the laboratory data given, consult laboratory forms (Chapter 13). Which results are out of normal range (if any)?

  Health Promotion Tip

To maintain a healthy heart:
- Eat nutritious foods, avoiding fat and cholesterol.
- Get regular daily exercise.
- Avoid smoking and secondhand smoke.
- Have regular physical assessments.
- Check blood pressure regularly.

CHAPTER 19

Respiratory System

Anatomy and Physiology of the Respiratory System

Function

The respiratory system provides the body tissues with oxygen and removes carbon dioxide.

Organs

All of the following are airways (see Figure 19.1).

nasal cavity (nā-zăl kăv-ĭt-ē) nose; nares (naris is singular); nasal septum divides cavity.

pharynx (făr-ĭnks) throat (through which air and food pass).

larynx (lăr-ĭnks) voice box; vocal cords.

trachea (trā-kē-ă) windpipe.

bronchi (bronchus) (brŏng-kī, brŏng-kŭs) one to each lung; lined with cilia (hairlike projections).

bronchioles (brŏng-kē-ōls) smaller divisions of bronchi.

alveoli (alveolus) (ăl-vē-ō-lī, ăl-vē-ō-lŭs) tiny air sacs at the ends of bronchioles that comprise lung tissue. In the alveoli, the gaseous exchanges take place (blood picks up oxygen, drops off carbon dioxide).

lungs right, three lobes; left, two lobes. *Apex* (plural is **a** pices) is the top of the lung; the *base* is the bottom. The lungs lie in the *pleural cavity* (tho **rac** ic cavity).

Other Terms

respiration (rĕs-pĭr-ā-shŭn) breathing; consists of *inspiration* and *expiration*. Air enters the nasal cavity and oral cavity and travels through the airways listed.

diaphragm (dī-ā-frăm) dome-shaped muscle that separates the pleural cavity from the abdominopelvic cavity. It *moves downward* on inspiration, creating suction in the chest to draw in air, expanding the lungs.

Accessory Structures

eustachian tubes (ū-stā-shŭn tūbs) (auditory tubes) tubes from pharynx to middle ear; they equalize pressure (see Figure 19.1).

epiglottis (ĕp-ĭ-glŏt-ĭs) flap that covers entrance to trachea; it closes during swallowing to prevent aspiration of food.

intercostal muscles (ĭn-tĕr-kŏs-tăl mŭs-ĕls) muscles between ribs.

paranasal sinuses (păr-ă-**nā**-săl **sī**-nŭs-ĕz) air spaces in cranium connected to nasal cavity (frontal, maxillary, ethmoid, sphenoid).

pleura (plŭr-ă) double mucous membrane that covers the lungs (**vis** ceral layer) and lines the thoracic cavity (pa **ri** etal) layer).

tonsils and **adenoids** (tŏn-sĭls, ăd-ĕn-ŏyds) part of the lymphatic system; act as filters (see Figure 19.1).

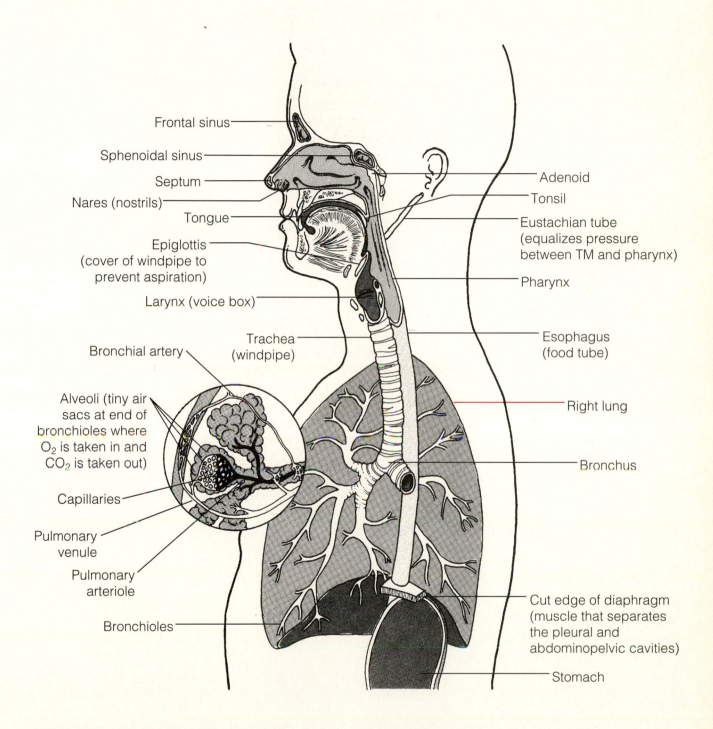

Frontal sinus

Sphenoidal sinus

Septum

Nares (nostrils)

Tongue

Epiglottis
(cover of windpipe to
prevent aspiration)

Larynx (voice box)

Trachea
(windpipe)

Bronchial artery

Alveoli (tiny air
sacs at end of
bronchioles where
O_2 is taken in and
CO_2 is taken out)

Capillaries

Pulmonary
venule

Pulmonary
arteriole

Bronchioles

Adenoid

Tonsil

Eustachian tube
(equalizes pressure
between TM and pharynx)

Pharynx

Esophagus
(food tube)

Right lung

Bronchus

Cut edge of diaphragm
(muscle that separates
the pleural and
abdominopelvic cavities)

Stomach

Figure 19.1. Lungs and airways showing the structures through which air passes on its way to the lungs. Capillaries and alveoli seen in inset.

uvula (ū-vū-lă)   muscle tissue that hangs down from the soft palate; it guards the opening from the nasal cavity, preventing food from entering. Many related terms use *staphyll/o* as the root word for *uvula*; for example, **staph** yloplasty.

Pathophysiology of the Respiratory System

Respiratory Diseases and Disorders

abscess (lung) (ăb-sĕs)   accumulation of pus (many causes).

allergy (ăl-ĕr-jē)   an acquired hypersensitivity to a substance (allergen).

asphyxiation (ăs-fĭk-sē-ā-shŭn)   suffocation due to interference with breathing.

asthma (ăz-mă)   usually due to allergy; dyspnea and wheezing due to spasm and swelling of airways.

atelectasis (ăt-ĕ-lĕk-tă-sĭs)   "incomplete dilatation" or collapsed lung; due to trauma, obstruction, or as a complication in lung disease.

bronchiectasis (brŏng-kē-ĕk-tă-sĭs)   "dilated bronchi" usually secondary to repeated early infections; foul pus discharge.

bronchitis (brŏng-kī-tĭs)   inflammation of bronchi; acute or chronic.

carcinoma (kăr-sĭ-nō-mă)   broncho **gen** ic carcinomas originate in bronchi: squamous, adenocarcinoma, and oat cell are types. Meta **stat** ic carci **no** ma of lung also occurs.

coccidioidomycosis (kŏk-sĭd-ĭ-ŏyd-ō-mī-kō-sĭs)   "valley fever," caused by fungus that lies dormant in spore form in hot, dusty climates; produces symptoms similar to pneumonia.

cor pulmonale (kŏr pŭl-mō-nă-lē)   heart failure due to pulmonary disease.

coryza (kŏ-rī-ză)   the common cold; caused by viruses.

cystic fibrosis (sĭs-tĭk fī-brō-sĭs)   mucovisci **do** sis; disorder of mucous glands leading to pancreatic insufficiency.

deviated septum (dē-vē-ā-tĕd sĕp-tŭm)   defect in wall between nostrils that can cause partial or complete obstruction.

diphtheria (dĭf-thē-rē-ă)   acute bacterial disease (immunization available).

effusion (ĕ-fū-zhŭn)   "flowing out" of liquid (see *pleurisy*).

emphysema (ĕm-fĭ-sē-mă)   distended or ruptured alveoli; irreversible condition characterized by severe dyspnea, especially exertional. Usually related to cigarette smoking, but can be due to an inherited deficiency of the protein AAT (alpha-1 anti **tryp** sin). Emphysema is one form of COPD (chronic obstructive pulmonary disease).

empyema (ĕm-pī-ē-mă)   pus in pleural cavity (abscess).

epistaxis (ĕp-ĭ-stăk-sĭs)   nosebleed caused by trauma, neoplasm, hypertension, or hormones.

fibrosis (fī-brō-sĭs)   abnormal formation of fibrous tissue (scar tissue in lungs), usually due to previous infections; may be referred to as idio **path** ic (cause unknown).

flail chest (flāyl)   erratic movement of chest due to multiple injuries of ribs or sternum.

"flu"   a term that has come to mean almost anything (used by laypeople).

hay fever   allergic coryza, pollin **o** sis.

hemothorax (hē-mō-thō-răks)   blood in thoracic cavity.

hiatal hernia (hī-ā-tăl hĕr-nē-ă)   diaphrag **mat** ic hernia; opening in diaphragm allows part of the stomach to move up into chest; usually treated conservatively with diet, antacids, and elevation of head when lying down.

hiccough, hiccup (hĭk-kŭp)   spasm of diaphragm due to many things; may involve phrenic nerve. Also called sin **gul** tus.

histoplasmosis (hĭs-tō-plăz-mō-sĭs)   fungus disease of lungs; lesions resemble TB.

hyaline membrane disease (hī-ă-līn) poorly developed alveoli leading to collapse of lungs in premature infants. Leading cause of neonatal deaths.

influenza (ĭn-flū-ĕn-ză) "la grippe"; group of virus-caused acute febrile pulmonary diseases, most serious in the very young or very old.

laryngitis (lăr-ĭn-jī-tĭs) inflammation of larynx (loss of voice or hoarseness).

laryngotracheobronchitis (lă-rĭng-gō-trā-kē-ō-brŏng-kī-tĭs) "croup"; so named because of croupy cough with air hunger (in young children).

pertussis (pĕr-tŭs-ĭs) acute febrile disease (whooping cough) caused by bacterial infection; immunization available in DTP.

pharyngitis (făr-ĭn-jī-tĭs) "sore throat," inflammation of the pharynx (can require pharyngeal culture to rule out strep).

pleurisy (plŭr-ĭ-sē) fluid discharged by inflamed pleural membranes (effusion), causing severe pain and dyspnea.

pneumoconiosis (nū-mō-kō-nē-ō-sĭs) any of the pulmonary disorders caused by irritating dusts, such as in asbes **to** sis and sili **co** sis, and other irritants (including chemicals) used in industry.

pneumocystis carinii (nū-mō-sĭs-tĭs kă-rī-nē-ē) an opportunistic pneumonia common in AIDS patients and other immunosuppressed patients.

pneumonias (nū-mō-nē-ăz) lung inflammation; many causes and types: bacterial and viral lung infection, aspiration and hypostatic pneumonia. May involve a lobe, a lung, or bronchial tubes.

rhinitis, rhinorrhea (rī-nī-tĭs, rī-nŏr-rē-ă) inflammation of nose; "runny nose" or "common cold" due to virus or allergy.

RSV or **RS virus** respiratory syncytial virus (sĭn-sĭ-shăl) type of myxovirus that causes formation of giant cells or syncytia. Common cause of epidemics of acute bronchiolitis, bronchopneumonia, and common colds in young children, and of sporadic episodes of acute bronchitis in adults. Can be fatal in young infants.

sinusitis (sī-nŭs-ī-tĭs) inflammation of paranasal sinuses; acute or chronic. (See Figure 19.2.)

streptococcal sore throat (strĕp-tō-kŏk-kăl) "strep throat;" communicable, may be asymptomatic; due to specific organism, characterized by sore throat; if not adequately treated with antibiotics may result in rheumatic fever and even rheumatic heart disease (all caused by streptococci).

tonsillitis (tŏn-sĭl-lī-tĭs) highly communicable; inflammation of tonsils with "crypts" of pus formation (usually); treated with antibiotics. T & A (tonsillectomy and adenoidectomy) may be indicated (but insurance guidelines usually require physician documentation of approximately four throat cultures positive for strep and/or four incidents of tonsillitis diagnosis in a one-year period in order to authorize payment).

tuberculosis (TB) (tū-bĕr-kū-lō-sĭs) infectious bacterial disease that produces "tubercles" in the lung (sometimes elsewhere also); caused by specific organism; treated with INH (isoniazid), PAS, and other drugs; patient need not be isolated if under treatment.

URI upper respiratory infection; general term for colds or what people call the "flu."

valley fever see *coccidioidomycosis*.

whooping cough (whū-pĭng cŏf) see *pertussis*.

Surgical, Diagnostic, and Treatment Terms

aerosol (ĕr-ō-sŏl) medication in spray form for relief of asthma symptoms.

anoxia (ăn-ŏk-sē-ă) without oxygen.

antihistamine (ăn-tĭ-hĭs-tă-mēn) medicine used to treat allergic reactions; counteracts histamine in the body.

apnea (ăp-nē-ă) temporary periods of not breathing.

bifurcation (bī-fŭr-kā-shŭn) separation into two branches, as with the bronchus.

biopsy (bī-ŏp-sē) excision of tissue to determine malignancy; lung biopsy is usually done with a bronchoscope.

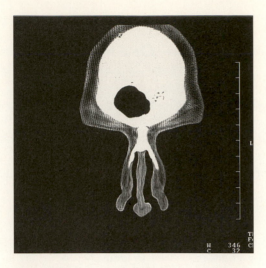 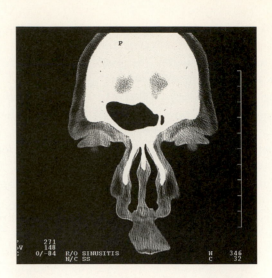

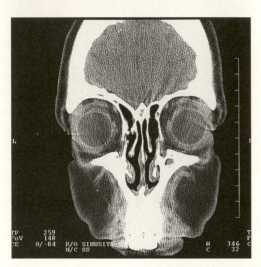 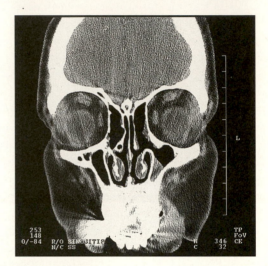

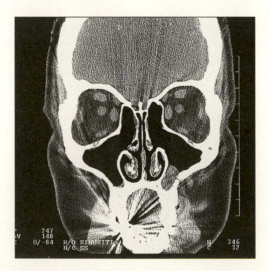

Figure 19.2 Excerpts from a CAT (CT) scan: computerized scan of some of the various axes/perspectives of the sinus (for example, to rule out sinisitis).

blood gases oxygen (O_2) and carbon dioxide (CO_2) quantities in arterial blood (laboratory test).

bronchodilators (brŏng-kō-**dī**-lā-tŏrs) medications to dilate bronchi.

bronchoscope (**brŏng**-kō-skōp) lighted instrument for viewing bronchi.

bronchoscopy (brŏng-**kŏs**-kō-pē) use of the above instrument.

bronchospasm (**brŏng**-kō-spăzm) contraction causing bronchi to constrict.

Cheyne-Stokes (chān stōks) irregular breathing; slow and shallow, increasing in rate and depth, then decreasing until breathing stops for 10–20 seconds; cycle repeats.

congestion (kŏn-**jĕs**-chŭn) "stuffy feeling" experienced with colds and other respiratory ailments, due to increased secretions of mucus in the respiratory tract. Also, excess fluid in chest cavity with lung infections.

consolidation (kŏn-sŏl-ĭ-**dā**-shŭn) solidification of lung tissue (in pneumonia).

cyanosis (sī-ă-**nō**-sĭs) condition of blueness due to insufficient oxygen, especially seen in nailbeds and skin.

dysphonia (dĭs-**fōn**-ē-ă) impaired voice.

dyspnea (**dĭsp**-nē-ă) difficulty breathing; may be parox **ys** mal nocturnal (PND), which is sudden and severe, or exertional (with exertion).

epinephrine (ĕp-ĭ-**nĕf**-rĭn) ("epi" or adrenaline) medication used to open bronchioles during unrelenting or severe asthma attack or allergic reaction.

expectorants (ĕk-**spĕk**-tō-rănts) medications that loosen secretions.

hemoptysis (hē-**mŏp**-tĭ-sĭs) expectoration of blood from lungs (frothy).

hiatus (hī-**ā**-tŭs) an opening, especially in diaphragm.

hilus (**hī**-lŭs) root of lung where vessels, nerves, and bronchi enter.

hypercapnia (hī-pĕr-**kăp**-nē-ă) increased CO_2 in blood.

hyperventilation (hī-pĕr-vĕn-tĭ-**lā**-shŭn) hyperp **ne** a; increased rate and/or depth of respiration; seen in anxiety states.

hyposensitization (hī-pō-sĕn-sĭ-tĭ-**zā**-shŭn) type of allergy treatment: increasing doses of the offending substance given to patient in an effort to build tolerance.

intubate (**ĭn**-tū-bāt) to insert an airway, in emergencies or in general surgery.

IPPB intermittent positive-pressure breathing, ventilator method used to assist breathing.

Kussmual breathing (**kūs**-mŏwl) deep, gasping type of breathing.

laryngectomy (lăr-ĭn-**jĕk**-tō-mē) excision of larynx, making it necessary for person to use esopha **ge** al speech or a pros **thet** ic larynx.

laryngoscopy (lăr-ĭn-**gŏs**-kō-pē) procedure of using la **ryn** goscope to view larynx.

lavage of sinuses (lă-**văzh**) washing out or irrigating sinuses.

lobectomy (lō-**bĕk**-tō-mē) excision of lobe of lung.

Mantoux (măn-**tū**) TB skin test.

mucolytic (mū-kō-**lĭt**-ĭk) type of medication to "dissolve" mucus.

orthopnea (ŏr-**thŏp**-nē-ă) able to breathe only in sitting position.

parenchyma (lung) (pă-**rĕn**-kĭ-mă) the "working part" of any organ is the parenchyma; in the lung the alveoli are the structures where gases are exchanged.

pneumothorax (nū-mō-thō-răks) introduction of air into thoracic cavity as a therapeutic measure or spontaneously as the result of an injury (puncture).

postural drainage (**pŏs**-tūr-ăl **drā**-năj) "postures" assumed by the patient to facilitate loosening and expectoration of secretions to improve ventilation.

productive cough a cough that produces sputum.

pulmonary function (**pŭl**-mō-nĕ-rē **fŭnk**-shŭn) various tests used to evaluate ventilation.

rales, rhonchi (răls, **rŏn**-kī) sounds in the chest indicating pathology.

rarefaction (răr-ē-**făk**-shŭn) term used to describe decreased density in x-ray films.

residual air (rĭ-**zĭd**-ū-ăl) air remaining in lungs after expiration; there is always some, but it is increased in some lung diseases.

respirators (ventilators) (rĕs-pĭr-ā-tŏrs)   mechanical assistance in breathing; Bird, Mark 7, and Bennett are some devices.

rhinoplasty (rī-nō-plăs-tē)   plastic surgery on nose; cosmetic and/or to improve breathing.

scan (lung, pleura)   use of radioactive isotopes to produce a "picture."

spirometer, spirometry (spī-**rŏm**-ĕt-ĕr, spī-**rŏm**-ĕ-trē)   instrument and its use in pulmonary function tests.

sputum (**spū**-tŭm)   secretions from bronchi; not saliva.

tachypnea (tăk-ĭp-**nē**-ă)   rapid breathing.

thoracentesis or **thoracocentesis** (thō-ră-sĕn-**tē**-sĭs) (thō-ră-**sĕn**-tē-sĭs)   "tapping" of chest to remove fluid.

thoracoplasty (**thō**-ră-kō-plăs-tē)   multiple rib resection to collapse diseased area of lung.

Tine test (tīn)   TB test.

tracheostomy (trā-kē-**ŏs**-tō-mē)   new permanent opening into trachea.

tracheotomy (trā-kē-**ŏt**-ō-mē)   incision into trachea when airway is obstructed.

transplant, heart-lung   donor organs substituted.

ventilators (**vĕn**-tĭ-lā-tŏrs)   see *respirators*.

vital capacity   amount of air that can be forcibly expelled from lungs after deep inspiration (pulmonary function test).

X-ray examination   routine, of chest; AP and lat (anteroposterior and side [lateral] view).

Specialists

Medical doctors involved in treating respiratory disorders include these specialists:
internist (pulmonary diseases), pulmonologist, ENT (ear-nose-throat; otolaryngologist), oncologist, thoracic surgeon, head and neck surgeon, radiologist.

Abbreviations

ARDS   acute, adult respiratory distress syndrome; "shock lung"; impaired gaseous exchange due to any cause (trauma, aspiration, etc).

CAT scan, CT scan   computerized (axial) tomography (see Figure 19.2).

CO   carbon monoxide; toxic gas

CO₂   carbon dioxide; gas expelled in expiration

COLD or **COPD**   chronic obstructive lung or pulmonary disease (emphysema, asthma, chronic bronchitis, etc.).

CPR   cardiopulmonary resuscitation; method of restoring circulation and breathing.

ET tube   endotracheal tube; intubation used during surgery and in emergency situations to establish a temporary airway.

IPPB   intermittent positive-pressure breathing (used as treatment with ventilator).

LAUP   laser-assisted uvula palatoplasty to cure snoring.

O₂   oxygen; gas inhaled and carried in the blood; administered as therapy by mask or cannulae.

P & A or **A & P**   percussion and auscultation; tapping and listening to the chest.

PPD   purified protein derivative (TB test).

RSV or **RS**   respiratory syncytial virus.

SMR   submucous resection (for deviation of septum); surgical procedure to correct defect.

SOB   shortness of breath or significant other at bedside.

SIDS   sudden infant death syndrome.

URI   upper respiratory infection (*not* urinary tract infection [UTI]).

Worksheet

Fill in the blank:

1. Cavity in which lungs are located (chest): _thoracic_____ or _____

2. Name the organs, *in order*, through which inspired air travels: _____

   _____   _____   _____

   _____   _____   _____

3. The muscle that separates the heart and lungs from the abdominal organs is the _____.
   When it contracts, it moves up/down (underline correct word), which makes more/less (underline correct word) room in the chest cavity. It contracts during inspiration/expiration (underline correct word).

4. The _____ keeps food from entering the larynx.

5. Where are the tonsils located? _____

   Where are the eustachian tubes? _____

   What do they do? _____

6. Define *alveoli*: _____

7. When the membrane that covers the lungs is inflamed, you have _____

8. Respiration includes the exchange of two gases. Name them and give the abbreviations: _____

   _____

9. The medical term for *nostrils* is _____ What is the dividing cartilage in the

   nose? _____

10. The top part of the lung is the _____. What is the plural form? _____

    What is the bottom or lower portion of lung? _____

11. Air spaces in the cranium are called _____

12. The trachea is in front of/in back of (underline correct phrase) the esophagus.

13. The physician who interprets X-ray films: _____

14. The physician who performs tonsillectomies: _____

15. _____ is a new permanent opening into the trachea.

16. A hiatal hernia is a hernia in the _____

17. A collapsed lung is called _____. Mantoux and Tine tests are tests

    for _____

18. What is meant by vital capacity? _____

    _____

19. COPD and COLD refer to chronic obstructive pulmonary disease. Name one such disease: _____

    _____

20. Difficult or labored breathing is called _____

21. _____ means "able to breath only when sitting upright."

22. A temporary cessation of breathing is called _____

23. Write all of the -itis words you can, using the organs in the respiratory system: _____

_____

Give the meaning of the following:

24. URI _____

25. SOB _____

26. IPPB _____

27. AP and lat (chest) _____

28. In the treatment of respiratory disorders several general kinds of medications are used. Name one

designed to loosen secretions: _____

Name a mist type: _____

29. Unusual chest sounds are also called _____

30. Name a malignant lung disease: _____

31. The plural of bronchus is _____

Define:

32. tachypnea   *fast breathing* _____

33. sputum _____

34. asthma _____

35. productive cough _____

36. spirometer _____

37. bronchoscope _____

38. inspiration _____

39. thoracocentesis _____

40. bilateral pneumonia _____

41. pneumocystis carinii _____

_____

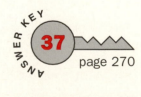

ANSWER KEY 37 page 270

Test p. 331
Alternate Test p. 333

■ Case Histories ■

CASE HISTORY 5

RADIOLOGY REPORT: Posteroanteior, lateral chest

Posteroanterior, Lateral Chest   There is opacity of the lower portion of the right hemithorax, apparently resulting from a large amount of fluid. The cardiac size is difficult to evaluate, but the heart may be somewhat enlarged, and the appearance of the visualized lung fields suggests passive congestion. The possibility of underlying fibrotic process in the right base cannot be exluded. There is calcification in the arch of the aorta.

CASE HISTORY 6

DISCHARGE SUMMARY: Bronchitis

Admitting Diagnosis   bronchitis.

Subjective Data   A 34-year old male admitted to the hospital because of a cough. He stated he was in his normal state of health until 1 week prior to admission when he began to experience a hacking cough that became extremely severe and was associated with malaise and sweating the night prior to admission.

Objective Data   CBC showed a leukocyt o sis of 19,000. Electrolytes, urinalysis, RPR were all WNL. Sputum for C & S grew out the usual upper respiratory tract flora. Noted on his rotochem was an elevated blood glucose; however, blood glucoses obtained after that showed the glucose to be within normal limits. Urine and blood cultures also were performed and revealed no growth. Alkaline phosphatase is 79, SGOT 38, SGPT 35, LDH 109, and a Gamma GT of 87. All of these are minimally elevated. ECG was totally WNL. Chest X-ray films were not helpful.

Hospital Course   The patient was admitted and treated with multiple antibiotic agents, mainly Keflex 500 mg qid; for his breathing Brethine 2.5 mg tid was used; however, he developed a drug reaction from Keflex and was changed to gentamicin sulfate 80 mg IV q12h, with Keflin 1 g q4h. Patient apparently did well on this medical regimen and after 10 days with medication was discharged from the hospital to be followed in the office in approximately 10 days.

CASE HISTORY 7

REPORT OF OPERATION: Bronchoscopy

Preoperative Diagnosis   bronchogenic carcinoma arising from the left upper lobe bronchus.

Operation   bronchoscopy; radical left upper lobectomy.

With the patient under satisfactory anesthesia, in the supine position and connected to the ECG monitor, a bronchoscopy was performed by introduction of 7 x 40 bronchoscope into the trachea. Epiglottis, vocal cords, trachea, right and left main bronchi were normal. There was a tumor originating 5 to 8 mm from the orifice of the left upper lobe with partial obstruction of the bronchus. A sample of bronchial washing was taken for C & S, and the bronchoscope was withdrawn.

The patient was then put in the thoracotomy position with the left side of the chest elevated and was connected to the ECG monitor. The skin of the chest wall was prepped with Betadine (bā-tă-dīn), and patient was draped and exposed. A costolateral thoracotomy incision was made. Muscle layers were transected with electrocautery. Chest was entered through the fifth intercostal space. Posterior thoracotomy was made through the fourth and fifth ribs to facilitate exposure. There was adhesion from the left upper lobe on the chest, which was lysed. The left superior hilum was reached. There was marked chronic inflammatory fibrosis of the pulmonary arteries and in the hilum, but, overall, there was no nodal involvement in this area. With considerable difficulty the branch of the pulmonary artery coming into the left upper lobe was dissected, ligating continuously, and transected. The superior segment of the left lower lobe was detached from the left upper lobe using a stapler. The superior pulmonary vein was dissected also, ligating continuously, and transected. All of the nodes were dissected toward the specimen, and the bronchus was dissected free of the adjacent structure. The bronchial artery was clipped.

At this point using the stapler and the transected upper lobe, cancer was noted in the stapler line. Again 2–0 stay sutures were placed over the main bronchus, and the remainder of the bronchus, which was about 8 mm in length, was cut flush with the left main bronchus. Bronchial closure was done using interrupted sutures of 4–0 silk. This closure was airtight. The second bronchial margin was negative for cancer.

After complete hemostasis, two chest tubes were inserted in the chest, exteriorized through the lower interspaces. The wound was then closed in layers, using interrupted sutures of No. 2 chromic, muscular layers with No. 1 chromic. The rest of the incision was closed in layers.

The patient tolerated the procedure well and was sent to the recovery room in satisfactory condition. Estimated blood loss was 4 units. The patient was transfused accordingly to keep up with the blood loss.

■ **Assignment:** The preceding reports were presented so that you experience the use of medical terminology in practice. Sometimes you will be able to understand a word you do not know simply because it becomes clear in context. Read the reports again and write the words you are not familiar with. Define them.

Health Promotion Tip

To prevent accidental injury to children, attending adults should be familiar with safety guidelines and know cardiopulmonary resuscitation techniques. In an emergency, brain damage or death could be prevented by dialing 911 and immediately employing appropriate CPR until help arrives.

Infant and toddler safety tips:

- To prevent asphyxiation and anoxia, be sure to keep cribs or beds a safe distance from windows (curtain strings could inadvertently get tangled around a child's neck during naptime, for example).

- To prevent aspiration, never give young children "choke foods" (such as grapes, popcorn, hard candy, and sliced hot dogs).

- To prevent tuberculosis, families (especially those with a member employed in an allied health field) should be sure to have annual physicals including a TB skin test, receive all immunizations that are appropriate, get daily exercise, have good nutrition and as much rest as possible, not smoke, and share affection. These factors promote optimal health and reduce the risk of TB, which is on the rise in the United States.

CHAPTER 20

Gastrointestinal System

Anatomy and Physiology of the Gastrointestinal System

Function

The gastrointestinal (GI) system (see Figure 20.1) provides for ingestion, digestion, and absorption of food or nutritive elements. It is also called the digestive system.

Gastrointestinal System Organs

The following are the organs of the alimentary canal, in order of digestive sequence.

mouth   oral cavity.

pharynx (făr-ĭnks)   throat.

esophagus (ē-sŏf-ă-gŭs)   tube to stomach, *behind* the trachea.

stomach (stŭm-ăk)   has the cardiac sphincter at entrance, py **lor** ic sphincter at exit. The greater and lesser curvatures are the large and small outer walls of the stomach. Do not confuse *stomach* and *abdomen*.

duodenum, jejunum, ileum (dū-ŏd-ĕ-nŭm, jē-**jū-**nŭm, **ĭl-**ē-ŭm)   the three parts of the small intestine. The *ileocecal valve* at the end prevents contents of large bowel from reentering small intestine.

cecum (sē-kŭm)   first part of large intestine; appendix attached.

ascending colon (ă-sĕnd-ĭng **kō-**lŏn)   large intestine.

transverse colon (trăns-vĕrs)   large intestine. *Splenic flexure* where transverse colon turns into

descending colon (dē-sĕnd-ĭng)   large intestine.

sigmoid colon (sĭg-mŏyd)   large intestine.

rectum (rĕk-tŭm)   large intestine.

anus (ā-nŭs)   anal sphincter (sphincter muscle is circular, like a purse string).

Accessory Organs

teeth   incisors (central and lateral); cuspids or canines; bicuspids or premolars; and molars (first and second); third are "wisdom" teeth.

tongue   muscular organ, covered with mucous membrane; taste buds are present on surfaces of papillae.

sal **ivary glands**   three pairs: pa **rot** id, sub **ling** ual, and subman **dib** ular.

pan **creas**   behind stomach; excretes pancreatic juice to duodenum (papilla of Vater); also secretes the hormone *insulin* into the blood (function of endocrine system).

liver   largest gland (RUQ); responsible for hundreds of chemical reactions.

1. Stores fats and sugars; makes proteins (albumin, globulins, cholesterol).
2. Secretes bile (essential for digestion of fats).
3. Regulates blood sugar.
4. Removes wastes from blood; detoxifies substances.

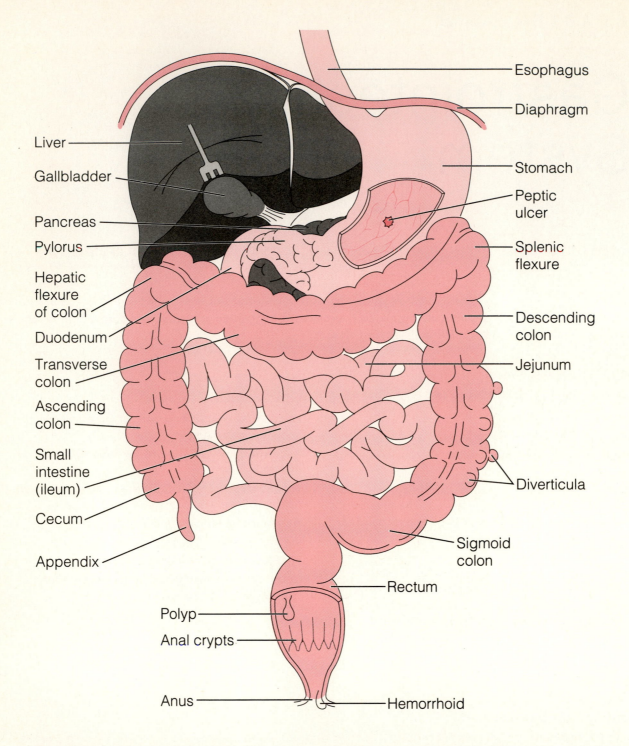

Liver

Gallbladder

Pancreas

Pylorus

Hepatic
flexure
of colon

Duodenum

Transverse
colon

Ascending
colon

Small
intestine
(ileum)

Cecum

Appendix

Esophagus

Diaphragm

Stomach

Peptic
ulcer

Splenic
flexure

Descending
colon

Jejunum

Diverticula

Sigmoid
colon

Rectum

Polyp

Anal crypts

Anus

Hemorrhoid

Figure 20.1 Gastrointestinal organs showing some pathologic conditions: peptic ulcer, diverticula, polyp, and hemorrhoid. The liver is being held back by a retractor so that the gallbladder is visible.

gallbladder (găhl-blăd-dĕr)   behind liver; stores and concentrates bile. *Hepatic ducts* drain bile from liver; *cystic duct* by which bile enters and leaves gallbladder; *common bile duct,* union of these two, into duodenum (by way of ampulla of Vater at sphincter of Oddi). The common bile duct and pancreatic duct meet to enter the duodenum (see Figure 20.2).

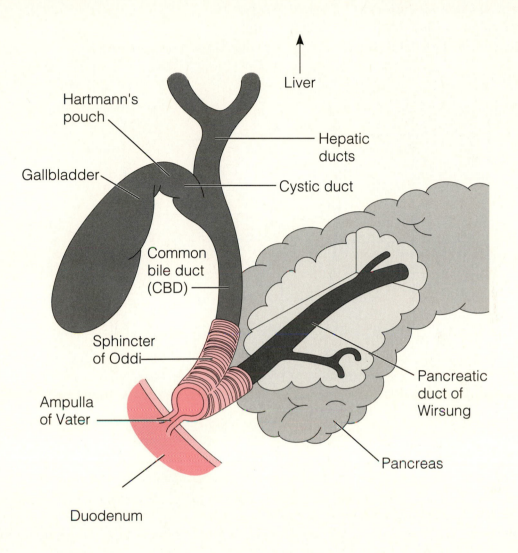

Figure 20.2   The gallbladder, its ducts, and their relationship to the pancreas and duodenum.

Areas of Abdomen

(See Figure 20.3.)

quad rants   four divisions: RUQ, RLQ, LUQ, and LLQ

divisions   nine sections:

1.	Right and left hypo **chon** dria	4.	Epi **gas** tric
2.	Right and left lumbar	5.	Um **bil** ical
3.	Right and left **ing** uinal or **il** iac	6.	Supra **pu** bic or hypo **gas** tric)

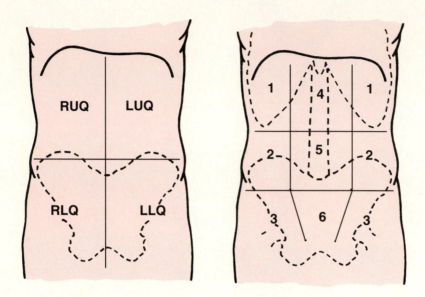

Figure 20.3   Areas of the abdomen.

Digestion

mechanical process   food is broken up, mixed with digestive juices. It is moved along by peri **stal** sis (rhythmic contraction of the intestines).

chemical process   food reacts with enzymes. Large molecules are broken down so they can pass through the mucous membrane into the blood and from there to the cells.

absorption   takes place in the small intestines. **Vil** li, which are tiny projections lining intestines, provide large surface area through which nutrients can be absorbed.

elimination   of solid wastes in the form of *feces.* Also called *fecal matter, excreta, stool,* and *bowel movement.*

metabolism (mĕ-**tăb**-ō-lĭzm)   the sum of all physical and chemical changes that take place within the body and all energy and transformations that occur within cells; change of food to mechanical energy or heat.

nutrients   food; proteins, fats, carbohydrates, plus vitamins and essential minerals. Proteins and carbohydrates (CHO) contain 4 calories per gram; fats contain 9. Protein is essential for growth and repair of tissue. Fats and carbohydrates provide heat and energy.

Essential vitamins: A, B_1 (thiamine), B_2 (riboflavin), niacin, B_6 (pyridoxine), B_{12} (cyanocobalamin), C (ascorbic acid), D, folic acid, and K.

Essential minerals: calcium, iron, iodine, zinc, copper, magnesium, potassium, phosphorus, sodium.

Pathophysiology of the Gastrointestinal System

Gastrointestinal Diseases and Disorders

adhesions (ăd-**hē**-zhŭns)   abnormal bands or fibers that bind one organ to another (especially intestines); can result from abdominal surgery or infection and may cause bowel obstruction. Surgical treatments are adhesi **ol** ysis, ahesi **ot** omy.

alcoholism (**ăl**-kō-hŏl-ĭzm)   addiction to alcohol, leading to malnutrition and liver damage (also brain damage and psychosociological problems).

anorexia (ăn-ō-**rĕk**-sē-ă)   a medical symptom noting that the patient is without appetite.

anorexia nervosa (ăn-ō-**rĕk**-sē-ă nĕr-**vō**-să)   a psychological disorder involving a distorted body image and an aversion to food which may result in severe weight loss, malnutrition, and possible death.

appendicitis (ăp-pĕn-dĭ-**sī**-tĭs)   inflammation of the appendix; ruptured appendix can lead to peritonitis.

atresias (ă-**trē**-zē-ăz)   **bil** iary: absence or closure of normal major bile ducts; esopha **ge** al; congenital failure of esophagus to develop.

botulism (**bŏt**-ū-lĭzm)   a severe type of food poisoning caused by anaerobic bacteria, leading to GI, eye, and neurologic symptoms; can be fatal.

bulimia (bŭ-**lē**-mē-ă)   eating disorder with binge eating followed by purge vomiting (most common in young women).

carcinoma (kăr-sĭ-**nō**-mă)   malignant tumor (may involve any GI organ).

cholecystitis (kōl-ĕ-sĭs-**tī**-tĭs)   inflammation of the gallbladder; acute usually caused by gallstones.

cholelithiasis (kōl-ĕ-lĭ-**thī**-ă-sĭs)   condition of gallstones.

cirrhosis (sĭr-**rō**-sĭs)   replacement of liver cells by fibrous tissue; occurs frequently in alcoholics.

cleft lip/palate (clĕft **păl**-ăt)   congenital failure of lip and/or palate to fuse. Treatment is surgical cheiloplasty (**kī**-lō-plăs-tē).

colitis (ulcerative, spastic) (kō-**lī**-tĭs)   inflammation of colon.

Crohn's (krōhnz)   inflammatory disease of the colon, more commonly found in the terminal ileum.

cryptitis (krĭp-**tī**-tĭs)   inflammation of "crypts," especially those in anus and penis.

diverticulitis, diverticulosis (dī-vĕr-tĭk-ū-**lī**-tĭs, dī-vĕr-tĭk-ū-**lō**-sĭs)   inflammation or condition of having diverticula that are "pouches," especially in the sigmoid colon (see Figure 20.1).

dysentery (**dĭs**-ĕn-tĕr-ē)   severe dehydrating diarrhea; types include ame **bi** asis, shigel **lo** sis, salmo **nel** la; slang term: Montezuma's revenge.

encopresis (ĕn-kō-**prē**-sĭs)   repeated, uncontrolled passage of feces (after 7 years of age).

esophageal varices (ē-sŏf-ă-**jē**-ăl **văr**-ĭ-sēz)   enlarged, incompetent veins in distal esophagus due to portal hypertension in cirrhosis.

esophagitis (ē-sŏf-ă-**jī**-tĭs)   inflammation of the esophagus (food tube).

food poisoning (gastroenteritis) (găs-trō-ĕn-tĕr-**ī**-tĭs)   acute nausea and vomiting, cramps, and diarrhea due to a variety of ingested toxins or bacteria.

gastric ulcers (peptic, duodenal) (**pĕp**-tĭk, dū-**ŏd**-ĕ-năl)   inflamed area with destruction of tissue; may cause bleeding and pain and may perforate.

gastritis (găs-**trī**-tĭs)   gastroenteritis; inflammation of stomach or entire GI tract; common in alcoholism.

glossitis (glŏs-**sī**-tĭs)   inflammation of the tongue.

hepatitis (hĕp-ă-**tī**-tĭs)   inflammation of the liver; type A, formerly called "infectious," and type B, formerly called "serum"; also non A and non B type. A vaccine is now available for hepatitis B high-risk groups.

hernia (**hĕr**-nē-ă)   many types: hi **a** tal, **ing** uinal (Figure 20.4), um **bil** ical, **fem** oral; protrusion of a part out of its natural place. *Hiatal* indicates that the stomach is pushed up through diaphragm into thoracic cavity; other types involve intestines and may cause bowel obstruction (strangulated hernia).

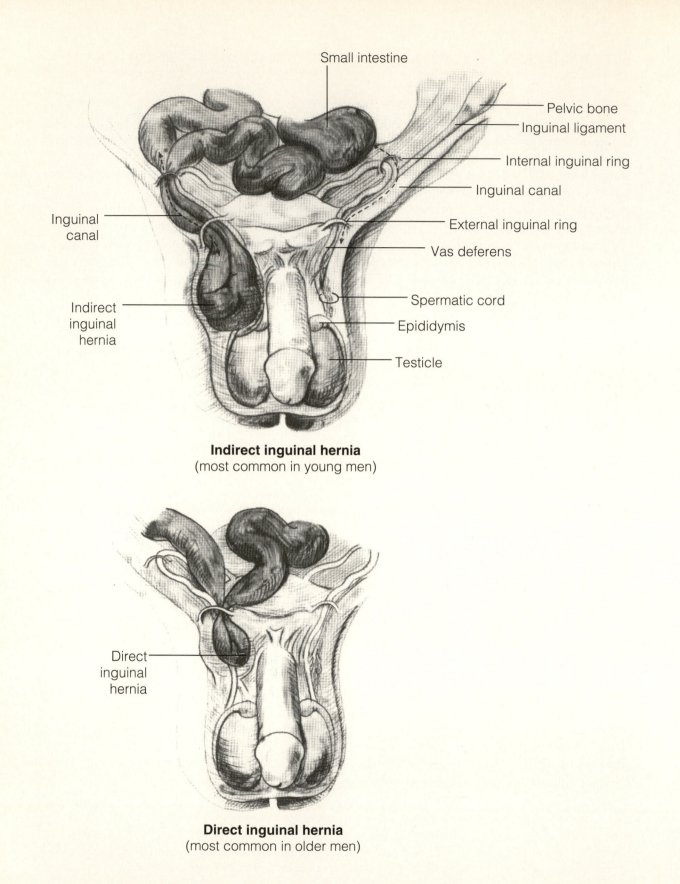

Indirect inguinal hernia
(most common in young men)

Direct inguinal hernia
(most common in older men)

Figure 20.4 Inguinal hernias, indirect and direct. (Adapted from Medical Times Patient Education Charts, Romaine Pierson Publishers, Inc., New York.)

impaction (fecal) (ĭm-**păk**-shŭn)   hard stool impacted in rectum that usually must be removed manually; this condition is a problem in elderly populations (especially in nursing homes) and is due to many factors, especially inactivity, low fiber or roughage intake, low fluid intake.

intussusception (ĭn-tŭs-ŭs-**sĕp**-shŭn)   telescoping of intestine (slides into itself), causing obstruction.

irritable bowel syndrome (IBS) (ĭr-rĭt-ăb-l **bŏw**-ĕl **sĭn**-drōm)   spastic bowel causing frequent, loose stools; often no organic cause can be found.

nausea and vomiting (**Năw**-sē-ă, **vŏm**-ĭt-ĭng)   N and V; common symptoms in many GI disorders.

obesity (ō-**bē**-sĭ-tē)   overweight: 20–30% above normal.

pancreatitis (păn-krē-ă-**tī**-tĭs)   inflammation of the pancreas.

peritonitis (pĕr-ĭ-tŏ-**nī**-tĭs)   inflammation of the peritoneal cavity, usually due to rupture of an organ (appendix, for example).

PKU, phenylketonuria (fĕn-ĭl-kē-tō-**nū**-rē-ă)   a congenital inability to metabolize phenyl **al** anine, which leads to mental retardation; treated with special diet.

polyposis (pŏl-ē-**pō**-sĭs)   condition of having polyps in colon (growths that hang from a thin stalk known as pedunculated polyp); familial and a precursor to cancer.

ptyalism (**tī**-ă-lĭzm)   excessive saliva production, due to pregnancy, disease, or medication.

pyloric stenosis (pī-**lŏr**-ĭk stē-**nō**-sĭs)   congenital condition; outlet of stomach is narrow and will not allow food to pass into duodenum, causing projectile vomiting.

rectocele (**rĕk**-tō-sēl)   hernia of rectum.

sialolith (sī-**ăl**-ō-lĭth)   stone in salivary duct.

stomatitis (stō-mă-**tī**-tĭs)   canker sores, sores in the mouth sometimes caused by dietary deficiencies or stress-related.

ulcers (**ŭl**-sĕrs)   see *gastric ulcers*.

xerostomia (zē-rō-**stō**-mē-ă)   dry mouth, common in many disease conditions; also a side effect of many medications.

■ **Note:** Treatment for many of the above conditions is surgery. Conservative treatment is often the treatment of choice in ulcers, colitis, diverticulosis, and hiatal hernia.

Diagnostic Procedures

biopsy (**bī**-ŏp-sē)   examination of living tissue; tissue may be taken from any of the GI organs, and this can be done through an endoscope usually. Needle biopsy may be done on liver.

blood chemistry (laboratory work)   tests for liver function; frequent tests done are bilirubin, alkaline phosphatase, SGOT and SGPT (enzymes); other helpful lab tests are gastric analysis, stool specimen examination for occult blood and parasites, and so on.

cholangiography (kō-lăn-jē-**ŏg**-ră-fē)   X-ray examination of the bile ducts using contrast medium (IV or, if during surgery, directly into ducts).

cholecystography and **choledochography** (kō-lē-sĭs-**tŏg**-ră-fē, kō-lĕd-ō-**kŏg**-ră-fē)   oral dye is ingested that outlines the gallbladder and bile duct so that X-ray detects stones; see *gallbladder series*.

colonoscopy (kō-lŏn-**ŏs**-kō-pē)   procedure of looking into the colon with a flexible, fiberoptic scope.

digital examination (**dĭj**-ĭ-tăl)   insertion of the gloved finger into the rectum.

endoscopic retrograde cholangiopancreatography (ERCP) (ĕn-dō-**skŏp**-ĭk **rĕt**-rō-grād kō-lăn-jē-ō-păn-krē-ă-**tŏg**-ră-fē)   a flexible tube is passed through the small intestine into the bile duct; after dye is injected, an X-ray is taken.

esophagogastroduodenoscopy (EGD) (ē-sŏf-ă-gō-găs-trō-dū-ŏd-ĕn-**ŏs**-kō-pē)   using scope to examine these structures.

flat plate of abdomen (**ăb**-dō-mĕn)   X-ray film of abdomen.

gallbladder series (GBS)   X-ray film is taken after patient has been given a dye that will outline a gallbladder; a second set of X-ray films is then taken after the patient has eaten a fatty meal.

gastrointestinal series (GI series) (găs-trō-ĭn-**těs**-tĭ-năl)   UGI (upper GI) or barium swallow; lower GI or barium enema (BE); an opaque substance called barium is given by mouth/enema and X-ray films are taken.

gastroscopy (găs-**trŏs**-kŏ-pē)   examining the stomach with a gastroscope.

percutaneous transhepatic cholangiography (PTC) (pěr-kū-**tā**-nē-ŭs trăns hě-păt-ĭk-kō-lăn-jē-**ŏg**-ră-fē) a thin needle is passed through the abdomen into the duct network of the liver to insert dye to enhance X-ray.

proctoscopy (prŏk-**tŏs**-kō-pē)   examining the rectum, sigmoid, with scope.

scan   using a special device, CT or CAT (computerized [axial] tomography), to produce a "picture" of any organ.

stool specimen (st ĕwl **spē**-sĭ-měn)   sent to laboratory for occult blood (guaiac) or for parasites, such as worms, amoebas.

ultrasonography (ŭl-tră-sō-**nŏg**-ră-fē)   using ultrasound method to obtain a "picture" of any organ; screening technique for gallstones; many other uses.

■ **Note:** Preparation may be vigorous for some of these procedures, for example NPO (nothing by mouth) at least 8 hours prior to test, laxatives and enemas until clear. Without such preparation the endoscopic and GI tests cannot be useful in diagnosis. Printed instructions are usually given to the patient.

Surgical Procedures

anastomosis (ă-năs-tō-**mō**-sĭs)   joining together two parts of intestine or common bile duct when portion has been removed; also called *resection*.

appendectomy (ăp-pĕn-**děk**-tō-mē)   excision of appendix.

biopsy (**bī**-ŏp-sē)   of any organ (diagnostic).

bypass (**bī**-păs)   removal of large portion of small intestine in cases of morbid obesity.

cheiloplasty (**kī**-lō-plăs-tē)   plastic surgery on lip, usually for cleft lip (cheilo = lip).

cholecystectomy (kō-lē-sĭs-**těk**-tō-mē)   excision of the gallbladder.

choledochoduodenostomy (kō-lěd-ō-kō-dū-ō-dē-**nŏs**-tō-mē)   new permanent opening between the common bile duct (choledoch/o) and duodenum.

choledocholithotomy (kō-lěd-ō-kō-lĭth-**ŏt**-ō-mē)   removal of gallstone through incision in the common bile duct (CBD).

colostomy (kō-**lŏs**-tō-mē)   new permanent opening of colon to surface of abdomen with a stoma.

gastrectomy (găs-**trěk**-tō-mē)   usually subtotal removal of stomach; Billroth I and II techniques, anastomosis between stomach and duodenum or jejunum.

hernioplasty or **herniorrhaphy** (**hěr**-nē-ō-plăs-tē, hěr-nē-**ŏr**-ră-fē)   surgical repair of hernia; many types; may use synthetic material for reinforcement.

ileostomy (ĭl-ē-**ŏs**-tō-mē)   new permanent opening into ileum; continent type holds contents until released by inserting tube.

laparotomy (lăp-ă-**rŏt**-ō-mē)   incision into abdomen, usually "exploratory."

lithotripsy (lithotriptor) (**lĭth**-ō-trĭp-sē)   shock wave lithotripsy uses external sound waves to fragment gallstones into small pieces. They may then pass spontaneously, or ursodiol taken orally may dissolve them.

MTBE   methyl-tertiary-butyl ether; chemical name of a stone-dissolving medication given by injection.

portacaval shunt (pŏr-tă-**kā**-văl shŭnt)   portal vein stitched to inferior vena cava to bypass the obstructed cirrhotic liver.

stomach stapling   staples across stomach to allow only very small amount of food to be eaten; used in cases of intractable obesity.

transplant   especially liver, usually performed on infants to correct biliary atresia. (Total liver, or part of parent's liver.)

ursodiol (ŭr-sō-**dī**-ōl)   a stone-dissolving drug, taken orally.

vagotomy (vā-**gŏt**-ō-mē)   cutting vagus nerve; a procedure sometimes used to treat ulcers.

Miscellaneous Terms

abdomen (**ăb**-dō-mĕn)   front of body between chest and pelvis; the belly area.

anasarca (ăn-ă-**săr**-kă)   severe, generalized edema.

ascites (ă-**sī**-tēz)   edema, collection of fluid in peritoneal cavity.

buccal (**bŭk**-ăl)   pertaining to the cheek.

cachexia (kă-**kĕk**-sē-ă)   severe malnutrition and wasting; emaci **a** tion.

calorie (**kăl**-ŏ-rē)   unit of heat; energy value of food.

cathartics/laxatives (kă-**thăr**-tĭks, **lăk**-să-tĭvs)   purgatives; any substance taken orally to induce bowel movement.

CBD(E)   common bile duct (exploration); union of hepatic and cystic ducts; choledoch/o = common bile duct; the CBD enters the duodenum through the ampulla of Vater.

cholesterol (kō-**lĕs**-tĕr-ŏl)   a chemical component of oils and fats; also synthesized in the liver and a normal constituent of bile. Includes high-density lipoprotein HDL ("good" cholesterol) and low-density lipoprotein LDL ("bad" cholesterol). LDL contributes to plaque formation in arteries.

deglutition (dē-glū-**tĭ**-shŭn)   swallowing.

emesis (emetic) (**ĕm**-ĕ-sĭs, ĕ-**mĕt**-ĭk)   to have an emesis is to vomit. Antiemetic drugs prevent vomiting.

enema (**ĕn**-ĕ-mă)   introduction of fluid into the rectum for cleansing and/or diagnostic purposes in preparation for barium enema, in which cases "enemas until clear" are ordered.

enzymes (**ĕn**-zīms)   more than 650 complex proteins manufactured by living tissue; they stimulate specific chemical changes, such as breakdown of starches to sugars (amylase enzyme), so that they can be absorbed by the intestines; most enzyme names end in -*ase* (exceptions are rennin, pepsin, and so on).

eviscerate (ē-**vĭs**-ĕr-āt)   internal organs come out (e.g., through a wound).

fistula (**fĭs**-tū-lă)   abnormal opening between two organs (rectovaginal) or to surface of skin.

flatus, flatulence (**flā**-tŭs, **flăt**-ū-lĕns)   excessive gas in the GI tract; may cause distension if severe.

Fleet's (enema)   prepackaged, disposable type of enema.

flexure (**flĕk**-shŭr)   a "turning" or angle, as the hepatic flexure of the colon near the liver.

fundus (**fŭn**-dŭs)   the body or larger part of a hollow organ, as the fundus of the stomach (also applies to the uterus and eye).

gamma globulin (**găm**-mă **glŏb**-ū-lĭn)   substance containing antibodies; used to provide passive (temporary) immunity in people who have been exposed to an infectious disease (infectious hepatitis, for example).

gavage (gă-**văzh**)   feeding by tube (especially premature infants).

glossal (**glŏs**-săl)   pertaining to the tongue.

hyperalimentation (hī-pĕr-ăl-ĭ-mĕn-**tā**-shŭn)   TPN (total parenteral nutrition) with a subclavian catheter.

lavage (lă-**văzh**)   to wash out, especially the stomach after ingestion of a poisonous substance.

lingual (**lĭng**-gwăl)   pertaining to the tongue; *sublingual* means "under the tongue."

nasogastric tube (nā-zō-**găs**-trĭk)   a soft, flexible tube introduced through the nose into the stomach for gavage, lavage, or suction.

NPO   "nothing by mouth" in preparation for tests and before and after surgery (until peristalsis is established again).

parotid (pă-**rŏt**-ĭd)   "near the ear"; parotitis or mumps results when the salivary glands near the ear become inflamed.

peritoneum (pĕr-ĭ-tō-**nē**-ŭm)   membrane lining the abdominal cavity. The *mesentery* is part of the peritoneum; it attaches intestines to the posterior body wall. The *greater and lesser omenta* are also part of the peritoneum; they connect abdominal viscera with the stomach.

stoma (**stō**-mă)   mouth or artificial abdominal opening following an -*ostomy* (e.g., colostomy or ileostomy).

viscera (**vĭs**-ĕr-ă)   internal organs.

Specialists

GI disorders may be treated by an internist (gastroenterologist), family practice specialist, general surgeon, oncologist, proctologist. Public health physicians are involved in cases of infectious hepatitis, food poisoning, and so on.

Treatment

Treatment is often surgical. Diet is often an important part of treatment in GI disorders. Bland diets and soft diets may still be used in some cases, but the trend recently has been toward more fiber in diets. Drugs that are important in treatment include antispasmodics, antacids, antinauseants, antiobesity anorexics (including amphetamines), antidiarrheals, laxatives, stool-softening drugs, as well as various antibiotics in the acute inflammatory disorders.

Abbreviations

BM   bowel movement

CBD   common bile duct

GBS   gallbladder series

GERD   gastroesophageal reflux disease

GI   gastrointestinal series (upper and lower)

HDL   high-density lipoprotein ("good" cholesterol)

IBS   irritable bowel syndrome

LDL   low-density lipoprotein ("bad" cholesterol)

LLQ   left lower quadrant

LUQ   left upper quadrant

N and V   nausea and vomiting

NG   nasogastric (e.g., tube)

NPO   nothing by mouth (no ice chips, water, food, etc.)

PKU   phenylketonuria

RLQ   right lower quadrant

RUQ   right upper quadrant

WNL   within normal limits

Worksheet

Fill in the blank:

1. Another name for the GI system is ___*digestive*___. The name of the cavity in which the GI viscera are contained is _____ or _____

2. Name an organ in the RUQ: _____ RLQ: _____

3. The six accessory GI organs that aid in the digestive process are _____

   _____

   _____

4. Name three sections of the small intestine, in order: _____

   _____

5. The tube from the pharynx through which food passes to the stomach is the _____ Food passage is assisted by muscular contraction called _____

6. Name all of the sections of the large intestine, in order: _____

   _____

   _____

7. The _____ is the opening to the outside of the body for solid wastes.

8. _____ and _____ and are other words for bowel movement.

9. Three X-ray procedures used in GI disorders are _____

   _____. Name three other procedures (not X-ray)

   _____

10. Where is bile produced? _____ Stored? _____

    What does it do? _____

    Name the three ducts connected to the gallbladder: _____

    _____

11. Give the root word for common bile duct: _____

    gallbladder: _____

    Name the procedure of X-raying common bile duct _____

    _____

Define:

12. enema _____

_____

13. villi _____

14. sphincter muscle _____

15. proctoscope _____

16. The three main food groups are _____

How many calories do each of these contain (per gram)? _____

17. Of these, which is important for growth and repair of tissue? _____

18. Draw and label the nine regions of the abdomen.

19. The mesentery is actually a part of the _____ membrane. The omenta are

attached to the stomach—to the _____ and _____ curvatures.

20. Gavage _____

21. Lavage _____

22. stomatitis _____

23. glossitis _____

24. cholecystectomy _____

25. colostomy _____

26. hepatitis _____

27. cholelithiasis _____

28. anorexia _____

Complete these sentences:

29. Nutrients are largely absorbed in the ___*small*___ intestine, which is lined with projections

    called _____ that increase the surface area.

30. Three surgical procedures on the GI tract not mentioned in the worksheet: _____

    _____

31. Name three diseases of this system, not already mentioned: _____

    _____

32. Define:

    cheiloplasty _____

    bulimia _____

    pyloroplasty _____

33. Identify:

    GBS _____

    NPO _____

    NG tube _____

    WNL _____

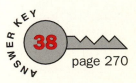

ANSWER KEY **38** page 270

Test p. 335
Alternate Test p. 337

■ Case Histories ■

CASE HISTORY 8

ADMISSION NOTE: Diverticulitis
Miller, John
Joseph Kantor, MD
Admitted: 7-10-96

Present Illness This is the third hospital admission of this 69-year old man with a past medical history of *essential hypertension, ischemic* heart disease with *angina, osteoarthritis* of the *lumbar* spine, and known *diverticulosis* with irritability of the *descending* and *sigmoid colon.* He was seen in my office with approximately a 4-day history of lower abdominal crampy pain, two or three bowel movements daily, which were soft in nature, *anorexia,* and some *dysuria.* He had noted an episode of *hematospermia* in June, which has continued until the present time. He denied, however, having mucus in the bowel movements. There were no complaints of *nausea,* temperature elevation, or food intolerances. Because of the amount of pain it was felt that hospitalization for investigation and treatment was warranted.

History Has been well reviewed in patient's old chart of 1994. It should be noted that recently the patient has been treated by J. Russell, MD, for his ischemic heart disease and hypertension.

Review of Systems See old chart.

Personal and Social History Patient's current medications include Apresoline, 25 mg *tid*; Inderal, 20 mg *tid ac,* plus hs; Esidrix, 50 mg *bid*; and Nitrostat, 0.4 mg *prn.* He states that in spite of his medications his B/P on his most recent visits to Dr. Russell has been running in the area of 200/100.

Physical Examination At the time of admission reveals a fellow of his stated age with a stoic appearance and complaints of lower abdominal pain. Temperature 98.6, pulse 72, respirations 18, B/P 184/88.

   skin Warm and dry with no evidence of rashes or eruptions.

   HEENT No evidence of recent cranial trauma. *Tympanic membranes* are grossly intact. *Conjunctivae* clear. Extraocular movements grossly intact. *Fundi* unremarkable. Nose and throat unremarkable. No notable lymph nodes in the usual areas. Thyroid does not appear to be enlarged.

   thorax There are equal and full respiratory excursions bilaterally. No spinal or *cva* tenderness noted.

   lungs All lung fields are clear to *A & P.*

   heart Regular sinus rhythm with no murmurs or rubs. No apparent *cardiomegaly.*

   abdomen No abdominal *organomegaly* or abdominal masses noted. Bowel sounds are normally active. Patient exhibits some right lower quadrant, suprapubic, and left lower quadrant *guarding* with no masses felt, along with moderate tenderness in these areas. No *rebound tenderness* referred to these areas, however.

   rectal Patient expresses a moderate amount of tenderness on rectal exam; prostate moderately enlarged, soft, tender and nonnodular.

   genitals *WNL.*

   neurologic WNL.

   impression Abdominal pain, probably secondary to *diverticulitis.*

CASE HISTORY 9

RADIOLOGY REPORT: Barium enema

Procedure Barium enema. There has been a history of surgical intervention in the large bowel. On the filled film there are *diverticula* present in the distal descending and sigmoid regions, as well as in the ascending colon. There is overlapping of bowel in the transverse colon, and whether this represents redundancy or a side-to-side *anastomosis* could not be determined either fluoroscopically or radiographically. On the evacuation film there is noted *contrast media* extending outside the bowel wall in the region of the sigmoid diverticula, and the possibility that these represent abscesses resulting from diverticulitis must be considered. The terminal *ileum* is visualized. No filling defects are seen.

CASE HISTORY 10

REPORT OF OPERATION: Cholecystectomy

Procedure Cholecystectomy. Under spinal anesthesia the patient was prepared and draped in the supine position. A right *subcostal* Kocher incision was made. The skin was incised and the incision carried down through the anterior rectus sheath, rectus muscle, posterior sheath, and *peritoneum*. Bleeders were clamped and ligated with 000 chromic suture.

The gallbladder was found to be markedly *edematous,* thickened, and *hyperemic*. It measured approximately 15 cm in length and 4 cm in diameter. There were numerous *adhesions* around the gallbladder, which were *lysed* by blunt dissection.

Exploration of the abdominal contents was normal. The finger could be inserted into the *foramen* of Winslow. The common duct was free of stones.

The gallbladder was removed using clamps to grasp the *fundus* and Hartmann's pouch. The cystic duct was then clamped, divided, and doubly ligated with 000 cotton. The cystic artery was likewise clamped, divided, and ligated with 00 cotton and the gallbladder removed. The gallbladder bed was oversewn with continuous locking 00 chromic. A medium-sized Penrose drain was placed into the foramen of Winslow and brought out through a separate stab wound in the abdomen. The peritoneum was closed using chromic. The fascia was closed in layers with cotton, the skin with Dermalon.

■ **Assignment:** Now that you have read these reports, define the italicized words.

Health Promotion Tip

To facilitate optimal weight and health, be nutrition conscious:

- Read labels on all foods to avoid heavy fat content and unnecessary preservatives.
- Eat limited portions with maximum nutrient content.
- Beware of "fat fear." Also beware of exhaustive exercise, eating for stress relief, rapid, *secret* junk food ingestion, food as a means to cope with life, or a distorted body image. These may signal eating disorders, which should not be ignored, denied, or kept as a secret. If any signal appears, seek professional counsel.

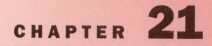

Urinary System

Anatomy and Physiology of the Urinary System

Function

The urinary system filters the blood. Urine is formed by the nephrons.

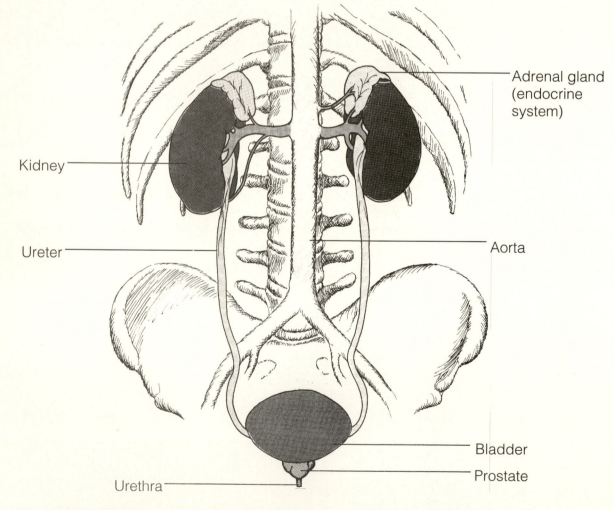

Figure 21.1 Normal urinary tract showing kidneys, ureters, bladder, and urethra, as well as their positions in relation to bony structures. The prostate gland is part of the male reproductive system but produces symptoms in the urinary system.

Urinary Organs

(See Figure 21.1).

kidneys (kĭd-nēz) two, lie behind the abdominal organs against muscles of the back (retroperitoneal) and are held in place by fat. The parts of the kidney include the following:

cortex (kŏr-tĕks) outer layer.

medulla (mĕ-dŭl-lă) inner portion.

nephrons (nĕf-rŏns) kidney cells and capillaries. The *glomerulus, Bowman's capsule,* and *renal collecting tubule* are all parts of the nephrons. The nephrons are the par **en** chyma (functioning parts) of the kidney.

renal pelvis (rē-năl **pĕl**-vĭs) the wide, upper end of the ureter (lies inside kidney).

ureters (ū-rĕ-tĕrs) two narrow tubes lined with mucous membrane. Urine passes from the kidneys through the renal pelvis and is moved through the ureters by peri **stal** sis.

urethra (ū-rē-thră) in female, one narrow short tube from bladder to exterior; in male, narrow long tube, carries urine and seminal fluid to exterior.

urinary bladder (blăd-dĕr) lined with mucous membrane; urine collects here, and bladder expands to hold urine.

urinary meatus (mē-ā-tŭs) opening of the urethra to exterior.

Pathophysiology of the Urinary System

Urinary Diseases and Disorders

calculus (renal) (kăl-kū-lŭs) kidney stones; cause blockage with severe, colicky pain.

cystitis (sĭs-tī-tĭs) inflammation of bladder; if not treated, will travel upward through ureters.

cystocele (sĭs-tō-sēl) hernia of the bladder.

"floating kidney" displaced and movable; **neph** ropexy may be done.

glomerulonephritis (glō-mĕr-ū-lō-nĕ-frī-tĭs) a form of nephritis involving glomeruli.

hydronephrosis (hī-drō-nĕ-frō-sĭs) collection of urine in pelvis of kidney due to obstructed outflow.

nephrolithiasis (nĕf-rō-lĭ-thī-ă-sĭs) see *calculus* (lith = stone); treatment is nephrolith **ot** omy.

nephroptosis (nĕf-rōp-tō-sĭs) prolapse or downward displacement of kidney; treatment is nephropexy.

pyelitis (pī-ĕ-lī-tĭs) inflammation of renal pelvis.

renal failure (rē-năl **fāyl**-ŭr) due to trauma or any condition that impairs flow of blood to the kidneys; also caused by some toxic substances.

uremia (azotemia) (ū-rē-mē-ă, ăz-ō-tē**-mē-ă) toxic condition (urine products in the blood); nitrogenous wastes not being excreted.

urethritis (ūr-ĕ-thrī-tĭs) inflammation of urethra (nonspecific or gonococcal); often spread through sexual contact.

Wilms' tumor (vĭlms tū-mŏr) nephroblas **to** ma, malignant tumor in children (ages 1–5); treated by surgery, radiation, and chemotherapy.

Surgical, Diagnostic, and Treatment Terms

albuminuria (ăl-bū-mĭ-nū-rē-ă) albumin (protein) in urine; abnormal.

anuria (ăn-ū-rē-ă) no urinary output.

bladder distention (blăd-dĕr dĭs-tĕn**-shŭn) full bladder; patient unable to void.

blood chemistries laboratory tests (see Chapter 13 section); especially BUN (blood urea nitrogen).

catheterization (kăth-ĕ-tĕr-ĭ-**zā**-shŭn)   emptying bladder with a catheter (tube); may be done to obtain a specimen, to relieve bladder distention, or to measure "residual" urine after patient has voided. Foley (retention) and French catheters are commonly used (see Figure 21.2).

Clinitest (also **Testape**) (**klĭn**-ĭ-tĕst)   convenient, inexpensive method of testing urine for glucose, acetone, albumin, and so on (tablet or specially treated paper are dipped into urine, and color changes occur; ranges are 1+ to 4+).

continent (**kŏn**-tĭn-ĕnt)   capable of controlling voiding and defecation.

cystogram (**sĭs**-tō-grăm)   the procedure of X-ray of bladder.

cystoscopy (sĭs-**tŏs**-kō-pē)   using a **cyst** oscope to examine the bladder.

dialysis (dī-**ăl**-ĭ-sĭs)   filtering blood with artificial kidney.

diuresis (dī-ū-**rē**-sĭs)   increased urinary output, due to medication with a diuretic drug.

dysuria (dĭs-**ū**-rē-ă)   difficult or painful urination.

enuresis (ĕn-ū-**rē**-sĭs)   bedwetting; not waking up to void.

extracorporeal shockwave lithotripsy (ĕks-tră-kŏr-**pŏr**-ē-ăl **shŏk**-wāv **lĭth**-ō-trĭp-sē)   patient partially submerged in a tub; lithotriptor (laser device) produces shock waves to pulverize stones.

frequency and urgency   frequent, urgent trips to bathroom, but voiding small amounts (painfully); symptoms occur with cystitis.

hematuria (hē-mă-**tū**-rē-ă)   blood in the urine (gross or microscopic); should always be investigated.

incontinent (ĭn-**kŏn**-tĭn-ĕnt)   general inability to control urination (and bowels); "stress" incontinence with coughing, sneezing, laughing.

lithotriptor (**lĭth**-ō-trĭp-tŏr)   see *extracorporeal shockwave lithotripsy*.

micturate (**mĭk**-tū-rāt)   urinate, void.

nephrorrhaphy (nĕf-**rŏr**-ră-fē)   surgical repair of kidney.

nocturia, nycturia (nŏk-**tū**-rē-ă, nĭk-**tū**-rē-ă)   getting up during the night to void.

oliguria (ŏl-ĭg-**ū**-rē-ă)   scanty output of urine.

percutaneous nephrolithotomy (pĕr-kū-**tā**-nē-ŭs nĕf-rō-lĭth-**ŏt**-ō-mē)   incision into kidney for removal of kidney stone.

pyuria (pī-**ū**-rē-ă)   pus in the urine.

renal transplant   transplanting donor kidney to recipient.

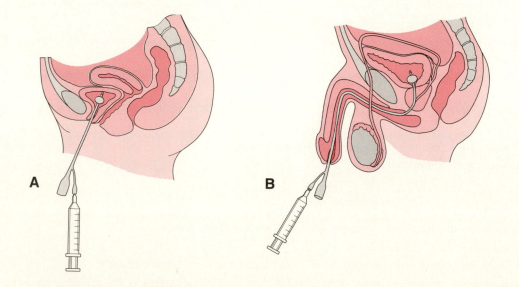

Figure 21.2   Foley catheter with balloon inflated, inserted into the bladder. (From Kozier, B., Erb, G., et al., 1995. *Fundamentals of Nursing,* ed. 5. Redwood City, CA: Addison-Wesley Nursing)

retrograde pyelogram (rĕt-rō-grād pī-ĕ-lō-grăm)   introduction of dye from below, through urethra, for X-ray examination of renal pelvis.

scan (renal)   "picture" of kidney after radioactive substance has been given intravenously; determines function and shape of kidney (renal = kidney).

ultrasonography (ŭl-tră-sŏn-ŏg-ră-fē)   using high-frequency sound waves directed into the body and reflected back onto a screen or diagrammed on paper to show organs.

ureterostomy (ūr-ē-tĕr-ŏs-tō-mē)   new opening for drainage of a ureter.

urinary retention (ūr-ĭ-nār-ē rē-tĕn-shŭn)   inability to void; many causes, including loss of muscle tone of bladder from anemia, old age, prolonged operation, psychogenic factors, medication with narcotics, and anesthetics.

vesico (vĕs-ĭ-kō)   combining form meaning *bladder*; for example, vesicovaginal = pertaining to the bladder and vagina.

void (vŏyd)   to empty (bladder).

Specialists

Male patients with urinary problems usually are treated by a urologist; female patients are often treated by gynecologists. *Nephrologist* is another term for urologist and is often combined with internal medicine (internist). Oncologists treats patients with urinary tract malignancies.

Treatment

Urinary tract infections are treated with medications. Dialysis is a treatment available to all regardless of ability to pay. Surgery and various methods of destroying stones are also used frequently. Kidney transplant is one of the most successful transplant surgeries. (One kidney is all that is needed for survival.)

Abbreviations

BUN   blood urea nitrogen, a blood chemistry test for determining kidney disorders.

ESRD   end-stage renal disease.

I & O   intake and output record of all liquids (IV or PO) taken in and voided, vomited, drained, or expressed over a 24-hour period or longer (see Figure 21.3).

Date: 7/15/99   **Intake** and **Output Chart**

	I	O
	30 cc water	10 cc emesis
	200 cc IV	50 cc urine
	5 cc soup	28 cc urine
	75 cc Coke	3 cc urine
24-hour total =	310 cc (I)	91 cc (H)

Figure 21.3 Twenty-four-hour intake and output chart (output may also include weight of chest tube dressing, infant's diaper, nasogastric drainage, loose stool, etc.).

IVP intravenous pyelogram; an IV dye is introduced for an X-ray of the renal pelvis.

KUB kidneys, ureters, bladder; usually refers to X-ray of them.

NSU nonspecific urethritis.

TUR(P) transurethral resection of the prostate; inserting device through urethra to prostate to remove prostatic tissue squeezing urethra.

U/A, Ua, or UA urinalysis; routine analysis of urine that generally includes pH, albumin, glucose, specific gravity (weight compared to water), and microscopic exam.

U/C, Uc, or UC urine culture; clean midstream urine sample is collected, swabbed onto a culture plate, incubated, and microscopically examined to identify suspected bacteria.

UTI urinary tract infection.

Worksheet

Fill in the blank:

1. Name four organs of the urinary system ___kidneys, ureters, bladder, urethra___

   _____

2. _Incontinent_ means _____

3. A catheter is used to _____

   or to _____

4. Inflammation of the renal pelvis is called _____

5. Renopathy means _____

6. Four terms for abnormal urination _____

   _____

7. UA means _____. Three tests done in routine UA:

   _____

8. Kidney cells are called _____

9. KUB stands for _____

Define:

10. void _____

11. diuretic _____

12. dialysis _____

   _____

13. uremia _____

_____

14. frequency and urgency _____

15. retrograde pyelogram _____

_____

Give a word for:

16. blood in the urine <u>hematuria</u> _____

17. no urinary output _____

18. bedwetting _____

19. surgical repair of the kidney _____

20. hernia of the bladder _____

Roots: Use the root word for these to write a complete word:

21. kidney <u>nephrolithiasis, nephrosis</u> _____

22. renal pelvis _____

23. ureter _____

Give the meaning of:

24. Foley catheter _____

_____

25. UTI _____

26. meatus _____

27. cystoscopy _____

28. pyelopathy _____

29. IVP _____

_____

30. pyuria _____

31. cystogram _____

32. lithotripsy _____

33. extracorporeal _____

34. Diagram KUB

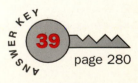

ANSWER KEY **39** page 280

Test p. 339
Alternate Test p. 341

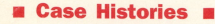

■ Case Histories ■

CASE HISTORY 11

RADIOLOGY REPORT: Intravenous pyelogram

Procedure Intravenous pyelogram. Examination of the KUB region shows the kidney and psoas muscle shadows to be normal. Serial study after IV administration of contrast medium shows a good nephrogram bilaterally. Prompt excretion of the dye is seen. A normal pelvis and ureters are seen bilaterally. The contour of the bladder is normal. Postvoiding film shows poor emptying of the bladder.

CASE HISTORY 12

DISCHARGE SUMMARY: Transitional cell carcinoma of the bladder

Discharge Summary This 70-year old married white male entered the hospital with marked lower urinary tract irritative symptoms. Nonfunction of the right kidney was found. A large bladder tumor involving the right side of the bladder was noted, and this was treated with open electroresection. The lesion was definitely stuck on the right side and on histologic examination proved to be grade IV transitional cell carcinoma. Shortly thereafter cobalt therapy was begun on an outpatient basis in this hospital.

Two days prior to admission the patient felt weak and fell down several times the day prior to admission. On the day of admission he had another episode of transient loss of consciousness. After the episodes he felt perfectly well. He was not incontinent and had no convulsive movements or tongue biting (according to the history). The patient had lost 15 pounds with the present illness.

Physical examination on admission revealed a chronically ill appearing man in no acute distress. Heart and lungs were normal. No abdominal masses were palpable. Rectal examination revealed a slightly enlarged prostate. An ill-defined mass was palpable above the prostate on the right. This mass appeared fixed.

Laboratory work: Hgb 9.1, and subsequently 8.2. Hct 30% and subsequently 27%. WBC 10,500 and 13,000. The red cells were described as normochromic and normocytic by the pathologist. Urine contained 15–20 red cells and was loaded with white cells. FBS was 98, 2 hr pp glucose was 138. BUN was 40 and creatinine 2.1. Blood type O positive.

Course in hospital: The patient continued to be unsteady and had difficulty walking and even fell down once. He experienced some diarrhea and nausea, which were controlled with Lomotil and Torecan. Irritative urinary symptoms were present but not troublesome. The patient was continued on Azo Gantanol, which he had taken prior to admission.

Radiotherapy was continued, and two units of whole blood were given. After this the patient did feel stronger and was much steadier on his feet. His Hgb was raised to 10.2 and Hct to 33% with this maneuver. On the twelfth day the radiologist decided to interrupt radiotherapy for a period of a few weeks because of radiation burns to the skin.

The patient was accordingly discharged on that day, to be followed by his urologist and to continue radiotherapy at a later date. Discharge medication included Azo Gantanol and pain medication the patient had at home.

Final diagnosis: Transitional cell carcinoma of the bladder, grade IV, with nonfunctioning right kidney.

■ **Assignment:** Read the cases aloud, then write and define all new or unfamiliar terms.

✔ Check Your Progress

You have now completed the first half of Part II. At this point you have learned a good deal about body systems and the terminology used to describe the components of these systems.

You may now be given a **review test** for Chapters 15–21, which can be found on page 343 in Appendix F. In this section, the beginning of Part 2, you have learned how to construct words that describe the anatomy, physiology, and pathology of the integumentary system, the musculoskeletal system, the cardiovascular system, the respiratory system, the gastrointestinal system, and the urinary system.

You will now move on to the last section of Part 2. This final section of the *Medical Terminology* text contains more body system terminology. Keep reviewing the completed Part 1 and Part 2 chapters so that you do not forget what you have learned.

▲ Health Promotion Tip

Awareness of possible symptoms of cystitis can assist in early detection and treatment. Symptoms include:

- dysuria (painful, burning sensation upon voiding)

- pyuria (pus, often visible in cloudy urine)

- hematuria (blood in urine, gross or microscopic)

- frequency and urgency

- enuresis (possible)

- incontinence

- oliguria

- lower abdominal discomfort

- fever (100° F or greater)

Tips to prevent urinary tract infections:

- Drink plenty of water and juice containing cranberry.

- Use good hygiene and proper wiping techniques after voiding (especially for females).

- Follow medical orders for sexual partner to obtain treatment if urethritis occurs; some cases result from sexual intercourse and recur if partner is not treated.

CHAPTER 22

Female Reproductive System, Neonatology, and Genetics

Anatomy and Physiology of the Female Reproductive System

Function

The female reproductive system functions to produce offspring by forming ova and, when an ovum is fertilized, by providing protection and nurture for the embryo until birth.

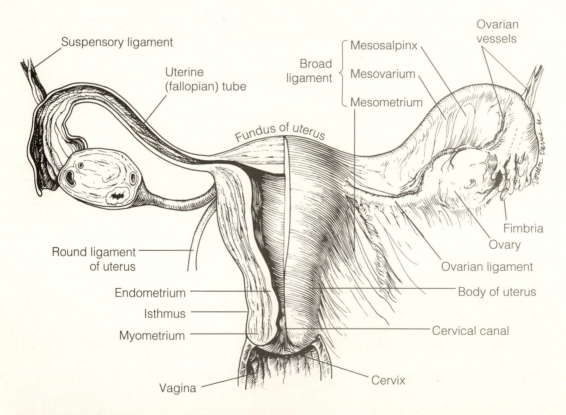

Figure 22.1 Structures of the female reproductive system as seen from behind. The posterior walls of the vagina, the left side of the uterus, the left uterine tube, and the entire left broad ligament have been removed. (From Spence, A. P., and Mason, E. B., 1987. *Human Anatomy and Physiology*, ed. 3. Menlo Park, CA: Benjamin/Cummings Publishing Co., p. 825.)

Female Reproductive (Genital) Organs

See Figure 22.1.

ovaries (ō-vă-rēz)   sex glands, located in pelvis. They form *ova* (ovum)—sex cells. In *ovu la tion*—ovum leaves ovary. The follicle that released the ovum secretes hormones: **es** *trogens* and *pro* **ges** *terones*.

ducts   fallopian tube, where fertilization occurs; fringe-like distal parts called *fimbriae*.

uterus (ū-tĕr-ŭs)   top part called the *fundus*; the neck (*cervix*) opens into the vagina.

vagina (vă-jī-nă)   birth canal; the *vaginal in* **tro** *itus* is the entrance to the vagina.

Bartholin's glands (băr-tō-lĭnz)   accessory mucous glands.

external genitals (jĕn-ĭ-tăls)   organs of generation; *vulva* or *pu* **den** *dum* (labia ma **jor** a and mi **nor** a).

breasts (brĕsts)   lactation controlled by hormones.

Pathophysiology of the Female Reproductive System

Female Reproductive Diseases and Disorders

abortion (ă-**bōr**-shŭn)   interruption of pregnancy before fetus is viable (able to live); may be spontaneous (as in miscarriage); see medical dictionary for other terms.

Bartholin's cyst or abscess (băr-tō-lĭnz)   inflammation of Bartholin's gland (chronic or acute).

Candida, **candidiasis** (**kăn**-dĭ-dă, kăn-dĭ-**dī**-ă-sĭs)   yeastlike fungus infection of vagina or other parts of body. Same as *Monilia*.

carcinoma (kăr-sĭ-**nō**-mă)   cancerous growth; may occur in any part of the uterus, ovaries; especially carcinoma in situ of cervix. Also breast cancer, with or without involvement of nearby lymph nodes.

cervical dysplasia (**sĕr**-vĭ-kăl dĭs-**plā**-zē-ă)   abnormal cell growth in cervix.

endometriosis (ĕn-dō-mē-trē-**ō**-sĭs)   cells of the inner lining of uterus spreading into pelvis (peritoneal cavity).

fibrocystic disease (fī-brō-**sĭs**-tĭk)   of the breasts; fibroadenoma: benign cysts in breasts.

fibroids (**fī**-brŏyds)   benign tumors of uterus.

fistula (**fĭs**-tū-lă)   an abnormal passageway, such as a vesicovaginal (between bladder and vagina) or vesicouterine (between bladder and uterus) fistula.

hydrosalpinx (hī-drō-**săl**-pĭnks)   fluid collection in fallopian tubes, causing distention.

leukorrhea (lū-kō-**rē**-ă)   white vaginal discharge.

miscarriage (mĭs-**kār**-ĭj)   see *abortion*.

Monilia, **moniliasis** (mō-**nĭl**-ē-ă, mō-nĭ-**lī**-ă-sĭs)   yeastlike fungus infection of vaginal or other parts of body). Same as *Candida*.

prolapse of uterus (prō-**lăps**)   or proci **den** tia; uterus dropping down into vagina.

salpingitis (săl-pĭn-**jī**-tĭs)   inflammation of fallopian tube; may cause sterility owing to adhesion formation.

Trichomonas, **trichomoniasis** (trĭk-ō-**mō**-năs, trĭk-ō-mō-**nī**-ă-sĭs)   parasite-caused vaginitis, with severe itching and foul discharge.

TSS   toxic shock syndrome; toxic symptoms produced by "blood poisoning" due to staphylococcus toxin. Symptoms: fever, rash, vomiting, diarrhea, hypotension, shock. Associated with super-absorbent tampons and individual susceptibility to "staph" (staphylococcal) infection.

Surgical, Diagnostic, and Treatment Terms

biopsy (bī-ŏp-sē)   of the cervix (cervical biopsy).

colporrhaphy (kŏl-**pŏr**-răf-ē)   surgical repair of vagina; also called A & P repair (anteroposterior); to correct cystocele, rectocele.

colposcopy (kŏl-**pŏs**-kō-pē)   procedure of using **col** poscope for magnified view of the cervix.

electrosurgical loop incision of the cervical transformational zone (ELECTZ)   a procedure to treat cervical dysplasia by shaving tissue away from the cervix.

hysterectomy (hĭs-tĕ-**rĕk**-tō-mē)   excision of uterus; HSO is hysterosalpingo-oophorectomy, excision of all reproductive organs (also called a panhysterectomy).

hysterosalpinogram (hĭs-tĕr-ŏ-săl-**pĭng**-gō-grăm)   "picture" of uterus and tubes to determine whether tubes are patent (open; **pā**-tĕnt); dye or air may be used.

laparoscope (**lăp**-ă-rō-skōp)   endoscope inserted through small abdominal incision to view and work on abdominopelvic (including reproductive) organs.

laparoscopic sterilization (lăp-ă-rō-**skŏp**-ĭk stĕr-ĭl-ĭ-**zā**-shŭn)   "Band-Aid surgery"; patency of tube is destroyed, as in tubal ligation.

mammogram, mammography (**măm**-ō-grăm, măm-**ŏg**-ră-fē)   X-ray of breasts to detect early cancer.

Marshall Marchetti (**măr**-shăl măr-**kĕt**-ē)   surgical repair of cystocele (for stress incontinence).

oophorectomy (ō-ŏf-ō-**rĕk**-tō-mē)   excision of ovary; removal of both is female castration.

pelvic exam (**pĕl**-vĭk)   using **spec** ulum to dilate vagina for inspection of cervix and to take sloughed-off cells for *Pap* (Papanicolaou) smear to detect early carcinoma.

salpingectomy (săl-pĭn-**jĕk**-tō-mē)   excision of fallopian tube; performed for ectopic pregnancy in tube.

tubal ligation (**tū**-băl lī-**gā**-shŭn)   "tying" fallopian tubes; sterilization.

tubal occlusion (**tū**-băl ŏk-**klū**-zhŭn)   with silicone; considered to be reversible.

vaginal speculum (**văj**-ĭn-ăl **spĕk**-ū-lŭm)   see *pelvic exam;* a dilating instrument.

Obstetrics, Neonatology, and Genetics

anesthesia (for OB) (ăn-ĕs-**thē**-zē-ă)   regional types (spinal, saddle, caudal); general anesthesia; local, pudendal block.

Apgar (**ăp**-găr) *10 points maximum;*   numerical expression of the condition of newborn infant; taken at 1 and 5 minutes following birth, maximum 2 points for each: appearance (color), pulse (rate), grimace (response to slap), activity (movement), respirations (breathing, crying, not breathing); for example, Apgar 4-9 (1 and 5 minutes).

bloody show (**blood**-ē shō)   bloody mucous plug usually passed during late labor.

(caesarean) cesarean (C section) (sē-**sār**-ē-ăn)   delivery by an incision into abdomen and uterus.

circumcision (sĭr-kŭm-**sĭ**-zhŭn)   cutting foreskin of newborn male; originally a Jewish rite but became universally done in the U.S.; now done less often.

Coombs' test (kōms)   blood test used to diagnose hemolytic anemias in newborn.

dystocia (dĭs-**tō**-shă)   difficult labor.

ectopic (extrauterine) (ĕk-**tŏp**-ĭk)   pregnancy outside of the uterus, usually the tube.

embryo (**ĕm**-brē-ō)   term used from 3rd to 8th week after fertilization.

episiotomy (ĕ-pĭs-ē-**ŏt**-ō-mē)   incision of perineum to facilitate delivery and avoid laceration (episi/o = vulva).

fertility (fĕr-**tĭl**-ĭ-tē)   ability to conceive.

fertilization (fĕr-tĭl-ĭ-**zā**-shŭn)   the fusion of two opposite-sex gametes to produce zygote (via insemination or intercourse).

fetus (**fē**-tŭs)   term used starting 9th week after fertilization.

forceps delivery (**fŏr**-sĕps)   low-forceps delivery is fairly routine and provides more control; mid- and high-forceps are complicated deliveries.

gestation (jĕs-**tā**-shŭn)   period of pregnancy (conception to birth or last menstrual period until birth); approximately 280 days.

gravida (**grăv**-ĭ-dă)   pregnant woman (gravid = pregnant).

induction (ĭn-**dŭk**-shŭn)   starting labor by artificial means; using medication or rupturing membranes to start contractions.

insemination (ĭn-sĕm-ĭn-**ā**-shŭn)   impregnating with sperm from mate or donor.

IVF (ĭn-**vē**-trō)   in vitro fertilization, procedure in which ovum is taken from ovary and subjected to sperm in a Petri dish; when conception takes place, ovum is implanted in uterus. (Thus, "test-tube baby" is a misnomer.)

lochia (**lō**-kē-ă)   vaginal discharge following delivery.

meconium (mĕ-**kō**-nē-ŭm)   first bowel movement passed by newborn; a black, tarry substance.

multipara (mŭl-**tĭp**-ă-ră)   woman who has borne more than one term infant.

neonatal period (nē-ō-**nā**-tăl **pēr**-ē-ŏd)   first 4 weeks of life.

OB index   Grav, Para, AB, SB (number of pregnancies, term deliveries, abortions, stillborn).

pelvimeter, pelvimetry (pĕl-**vĭm**-ĕ-tĕr, pĕl-**vĭm**-ĕ-trē)   instrument to estimate pelvic diameter for delivery (CPD = cephalopelvic disproportion); X-ray pelvimetry and ultrasound are also done.

placenta (plă-**sĕn**-tă)   the afterbirth; placenta **pre** via and ab **rup** tio placentae are complications of pregnancy (placenta lying low and "coming first" and premature separation of placenta).

postpartum (pŏst-**păr**-tŭm)   six-week period following childbirth.

prenatal (prē-**nā**-tăl)   before birth; important time for care of pregnant woman, for her and the infant.

presentation (prĕ-zĕn-**tā**-shŭn)   position infant is in for delivery: *vertex* is head first (LOA, ROA, left or right occiput anterior; LOP, ROP, left or right occiput posterior); *breech* is usually buttocks first but may be footling also.

primipara (prī-**mĭp**-ă-ră)   woman who is bearing her first child.

sonogram (**sŏn**-ō-grăm) (or ultrasound)   a record of ultrasonic echoes as they locate tissues of varying densities (see Figure 22.2).

sterility (stĕr-**ĭl**-ĭ-tē)   inability to conceive.

stillborn (sb) (**stĭl**-bŏrn)   fetus dead at birth.

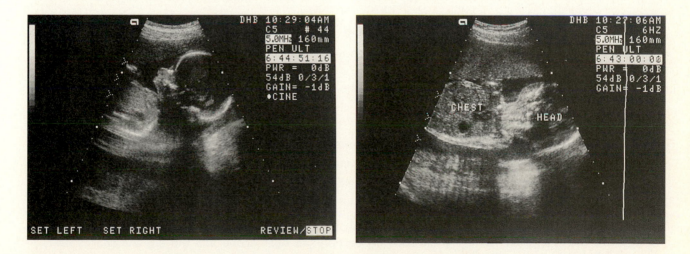

Figure 22.2   Two sonograms of a fetus. (Adapted from Olds, S.B., London, M.L., et al., 1996. *Maternal-Newborn Nursing,* ed. 5. Menlo Park, CA: Addison-Wesley Nursing.)

"test-tube baby"   see *in vitro fertilization*.

toxemia (tŏk-**sē**-mē-ă)   of pregnancy (also called pre-eclampsia [prē-ē-**klămp**-sē-ă]); characterized by hypertension, edema, sudden weight gain; a serious complication that may be fatal to mother and child if not treated (called *eclampsia* only if seizure occurs).

trimester (**trī**-měs-těr)   three-month periods in pregnancy; first trimester is the period when virus infections such as rubella can produce fetal anomalies.

vernix caseosa (**věr**-nĭks kā-sē-**ō**-să)   cheesy white substance on the skin of newborn.

Miscellaneous Terms

alpha-fetoprotein (**ăl**-fă-fē-tŏ-**prō**-tēn)   a blood screening test done at 15–20 weeks of pregnancy to measure the amount of AFP transversing from fetal circulation into the maternal bloodstream (a low AFP correlates with an increased risk of Down syndrome and trisomy; a high AFP correlates with anencephaly, open spinal bifida, and some ventral wall defects).

amniocentesis (ăm-nē-ō-sĕn-**tē**-sĭs)   obtaining a sample of amniotic fluid by abdominal needle extraction into a syringe of cells sloughed off by the fetus into the amniotic fluid. These cells are then cultured and grown for about three weeks to increase the number of cells for subsequent chromosomal and biomedical analyses to rule out genetic defects.

chorionic villus sampling (CVS) (kō-rē-**ŏn**-ĭk **vĭl**-ŭs)   collecting chorionic cells that surround the human embryo via a catheter through the vagina to the uterus. Because chorionic cells are the same genotype (type of gene) as the embryo and this procedure may be performed at 8 or 9 weeks of pregnancy, CVS is sometimes recommended instead of amniocentesis, done at 16 weeks, especially with high-risk pregnancies.

chromosome (**krō**-mō-sōm)   a linkage structure of specific genetic information.

chromosome engineering   the incorporation of parts of or whole alien chromosomes into a given set of chromosomes.

gamete (**găm**-ēt)   one of two cells (male and female) whose union is needed for sexual reproduction.

genetic counseling (jĕ-**nĕt**-ĭk)   a service providing people with information regarding the relative risk of having a genetically abnormal progeny.

genetic engineering   DNA manipulation with in vitro techniques within or between species for deliberate gene changes for genetic analysis or improvement (e.g., gene transfer or cloning).

genetics   the science of heredity and variation of genes (human, virus, plant, or animal).

genetic therapy   addition of a functional gene or group of genes to a cell by gene insertion to correct a hereditary disease.

in vitro (ĭn **vē**-trō)   "in glass"; studies under artificially controlled conditions outside the organism.

menarche (mĕn-**ăr**-kē)   onset of menses.

menopause (**mĕn**-ō-păwz)   change of life, climacteric; cessation of menses.

menstruation (mĕn-strū-**ā**-shŭn)   the flow from the uterus when conception does not take place; approximately every 28 days, but varies somewhat.

mutation (mū-**tā**-shŭn)   any heritable alteration in the genetic material of a living cell or virus.

progeny (**prŏj**-ĕ-nē)   offspring from a given mating.

spermicide (**spĕr**-mĭ-sīd)   sperm-killing agent.

viable (**vī**-ă-bl)   capable of survival; standard for premature infants.

zygotes (**zī**-gōts)   a cell resulting from the union of male and female gametes.

Alternative Fertilization Techniques

in vitro fertilization (IVF)   the ovaries are stimulated (with medication) to produce more than one egg. The eggs are then retrieved via vaginal ultrasound direction and laparoscope, and the egg and sperm are mixed in a Petri dish, where fertilization occurs. The resulting embryos are delivered via cervical catheter to the uterus two days later.

gamete intrafallopian transfer (GIFT) (găm-ēt ĭn-tră-fă-lō-pē-ăn) used only in women with normal, unobstructed fallopian tubes. Eggs are retrieved with laparoscope and vaginal ultrasound, mixed with sperm in a catheter, and injected into the fallopian tubes, where natural fertilization occurs.

zygote intrafallopian transfer (ZIFT) (zī-gōt) like GIFT, except the eggs are fertilized by the sperm in a Petri dish. Embryos are placed in the fallopian tubes via laparoscopy one or two days thereafter.

intrauterine insemination (IUI) (ĭn-tră-ū-tĕr-ĭn ĭn-sĕm-ĭn-ā-shŭn) at ovulation, sperm is delivered via catheter through the cervix to the uterus. The man collects semen in the andrology lab several hours prior to the insemination, and the sperm is washed (to increase function).

artificial insemination with donor sperm (AID) frozen (cryopreserved) sperm from donors, screened for many hereditary and infectious diseases, injected into female reproductive tract.

intracytoplasmic sperm injection (ICSI) (ĭn-tră-sī-tō-plăz-mĭk) helps sperm enter eggs by using a microneedle to pierce each egg's outer shell, then injecting one sperm into the center of the egg. The fertilized eggs are placed in a Petri dish, and resulting embryos are inserted in the uterus two days later.

assisted hatching helps embryo hatch from its early protective membrane to increase chances of uterine implantation; membrane is pierced with a microneedle and embryo is transferred to uterus.

cryopreservation (krī-ō-prĕz-ĕr-vā-shŭn) freezing of tissue for future use. Cryopreserved embryos produced by IVF can be used later if an earlier pregnancy attempt fails.

donor egg program using eggs donated by relatives or other women undergoing IVF (who had extra eggs). Eggs are screened for congenital and communicable diseases.

donor embryo program using embryos donated by women who underwent IVF. Embryos screened for hereditary and infectious diseases.

Specialists

Obstetricians care for women during and following pregnancy and deliver the infants. As soon as the infant is born, a pediatrician or neonatologist examines it. Other specialists may be involved as needed, especially neurologists when premature infants are delivered. Many congenital defects are corrected by various surgeons. Midwives may also deliver babies and handle uncomplicated cases. Reproductive specialists perform in vitro fertilization. Gynecologists perform surgery on women (reproductive organs).

Abbreviations

AB abortion (spontaneous or therapeutic); interruption of pregnancy before fetus becomes viable (able to live).

AFP alpha-fetoprotein; pregnancy blood test.

AI artificial insemination.

ART assisted reproductive technologies.

CIN cervical intraepithelium neoplasia; Pap smear result (CIN 1: mild, CIN 2: moderate).

CVS chorionic villus sampling; to test for possible birth defects.

D & C dilation and curettage; dilating the cervix and scraping the inner surface of the uterus with a curette in order to abort the fetus, diagnose uterine disease, or after an incomplete abortion.

EDC or EDA estimated date of confinement or arrival; due date.

ELECTZ electrosurgical loop incision of the cervical transformational zone (a procedure in which tissue is shaved away from the cervix to treat cervical dysplasia).

FHT fetal heart tones heard via a fetoscope or fetal monitor.

GIFT gamete intrafallopian transfer; egg and sperm put inside fallopian tube to fertilize and move to uterus.

ICSI intracytoplasmic sperm injection; one sperm is injected into one egg, which is transferred to uterus.

IUI intrauterine insemination.

IVF   in vitro fertilization.

LMP   last menstrual period.

PDD   premenstrual dysphoric disorder; remarkable depressed mood, anxiety, affective lability, and lack of interest that has occurred most months in the past year but remits within a few days of the onset of menses, as well as the week following menses.

PID   pelvic inflammatory disease (may lead to scar tissue accumulation and subsequent sterility).

PMS   premenstrual syndrome; produces symptoms of irritability, breast tenderness, weight gain, and bloating from water retention.

TSS   toxic shock syndrome; blood poisoning due to staphylococcus toxin; correlates with use of super-absorbent tampons and susceptibility to staph infection. Symptoms are: fever, rash, vomiting, diarrhea, hypotension, and shock.

VBAC   vaginal birth after caesarean (cesarean).

ZIFT   zygote intrafallopian transfer; fertilized eggs are incubated 24 hours prior to being put into the fallopian tube.

Worksheet

Fill in the blank:

1. Female sex cell _ovum_____ ; female sex gland _____

2. "Neck" of the uterus _____ ; body (top part) of the uterus _____

3. Fertilization occurs in _____

4. The afterbirth is the _____

5. Common carcinoma in the female occurs in the _____

6. Female sterilization is called _____

7. Abdominal incision to deliver infant is _____

Spell out and explain:

8. D & C _dilation and curettage; dilating cervix and scraping uterus lining_____

9. EDC _____

10. FHT _____

11. LMP _____

12. LOA, ROA _____

_____

13. ZIFT _____

14. Para V Grav VII _____

Define:

15. Pap _____

16. trimester _____

17. ovulation _____

18. breech _____

19. Apgar _____

_____

20. mammoplasty _____

_____

Write a word that means:

21. excision of fallopian tube _____

22. excision of uterus _____

23. incision into the perineum (to facilitate delivery) _____

24. instrument for measuring pelvis _____

25. pregnancy outside of the uterus _____

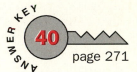

ANSWER KEY **40** page 271

Chapter 22 and 23 combined Test p. 347
Alternate Test p. 351

■ Case Histories ■

CASE HISTORY 13

REPORT OF OPERATION: Hysterectomy with salpingo-oophorectomy

Preoperative adenocarcinoma of the endometrium, post progesterone therapy.

Postoperative same, plus extensive abdominal adhesions.

Procedure Under general anesthesia, the vagina was prepped. The patient was placed in the lithotomy position and the cervix closed with a figure-of-eight suture of #1 chromic. A Foley catheter was then inserted into the bladder, the abdomen was prepped and draped in the usual manner. A midline incision was made on the skin, excising an old scar. The incision was carried vertically through the recti muscles. The recti muscles were then separated along the midline, the peritoneum opened vertically. Omental adhesions, parietal peritoneum, were encountered and were lysed by sharp and blunt dissection. The bleeding points were tied with 3-0 chromic.

Examination of the pelvis revealed an antiverted, slightly enlarged uterus for the patient's stated age of 61. There were dense adhesions between the rectal sigmoid and the left adnexa. There was surgical absence of the left tube and ovary. The adhesions were released by sharp dissection. The right ovary was atrophic and the tube normal. The right infundibulopelvic ligament was clamped, cut, and ligated with #1 chromic. The left round ligament was clamped, cut, and ligated with #1 chromic. The uretervesical reflection of peritoneum was incised transversely and the bladder reflected from the cervix. The uterine vessels, cardinal ligaments, and uterosacral ligaments were then successfully clamped, cut, and ligated with #1 chromic. The vaginal vault was opened anteriorly and the cervix excised from the vagina. Vaginal mucosa was run with continuous-locking 2-0 Dexon, and ¼-inch Penrose drain placed through the cuff.

The pelvis was peritonealized with continuous 2-0 chromic. Extensive adhesions of small bowel were lysed, freeing the small bowel completely from the ileocecal valve up to the ligament of Treitz. Palpation of the liver, gallbladder revealed no abnormalities. There were a few adhesions around the right kidney and also in the left gutter. The abdomen was irrigated with saline. One unit of Dextrane 40 and physiological saline was placed in the peritoneal cavity; 100 mg ampicillin was added to this.

The abdomen was then closed in layers, using continuous chromic 0 on the peritoneum, interrupted figure-of-eight sutures of #1 chromic in the fascia, continuous 3-0 chromic subcutaneously; the skin was approximated with clips and 4-0 Dexon retention sutures. Estimated blood loss was 400 cc. The patient tolerated the procedure well and was taken to the RR in good condition.

CASE HISTORY 14

REPORT OF OPERATION: Vaginal hysterectomy

Preoperative Diagnosis cystocele, rectocele, uterine prolapse.

Postoperative Diagnosis same.

Operation vaginal hysterectomy, anterior and posterior vaginal repair.

Procedure Under general anesthesia the patient was placed in lithotomy position, prepped and draped in the usual manner. With traction on the cervix, the cervix came easily into the introitus. An elliptical incision was made around the cervix. Bladder was reflected anteriorly, and the peritoneum was opened. The cul-de-sac was then opened. Approximately 10–20 cc of clear fluid escaped from the cul-de-sac at this point, which was compatible with pelvic congestion.

Vaginal hysterectomy was carried out. The uterine ligaments were clamped, cut, and suture-ligated with #1 chromic. The tubes and ovaries were normal, and were not removed. There was recent evidence of corpora lutea and ovulatory function bilaterally. The pelvis was then irrigated with 10% Betadine, left in for two minutes. One suture of 2-0 Ethibond was used to plicate the uterosacral ligaments. The peritoneum was closed transversely with continuous chromic 0. The sponge count was correct.

An elliptical incision was made in the anterior vaginal wall removing the redundant vaginal mucosa. The underlying pubovesicocervical fascia was plicated with interrupted chromic 0, and incision was closed with the same. The vaginal vault was closed transversely with continuous locking 2-0 chromic, the midportion left open for drainage. Posterior colporrhaphy was then carried out. An elliptical incision was made in the posterior vaginal wall, removing the redundant vaginal mucosa. The fascia was freed from the mucosa by sharp and blunt dissection. A finger was placed in the rectum to guide the sutures. Three interrupted sutures of 2-0 Ethibond were placed in the perirectal fascia to correct the cystocele. The vaginal mucosa and perivaginal fascia were then plicated in one layer with continuous-locking chromic 0. There is good vaginal depth. Hemostasis complete.

The bladder was filled with 300 cc of saline, and cystocath, 8 French, introduced suprapubically. The urine is clear. Estimated blood loss, 100 cc. No drains or packing were placed in the wound. Patient tolerated procedure well; taken to recovery in good condition.

CASE HISTORY 15

DISCHARGE SUMMARY: Premature infant

Chief Complaint This is the first Duke Hospital admission for a newly born, first of twins, infant admitted for prematurity.

Present Illness Called to delivery room for the first of twins, 1770 g white male product of a 34-week gestation of a 23-year-old, para O-O-O, A positive, STS negative, GC negative, married white female. Pregnancy was complicated by questionable leakage of membranes three days prior to delivery. It was also complicated by premature labor and premature rupture of membranes 16 hours prior to delivery. There was no meconium staining, foul smell, or maternal fever. Labor was spontaneous with an elective low-forceps delivery. Breathing and crying time were stat, with an Apgar of 8–9. Resuscitation given with bulb syringe and oxygen, and the patient was transferred to the ICN.

Physician Exam Patient is a small, but well-formed preterm white male infant in no acute distress, active and pink. Pulse 140, resp 56, B/P 42/22, temp 36.1, length 44 cm, weight 1770 g, head circ 30.6 cm.

Head: moderate molding. Ears: decreased cartilage. Breast tissue 2–3 mm in diameter. Abdomen: liver down 1.5 cm. Genitals: normal uncircumcised male with testes descended bilaterally; however, right testicle was in the lower part of the canal and not quite in scrotum. The rest of the exam was completely WNL.

Accessory Laboratory Data Venous hct 44%; capillary hct 56%; Dextrostix 90–130; blood gas: pH 7.16, bicarb 21 mEq/L, PCO_2 of 60; gastric aspirate gram stain showed rare polys and no bacteria. CBC: Hgb 15.3; Hct 50%; white cell count 7900; 53 polys; 21 lymphs; 16 monos; 5 eos; 4 stabs; 1 metamyelocyte; 5.8% reticulocytes. Micro chem 12; glucose 130; BUN 9; sodium 140 mEq/L; potassium 5.1 mEq/L; chloride 100 mEq/L; CO_2 of 27 mm/L; total protein 4.4; albumin 2.9; calcium 7.6; phosphorus 5.6; total bilirubin 3.4; direct bilirubin 0.1. Urinalysis was unremarkable; blood type, A negative; direct Coombs, negative.

HOSPITAL COURSE

Impression

1. Preterm infant, 34 weeks GA first of twins.
2. Status/post intrapartum hemorrhage, with secondary hypotension, resolved.
3. Hypocalcemia.
4. Metabolic acidosis.
5. Right corneal opacity

Disposition

1. Continue 20 cal Enfamil gavage feedings 45 mL q3h.
2. Neo-Calglucon 250 mg tid po.
3. Sodium bicarbonate 1 mL tid po.
4. Return to special care clinic in one month and be seen by ophthalmology for corneal opacity.

■ **Assignment:** Read the preceding three cases aloud, then write and define all new or unfamiliar terms.

▲ **Health Promotion Tip**

To promote a healthy pregnancy:
- Seek early prenatal care.
- Be completely honest in giving the doctor your history.
- Avoid contact with any environmental contagion or chemical agent.
- Avoid cigarette smoke and ingestion of drugs or alcohol.
- Maintain a healthy diet and regular exercise, if obstetrician recommends continued exercise.
- Wear appropriate car seat belt.

CHAPTER 23

Male Reproductive System and Sexually Transmitted Diseases

Anatomy and Physiology of the Male Reproductive System

Function

The male reproductive system functions to produce offspring by making sperm and delivering them to the female reproductive tract, where one sperm may fertilize an ovum.

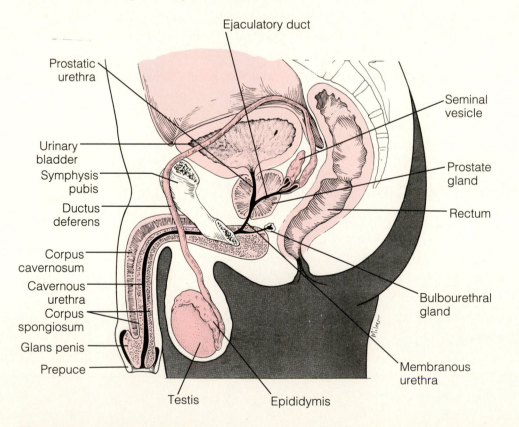

Figure 23.1 Median sagittal section of the male pelvis with a portion of the left pubic bone attached to illustrate the path of the ductus deferens. (From Spence, A. P., and Mason, E. B., 1987. *Human Anatomy and Physiology,* ed. 3. Menlo Park, CA: Benjamin/Cummings Publishing Co., p. 817.)

Male Reproductive (Genital) Organs

(See Figure 23.1.)

testes (testis) (**tĕs**-tēz, **tĕs**-tĭs)   also called *testicles*; sex glands, located in *scrotum*. They form spermatozoa (sex cells) and secrete the hormone *tes **tos** terone*.

ducts

  epididymis (ĕp-ĭ-**dĭd**-ĭ-mĭs)   at top of each testis; spermatozoa are stored in these ducts.

  vas deferens (văs **dĕf**-ĕr-ĕns)   ductus deferens; excretory duct of the testis.

  seminal duct (**sĕm**-ĭn-ăl dŭkt)   excretory duct of the seminal vesicle.

  ejaculatory duct (ē-**jăk**-ū-lă-tŏr-ē dŭkt)   canal formed by union of ductus (vas) deferens and the excretory duct of the seminal vesicle.

  urethra (ū-**rē**-thră)   opening for sperm and urine passage.

accessory glands   secrete alkaline secretions that together with sperm make up *seminal fluid*.

prostate gland (**prŏs**-tāt glănd)   surrounds urethra; secretes alkaline fluid that forms part of semen. Tends to enlarge in older men and may block flow of urine.

external genitalia (ĕks-**tĕr**-năl jĕn-ĭ-**tāl**-ē-ă)   *scrotum* and *penis*.

Pathophysiology of the Male Reproductive System

Male Reproductive System Diseases and Disorders

carcinoma (kăr-sĭ-**nō**-mă)   cancerous growth; in male genitals occurs especially in prostate.

cryptorchidism (krĭpt-**ŏr**-kĭd-ĭzm)   "hidden testes"; undescended.

epididymitis (ĕp-ĭ-dĭd-ĭ-**mī**-tĭs)   inflammation of epi **did** ymis (ducts where sperm are stored).

hydrocele (**hī**-drŏ-sēl)   hernia (of fluid) in scrotum.

orchitis (ŏr-**kī**-tĭs)   inflammation of testes; may be due to trauma, mumps, or infection elsewhere in body.

varicocele (**văr**-ĭ-kō-sēl)   varicose veins near testes; common cause of male infertility; may be corrected with surgery.

Surgical Terms

biopsy (**bī**-ŏp-sē)   can be done on prostate through cytoscope.

circumcision (sĭr-kŭm-**sĭ**-zhŭn)   cutting around head of penis, removing foreskin.

orchiectomy (ŏr-kē-**ĕk**-tō-mē)   excision of a testicle, castration.

orchiopexy (ŏr-kē-ō-**pĕk**-sē)   operative transfer of undescended testis into scrotum and suturing it there; also called **or** chidopexy, **or** chidoplasty, orchi **or** rhaphy.

prostatectomy (prŏs-tă-**tĕk**-tō-mē)   excision of prostate; may be done in several ways: transu **reth** ral, TUR(P), supra **pub** ic, peri **ne** al.

vasectomy (vă-**sĕk**-tō-mē)   male sterilization procedure.

vasovasostomy (văs-ŏ-vă-**sŏs**-tō-mē)   rejoining of vas deferens postvasectomy (vasectomy reversed).

Specialists

Urologists usually perform male reproductive organ surgery.

Sexually Transmitted Diseases (STDs)

General Information

See Table 23.1.

transmission   via sexual intercourse (vaginal, anal).

prevention   (1) use of condoms; (2) avoidance of multiple sex partners; (3) maintenance of a monogamous relationship; (4) abstinence.

multiple diseases   may be contracted at the same time.

remissions and exacerbations   occur in many.

no vaccine available

no immunity occurs   may contract STDs many times.

symptoms   may be less evident in the female. All contacts should be notified and treated if necessary.

■ **Note:** All of these sexually transmitted diseases are dangerous. Not all are as life threatening as AIDS, but if untreated, most will lead to sterility and pain and in pregnant women can cause severe fetal abnormalities.

HIV, Human Immunodeficiency Virus, and AIDS, Acquired Immune Deficiency Syndrome

History   first reported in 1981.

Those affected   no one is immune to this disease. The greatest growth rate from 1985 to 1995 was in the heterosexual population; other populations that have been greatly affected are homosexual and bisexual men, hemophiliacs, people who received blood transfusions prior to the time when antibody tests were done on donated blood, infants born to mothers with HIV, and intravenous drug users and their sex partners.

Specific cause   HIV virus (human immunodeficiency virus); also called HTLV-III (human T-lymphotropic virus, type III) and LAV (lymphadenopathy-associated virus).

The danger in AIDS is not the virus itself, but the damage it does to the body's natural immune system. The human body does develop antibodies against this virus (that is the basis of the test for AIDS). Why then is the body unable to survive this viral attack? No one knows the answer. The antibodies produced by the HIV virus are ineffective and cannot check the damage caused by the virus.

Opportunistic diseases   OIs—opportunistic infections, namely pneumocystis carinii pneumonia (PCP) and Kaposi's sarcoma (KS), are generally the cause of death in AIDS patients. These are diseases that would not be common or severe in persons whose immune systems were not compromised.

Treatment   no curative treatment is available, but some drugs are being used to treat the opportunistic diseases. AZT was used initially for patients with AIDS, but now is more commonly given to individuals before they develop AIDS—for example, those who test HIV positive. There are now many experimental drugs being used.

Abbreviations

AIDS   acquired immune deficiency syndrome.

ARC   AIDS-related complex, (person tests positive for HIV but no severe symptoms are present).

AZT   azidothymidine (drug used in AIDS treatment).

BPH   benign prostatic hypertrophy.

EIA/ELISA   enzyme immunosorbent assay or enzyme-linked immunosorbent assay (detects presence of HIV antibodies); screening test only.

GC   gonococcus, gonorrhea.

HIV   human immunodeficiency virus.

Disease	Cause	Symptoms	How Detected	Treatment	Complications, Sequelae
AIDS	HIV virus	severe wasting (weight loss); adenopathy; loss of immunity to OIs	ELISA test Western blot	AZT Retrovir (zidovudine)	Kaposi's sarcoma PCP death
gonor *rhe* a (GC)	*Neisseria gonorrhoeae* (bacterium)	discharge, burning	smear, culture	Penicillin	PID sterility (newborn-eye infections)
***syph* ilis (also called *lues*)**	*Treponema pallidum* (spirochete)	*Stages* 1. painless chancre 2. rash 3. dementia	serum test: VDRL, RPR & others	PCN ceftriaxone and doxycycline or tetracycline for penicillin-resistant organisms (CDC recommendation)	*Stages* 1. clears 2. clears 3. severe mental illness; newborn-congenital syphilis
chla *myd* ia and nonspecific urethritis (NSU)	bacteria	similar to GC	smear	tetracycline	same list as gonorrhea
***her* pes geni *tal* is**	viruses: HSV-2 HSV-1	blisterlike lesions, pain, burning	lesions	Zovirax (acyclovir)	no cure; remissions and exacerbations; newborn severe neurological damage
ve *ne* real warts (ver *ru* cae)	virus	warts genital area	clinical signs	topical or cautery	need to biopsy to exlude carcinoma or syphilis lesions
tricho *moni* as	flagellate protozoon	itching, burning, foul discharge	smear	oral medication (Flagyl); douches suppositories	check for diabetes; often associated with antibiotic treatment which changes "flora."
candi *di* asis (moni *li* asis)	*Candida albicans* (yeast)	itching, burning	smear	douches, suppositories	newborn may contract in birth canal (thrush)
crab lice (pedicu *lo* sis)	louse	severe itching	clinical signs, louse present	various "local" products: Kwell, RID (OTC)	could be transmitted in bedding

Table 23.1 Sexually Transmitted Diseases (STDs)

HSV-2   herpesvirus genitalis.
HTLV-III   human T-lymphotropic virus, type III, same as HIV.
IVDU   intravenous (IV) drug user.
KS   Kaposi's sarcoma.
LAV   lymphadenopathy-associated virus, same as HIV.
NSU, NGU   nonspecific urethritis, nongonorrheal urethritis.
OI   opportunistic infection.
PCN   penicillin.
PCP   pneumocystis carinii pneumonia.
PID   pelvic inflammatory disease.
PSA   prostate-specific antigen; blood test for early prostate malignancy.
PWA   person with AIDS.
RPR   rapid plasma reagin (syphilis test).
STD   sexually transmitted disease.
STS   serological test for syphilis.
VDRL   Venereal Disease Research Laboratory.

Worksheet

Fill in the blank:

1. Male sex cell _____; male sex gland _____

2. Common carcinoma in the male occurs in the _____

3. Pneumocystis pneumonia is an opportunistic infection often seen in _____ patients.

4. Male sterilization is called _____

5. Name two structures located in the scrotum: _____

6. STD means _____

    _____

7. PSA means _____

    and is used in _____

Write a word that means:

8. "hidden testes" (undescended) _____

9. excision of prostate _____

10. "cutting around" penis (foreskin) _____

11. Name 3 sexually transmitted diseases:

    _____

    _____

12. Choose one STD and tell the cause, the symptoms, the treatment if any, and the sequelae and prognosis.

_____

_____

_____

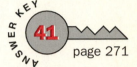

Chapter 22 and 23 combined Test p. 347
Alternate Test p. 351

■ Case History ■

CASE HISTORY 16

REPORT OF OPERATION: Circumcision

Preoperative Diagnosis phimosis.

Anesthetic general.

Procedure Circumcision. The patient was premedicated and taken to the operating room, where a general anesthetic was administered by Dr. Andrews. The genitalia were prepped and draped in the usual manner, the foreskin was grasped and a dorsal slit made, and the foreskin retracted. Next, the Bell clamp was applied, and the foreskin removed. This was reinforced by interrupted 3-0 plain chromic stitches, approximately one dozen being placed around the penis. A Vaseline gauze dressing was applied. The patient withstood the procedure well and was returned to the recovery room in good condition with minimal blood loss.

■ **Assignment:** Read the case aloud, and write down and define all unfamiliar terms.

▲ **Health Promotion Tip**

To prevent sexually transmitted diseases:

• Practice abstinence (if appropriate) or maintain a mutually monogamous relationship.

• Use a condom!

• Maintain good hygiene.

• Avoid contaminated needles (or partners who use them).

CHAPTER 24

Nervous System and Psychiatric Terms

Anatomy and Physiology of the Nervous System

Function

The central nervous system (CNS) coordinates and controls all of the body's activities and, together with the endocrine system, helps to maintain homeostasis. The autonomic nervous system (or peripheral nervous system) controls, regulates, and coordinates organ and gland function.

Central Nervous System (CNS)

brain (brān)   See Figure 24.1.

> **cerebrum** (**sĕr**-ē-brŭm)   largest part. *Lobes*: frontal, pa **ri** etal, **tem** poral, and oc **cip** ital. *Function*: consciousness, mental processes, sensations, emotions, and voluntary movement.

> **cerebellum** (sĕr-ĕ-**bĕl**-lŭm)   occupies posterior cranial fossa (shallow depression) behind brain stem. *Function*: maintains equilibrium, normal postures, coordination.

> **brain stem**   pons and me **dul** la oblon **ga** ta. An enlarged extension of the spinal cord. Contains the vital centers: cardiac, vasomotor, and respiratory centers. *Function*: controls rate and strength of heartbeat, constriction and dilatation of blood vessels, and rate and depth of respirations.

spinal cord (**spī**-năl kŏrd)   lies inside the spinal column (**ver** tebral column) from the oc **cip** ital bone through the fo **ra** men **mag** num down to the first lumbar vertebra. *Function*: conducts impulses between the brain and other parts of the body and serves as a center for reflexes.

meninges (singular, **men** inx) (mĕn-**ĭn**-jēz)   membranes that cover the spinal cord and brain (see Figure 24.2 on p. 220.)

> **duramater** (**dū**-ră **mā**-tĕr)   tough outer covering.

> **arachnoid** (ă-**răk**-nŏyd)   middle layer.

> **piamater** (**pē**-ă **mā**-tĕr)   internal layer, directly covering brain and cord.

cerebrospinal fluid (CSF) (sĕr-ĕ-brō-spī-năl **flū**-ĭd)   fluid that circulates around the cord and the brain, in the suba **rach** noid space (see Figure 24.1).

Autonomic Nervous System (Peripheral Nervous System)

The **autonomic** (ăw-tō-**nŏm**-ĭk)   **nervous system (ANS)** is called "involuntary" because we do not control it; an example is circulation. (*Autonomic* means "self-governing.") The ANS conducts impulses out from

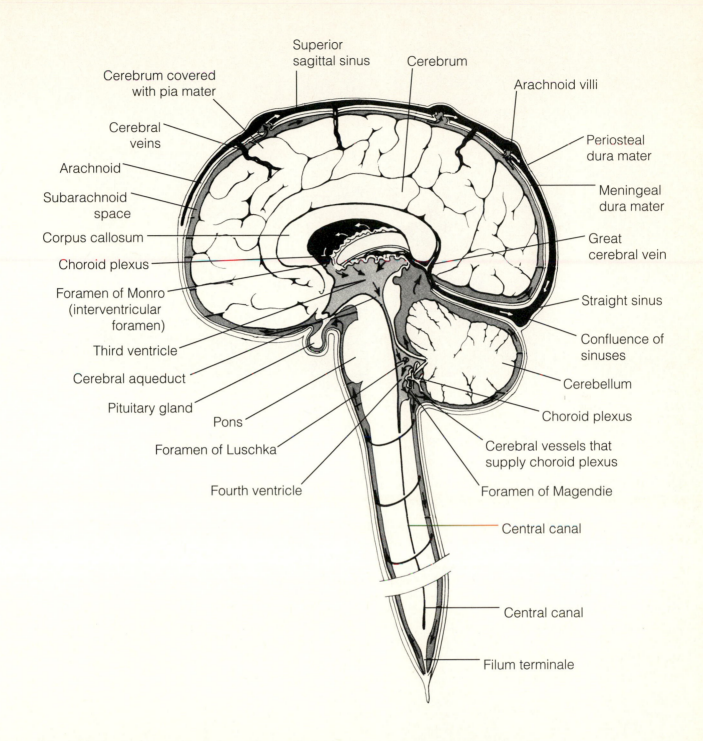

Labels (clockwise from top):

Superior sagittal sinus

Cerebrum

Cerebrum covered with pia mater

Arachnoid villi

Cerebral veins

Periosteal dura mater

Arachnoid

Meningeal dura mater

Subarachnoid space

Corpus callosum

Choroid plexus

Great cerebral vein

Foramen of Monro (interventricular foramen)

Straight sinus

Third ventricle

Confluence of sinuses

Cerebral aqueduct

Cerebellum

Pituitary gland

Choroid plexus

Pons

Cerebral vessels that supply choroid plexus

Foramen of Luschka

Fourth ventricle

Foramen of Magendie

Central canal

Central canal

Filum terminale

Figure 24.1 The brain and spinal cord and the location of the cerebrospinal fluid that surrounds them. The arrows indicate the direction of flow of the fluid. (From Spence, A. P., and Mason, E. B., 1987. *Human Anatomy and Physiology,* ed. 3. Menlo Park, CA: Benjamin/Cummings Publishing Co., p. 355.)

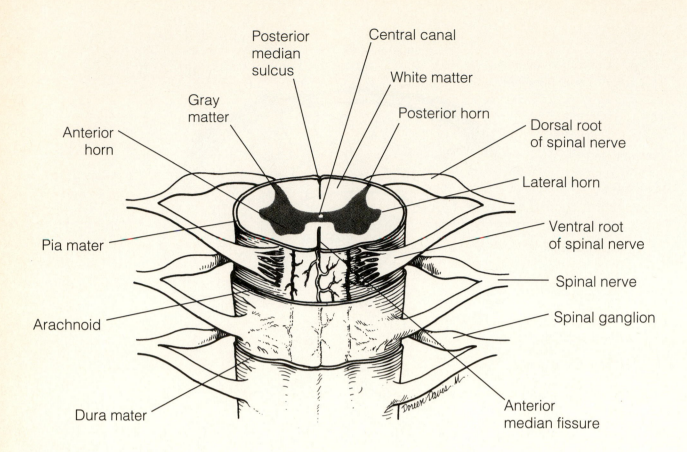

Figure 24.2 The meninges that surround the spinal cord. (From Spence, A. P., and Mason, E. B., 1987. *Human Anatomy and Physiology*, ed. 3. Menlo Park, CA: Benjamin/Cummings Publishing Co., p. 361.)

the brain stem or spinal cord to smooth muscle, cardiac muscle, and so on. Thus, it is peripheral to the CNS and is also called the **peripheral** (pĕr-ĭf-ĕr-ăl) **nervous system (PNS).** Parts of the ANS include:

cranial nerves 12 pairs:

1. Olfactory (ŏl-**făk**-tō-rē)   sense of smell.

2. Optic (**ŏp**-tĭk)   vision.

3. Oculomotor (ŏk-ū-lō-**mō**-tŏr)   movement of eyes.

4. Trochlear (**trŏk**-lē-ăr)   muscle of eyes.

5. Trigeminal (trī-**jĕm**-ĭn-ăl)   facial movements.

6. Abducens (ăb-**dū**-sĕnz)   eye muscles that turn eye outward.

7. Facial (**fā**-shăl)   muscles of face, ears, scalp.

8. Auditory (**ăw**-dĭ-tō-rē)   hearing and equilibrium.

9. Glossopharyngeal (glŏs-ō-fă-**rĭn**-jē-ăl)   secretion of parotid gland, taste.

10. Pneumogastric, vagus (nū-mō-**găs**-trĭk, **vā**-gŭs)   voice and swallowing.

11. Spinal (**spī**-năl)   neck muscles.

12. Hypoglossal (hī-pō-**glŏs**-săl)   tongue.

A mnemonic to help memorize these: "On old Olympus', torrid top, a Finn and German picked some hops."

spinal nerves (spī-năl něrvs) 31 pairs attached to spinal cord. Numbered according to the section of the spinal column; for example, C-1 is first cervical, T-8 is eighth thoracic, and so on. Co is the coccyx.

plexus (plěk-sŭs) a network of nerves (or blood or lymph vessels). Example: *solar plexus*, located behind the stomach. Taber's dictionary lists all of the plexuses in an appendix.

The two subdivisions of the autonomic nervous system:

sympathetic (sĭm-pă-thět-ĭk) cell bodies originate in thoraco **lum** bar sections T-1 to L-2. Assists the body in emergencies, defense, and survival. *Adre **ner** gic* refers to sympathetic nerve fibers that produce an adrenaline-like substance.

parasympathetic (păr-ă-sĭm-pă-thět-ĭk) cell bodies originate in cranio **sac** ral sections. Brings the body functions back to normal after a stressful situation has ended. *Choli **ner** gic* refers to nerve fibers or agents that produce the effect of acetylcholine to block the action of parasympathetic nerves.

In general, these two divisions have opposing functions; they are important in maintaining the body's homeo **stat** ic condition. Following are *some* examples of their action:

Sympathetic (adrenergic nerves)		Parasympathetic (cholinergic nerves)
Constrict	Cerebral arteries	Dilate
Dilate	Pupils	Constrict
Increased	Metabolic rate	No action
Dilate	Branchi	Constrict
Constrict	Pulmonary arterioles	Dilate
Rate increased	Heart	Rate decreased
Decreased	Stomach/GI motility	Increased

■ **Note:** Although it has been thought that we have no control over the autonomic functions, experience with bio **feed** back in recent years has shown that blood pressure, body temperature, and some other "involuntary" functions can be altered somewhat.

Nerve Cells (Neurons)

Neurons (nū-rŏnz) respond to stimuli (stimulus-response) and specialize in transmitting impulses. Nervous tissue is extremely delicate and is well protected by bones of the cranium and spinal column. Further protection is provided by the membranes (meninges) and the cerebrospinal fluid.

Pathophysiology of the Nervous System

Nervous System Diseases and Disorders

abscess (brain) (ăb-sĕs) secondary to infection in body (ear, sinuses, for example).

ALS (amyotrophic lateral sclerosis) (ă-mī-ō-trō-fĭk lăt-ĕr-ăl sklĕ-rō-sĭs) progressive disease, cause unknown, starting with loss of coordination and leading to extensive disability.

Alzheimer's disease (presenile dementia) (ăltz-hī-mĕrz, prē-sē-nīl dē-měn-shē-ă) early senility, cause unknown, leading to severe deterioration.

anencephaly (ăn-ĕn-sĕf-ă-lē) congenital absence of brain ("monster"); always die in 1–2 days. One of the possible results of *neural tube defects (NTDs)*, defective closure of the embryonic form of the brain and spinal cord. Other NTDs are spina bifida and meningoceles.

Bell's palsy (bĕlz **pǎwl**-zē)   paralysis of one side of face, inflammation of seventh cranial nerve.

botulism (**bŏt**-ū-lĭzm)   caused by toxin in food, produced by anaerobic organism (*Clost rid ium botu lin um*); GI symptoms, leading to difficulty swallowing and respiratory paralysis. Treatment: antiserum.

cerebral palsy (**sĕr**-ĕ-brăl **pǎwl**-zē)   paralysis resulting from developmental defects or trauma; variety of symptoms; may be spastic, flaccid, athetoid (writhing movements).

concussion (kŏn-**kŭsh**-ŭn)   injury to brain due to blow to head; may involve loss of consciousness; bleeding and swelling may follow, putting potentially fatal pressure on the brain.

convulsion (seizure) (kŏn-**vŭl**-zhŭn, **sē**-zhūr)   sudden disturbances in mental functions and body movements, some with loss of consciousness; may be due to epilepsy, high fever (febrile convulsion), or CVA.

CVA (cerebrovascular accident) (sĕr-ē-brō-**vǎs**-kū-lǎr)   any interruption of blood supply to the brain causes brain damage, with resulting neurologic symptoms (such as numb sensation, tingling, loss of grip, interruption/distortion of speech or vision, incontinence, unconciousness, convulsion/seizure, and/or severe headache). Damage occurs either when blood vessel ruptures and bleeds into the brain or skull resulting in pressure on surrounding tissue (also known as hemorrhagic stroke) or when artery is blocked by embolism or clot.

encephalitis (ĕn-sĕf-ă-**lī**-tĭs)   inflammation of the brain; many types. Can be caused by bacterial or viral infection; some types borne by mosquito; can occur following some vaccinations.

epilepsy (**ĕp**-ĭ-lĕp-sē)   seizure disorder; may be caused by injury, but often the cause is unknown. Treated but not cured with medication. *Grand mal* and *petit mal* are terms to describe type of seizure.

fracture (skull) (**frǎk**-chūr)   usually comminuted with bony fragments in brain, making surgery imperative. Trauma to the skull may be due to birth injury, falls or blows to the head, gunshot wounds, and so on.

Guillain-Barré syndrome (gē-**yǎn**-bă-**rā**)   acute, rapidly progressive polyneuropathy with muscular weakness and sensory loss, usually following infection or immunization.

hematoma (hē-mă-**tō**-mă)   "blood tumor" (clot), may be sub **du** ral, suba **rach** noid, epi **du** ral or intra **cer** ebral; if large enough to cause pressure on brain, it must be removed.

herpes zoster (**hĕr**-pēz **zŏs**-tĕr)   "shingles": an acute inflammatory reaction in spinal or cranial nerve due to dormant viral infection in body; common in older people and with some carcinoma patients.

Huntington's chorea (**hŭn**-tĭng-tŏns **kō**-rē-ă)   hereditary disorder due to a gene on chromosome 4; onset usually between ages 30–40; purposeless movements, constant and uncontrolled, leading to dementia.

hydrocephalus (hī-drō-**sĕf**-ă-lŭs)   "water in the head": increased accumulation of CSF in ventricles of the brain; may be due to trauma, tumor, anomaly, or infection; causes mental retardation.

Korsakoff's syndrome (**kŏr**-să-kŏfs)   deficiency of vitamin B complex (specifically thiamine and B_{12}), usually secondary to alcoholism; characterized by memory deficits progressing to complete amnesia.

Lyme disease (līm)   caused by a spirochete through a tick bite. Symptoms are skin, neuro, and cardiac abnormalities, arthritis. Treatment: antibiotics. Diagnosis by laboratory test for antibodies.

meningitis (mĕn-ĭn-**jī**-tĭs)   inflammation of meninges due to bacterial, viral, or fungal infection; may be secondary to disease of sinuses, ear, mastoid; aseptic meningitis is a nonpurulent form.

meningocele (myelomeningocele) (mĕ-**nĭn**-jō-sēl, **mī**-ĕ-lō-)   hernia of meninges (and cord) to surface of the back; a congenital anomaly. May be repaired surgically, but some disability will remain.

multiple sclerosis (MS) (**mŭl**-tĭ-pl sklĕ-**rō**-sĭs)   brain and cord contain areas of degenerated myelin; symptoms and course of the disease are variable, but visual problems are common; manifested by tremors, slurred speech, eventual disability. No really effective treatment; age of onset usually 30–40.

neurofibromatosis (nĕ-rŏ-**fī**-brō-mă-tō-sĭs) (or von Recklinghausen's disease)   hereditary peripheral nerve disorder.

neuropathy (neuritis) (nĕ-**rŏ**-păth-ē)   disease of peripheral and cranial nerves; motor, sensory, and reflex impairment.

organic brain syndrome (chronic brain syndrome) group of symptoms of the senile variety; these diagnoses are used when nothing else "fits," and the patient has brain damage (possibly due to alcoholism or syphilis).

Parkinson's disease (**păr**-kĭn-sŏns) usually occurs after age 50 years; manifested by expressionless face, slow movement, muscular tremors, stooped posture, shuffling-type gait, rigidity. L-dopa medication helpful. Usually cause is unknown, but occasionally it is a sequela to encephalitis.

poliomyelitis (pō-lē-ō-mī-ĕ-**lī**-tĭs) viral infection affecting all areas of the brain, brain stem, and cord; paralytic type is most severe. Prevention is the key with vaccination of the oral type (Sabin).

Reye's syndrome (rīz) acute encephalopathy following viral infection.

sciatica (sī-**ăt**-ĭ-kă) severe pain in the leg along the course of sciatic nerve, felt at back of thigh running down inside of the leg; may be associated with herniated disk.

spina bifida (**spī**-nă **bĭf**-ĭ-dă) see *meningocele*.

spinal cord injuries three types: compression or transection inevitably leave permanent dysfunction depending on the level of cord damage; contusion (rapid edematous swelling of cord) *may* leave some residual disability (paraplegia, quadriplegia).

tetanus (**tĕt**-ă-nŭs) commonly called lockjaw; caused by toxin produced by anaerobic organism (*Clost* **rid** *ium* **tet** *ani*) in puncture-type wound; dysphagia, irritability, stiffness progressing on to convulsions, asphyxia, exhaustion, and usually death. Prevention: tetanus immunization, DTP, DT with booster every 10 years.

Tourette's syndrome (tŏŏ-**rĕts**) genetic disorder characterized by uncontrolled blinking, facial twitching/tics, and/or obscenity spoken.

transient ischemic attack (TIA) (**trăn**-zē-ĕnt ĭs-**kē**-mĭk) (or "mini" stroke) temporary occlusion resultnig in impairment of blood flow to the brain (due to clot/thrombus or embolism). Symptoms include loss of sensation or tingling (for no apparent reason and lasting 1–2 minutes or more), sudden inability to communicate, drooped facial expression, visual disturbance, vertigo, or disturbed gait for 5 minutes or more.

tumors (cord, brain) benign or malignant, primary or metastatic; may be classified by location, tissue type, or degree of malignancy (grades I to IV); may be intracerebral, extracerebral, intradural, extradural; detailed discussion is beyond the scope of this text. Some common tumors are gli **o** mas (astrocy **to** ma, glioblas **to** ma, oligodendrogli **o** ma, ependy **mo** ma), hemangioblas **to** ma, medulloblas **to** ma, spongioblas- **to** ma, meningi **o** ma, neu **ro** mas (schwann **o** ma, neurilem **mo** ma, neurofi **bro** ma, neuri **no** ma). Metastatic lesions often come from lung, breast, prostate. All tumors, benign or malignant, may be life threatening because they may be inaccessible surgically.

"whiplash" imprecise term for injury to cervical vertebrae and adjacent soft tissues (sudden jerking producing hyperextension of neck).

Surgical, Diagnostic, and Treatment Terms

angiogram (arteriogram), cerebral (**ăn**-jē-ō-grăm, ăr-**tē**-rē-ō-grăm) radiopaque substance is injected into arteries in neck, then X-ray films are taken.

angioplasty (**ăn**-jē-ō-plăs-tē) balloon inflated in artery or tube (stent) inserted in artery and inflated to open the artery by squishing the plaque.

Babinski's sign (bă-**bĭn**-skēz) reflex response; when sole of the foot is stroked, big toe turns up instead of down (normal in newborn, but pathologic later on).

brain scan radioactive element is given and later observed in brain tissue.

burr holes small openings made with a trephine (cylindrical saw) in the bone of the skull to permit access, obtain biopsy, evacuate hematoma, and for insertion of drains or monitoring devices.

carotid endarterectomy (kă-**rŏt**-ĭd ĕn-dăr-tĕr-**ĕk**-tō-mē) surgically cleaning the carotid artery; especially successful with 70–99% of blocked vessels.

cordotomy (kŏr-**dŏt**-ō-mē) cutting of nerve fibers to relieve intractable pain.

craniotomy (krā-nē-**ŏt**-ō-mē) incision to gain access to the brain when burr holes are not adequate for the procedure.

CT, CAT scan computerized (axial) tomography, a noninvasive technique used in X-ray. Information produced is similar to PEG but no discomfort involved.

EEG (echoencephalogram) (ĕk-ō-ĕn-**sĕf**-ă-lō-grăm)   use of ultrasound to show displacement of brain structures.

EEG (electroencephalogram) (ē-lĕk-trō-ĕn-**sĕf**-ă-lō-grăm) record of electrical activity of the brain. There are four classifications of electrical activity, or brain waves; *alpha*, calm and awake; *beta*, alert; *theta*, early sleep and dreaming; *delta*, deep sleep, not usually included in an EEG report. Both EEGs are useful in seizure disorders and in locating area of damage.

laboratory procedures   examination of cerebrospinal fluid (cell counts, cultures, blood, and so on).

laminectomy (lăm-ĭ-**nĕk**-tō-mē)   excision of the arches of vertebrae to view spinal cord.

lobotomy (prefrontal) also **amygdalotomy** (lō-**bŏt**-ō-mē)   an operation that used to be performed for severe mental illness. *Amygdaloid* means "almond shaped"; the amygdaloid nucleus, a small part of the temporal lobes of the brain, is involved in a wide variety of behavior patterns; its removal was meant to help control behavior and appropriate responses.

lumbar puncture (LP), spinal tap (**lŭm**-băr **pŭnk**-chūr, **spī**-năl tăp)   insertion of needle into subarachnoid space to measure pressure, get lab sample, inject dye for myelography, and administer regional anesthesia.

lumbar sympathectomy (**lŭm**-băr sĭm-pă-**thĕk**-tō-mē)   cutting fibers of sympathetic nerves that contract walls of blood vessels of the lower leg to relieve poor peripheral circulation.

myelogram (myelography) (**mī**-ĕl-ō-grăm, mī-ĕ-**lŏg**-ră-fē)   a "picture" produced after the injection of a dye into subarachnoid space to detect tumors or herniated disks.

nerve block   injection of anesthetic into nerve to produce loss of sensation.

pneumoencephalogram (PEG)   "picture" of brain after air has been injected into subarachnoid space by lumbar puncture; useful in diagnosis of hydrocephalus, tumors, abscesses, blood clots, or atrophy of the brain. An unpleasant test compared to the CT scan, which does not have side effects.

rhizotomy (rī-**zŏt**-ō-mē)   cutting roots of spinal nerves to relieve incurable pain.

Romberg test (**rŏm**-bĕrg)   checking balance by having person touch tip of nose with index finger with eyes closed; arms are outstretched with eyes closed; observer watches for "drift."

scan   see *CT scan* and *brain scan.*

shunts (shŭnts)   types of bypass, via catheter, for drainage of CSF from the ventricles in the brain to the spinal canal or the thoracic cavity; for example, ventriculo **pleur** al, ventriculocistern **os** tomy, ventriculo **at** rial; used in treating hydrocephalus.

spinal tap (**spī**-năl tăp)   see *lumbar puncture.*

trephination (trĕf-ĭ-**nā**-shŭn)   drilling hole in skull to evacuate clots or inject air for diagnostic procedure.

vagotomy (vā-**gŏt**-ō-mē)   cutting vagus nerve as treatment for peptic ulcer (lessens secretion of hydrochloric acid in stomach).

ventriculography (vĕn-trĭk-ū-**lŏg**-ră-fē)   injection of air directly into ventricles when PEG cannot be done because of massive lesion or increased intracranial pressure.

Specialists

Patients with neurological disorders or injury to the brain or cord are usually treated by neurologists and neurosurgeons. Other involved specialists are internists, radiologists, psychiatrists, and physiatrists.

The Neurological Examination

mental status   intellect; **af** fect (mood or emotional state); orientation as to time and place; disordered thought, such as delusions, hallucinations, illusions; insight; consciousness; language function.

cranial nerves   tested separately for taste, touch, temperature, visual acuity, position sense, and so on.

spinal cord and peripheral nerves

1. Motor function: muscles, adequate strength, quick contraction, prompt relaxation; flaccid and spastic paralysis.
2. Sensory function: touch, pain, position, vibration.
3. Complex functions: involved movement, coordination, reflexes (including Babinski), balance (Romberg).

Miscellaneous Terms

aphasia (ă-**fā**-zē-ă)   loss of ability to speak; "without speech."

ataxia (ă-**tăk**-sē-ă)   lack of muscle coordination.

biofeedback (bī-ō-**fēd**-băk)   training to develop ability to control autonomic nervous system (B/P, heart rate, and so on).

cauda equina (**căw**-dă ē-**kwīn**-ă)   "horse's tail": the end of the spinal cord or the sacrococcygeal area; also, the group of nerves that supply the rectal area (below L-2.) *Caudal* refers to this area (caudal anesthesia, for example).

comatose (**kō**-mă-tŏs)   in a deep stupor; cannot be aroused.

contrecoup (kŏn-tr-**kŏŏ**)   occurring on the opposite side; injury in which brain literally bounces back and forth, causing injury to side opposite the blow to the head.

DTR (deep tendon reflex)   body movement at unconscious level.

encephalon (ĕn-**sĕf**-ă-lŏn)   the brain.

fissure (**fĭsh**-ŭr)   deep furrow in the brain (*fissure* also has other meanings).

flaccid (**flă**-sĭd)   flabby; poor muscle tone, seen in paralysis.

foramen magnum (fō-**rā**-mĕn **măg**-nŭm)   opening in occipital bone through which cord passes.

ganglion (**găng**-lē-ŏn)   a "knot" of many cell bodies outside the cord and brain.

gyrus, gyri (plural) (**jī**-rŭs, **jī**-rī)   convolutions of the cerebrum.

hemiplegia (hem-i-**plē**-jē)   paralysis of only one side of the body.

hemisphere (**hĕm**-ĭs-fēr)   either half of the brain.

ipsilateral (ĭp-sĭ-**lăt**-ĕr-ăl)   on the same side; affecting the same side.

limbic system (**lĭm**-bĭk)   "edge or border of a part," refers to that part of the brain having to do with emotional behavior and attitudes.

manometer (măn-**ŏm**-ĕt-ĕr)   apparatus to measure pressure (of spinal fluid), in mm of H_2O (70–200 mm in adult).

myelin (**mī**-ĕl-ĭn)   white fatty substance that surrounds certain nerve fibers (white matter).

neurilemma (sheath of Schwann) (nū-rĭ-**lĕm**-mă)   membrane enveloping peripheral nerves.

paralysis (pă-**răl**-ĭ-sĭs)   inability to use muscles due to nerve damage.

paresis (pă-**rē**-sĭs)   incomplete or partial paralysis.

paresthesia (păr-ĕs-**thē**-zē-ă)   abnormal sensation, such as numbness and tingling without apparent cause; heightened sensitivity; occurs in central and peripheral nerve lesions/disorders.

plexus (**plĕk**-sŭs)   a network of nerves (or blood vessels).

reflex (**rē**-flĕks)   involuntary response to stimulus.

spastic (**spăs**-tĭk)   having forceful uncontrollable contractions.

stimulus (**stĭm**-ū-lŭs)   anything that brings about a response; an irritant such as a pinprick.

sulcus, sulci (plural) (**sŭl**-kŭs, **sŭl**-kī)   deep furrow in the brain (groove).

syncope (**sīn**-kō-pē)   fainting; loss of consciousness.

ventricle (brain) (**vĕn**-trĭk-l)   cavity in the brain; there are four.

Psychiatric Terms

affect (ăf-fĕkt)   emotional reaction; may be normal, inappropriate, or completely absent (e.g., *flat affect*: no reaction following a trauma).

aggression (ă-grĕsh-ŭn)   hostile attitude; may be due to insecurity or feeling of inferiority.

ambivalence (ăm-bĭv-ă-lĕns)   opposing feelings, such as love and hate occurring simultaneously and negatively affecting daily function.

amnesia (ăm-nē-zē-ă)   loss of memory.

anorexia nervosa (ăn-ō-rĕk-sē-ă nĕr-vō-să)   an eating disorder; occurs mostly in thin young women. Symptoms include excessive weight loss, extreme fear of becoming fat (despite reality of not being fat, even to the point of emaciation), depression, fatigue, denial of hunger, hormonal imbalance, irregular (or cessation of) menstruation, osteoporosis, and possible death.

anxiety (ăng-zī-ĕ-tē)   excessive and long-lasting apprehensive expectation about upcoming life events that a person feels unable to control.

autism (ăw-tĭzm)   complete withdrawal; not able to communicate.

binge eating disorder (bĭnj)   an eating disorder; occurs in obese people. Symptoms are eating large amounts of food when not hungry (binging but not purging), eating alone to conceal unusually large portions ingested, eating quickly, and feeling guilty or disgusted after eating. Binging increases risks of diabetes, high cholesterol, heart disease, and hypertension.

bipolar affective disorder (bī-pōl-ăr ă-fĕk-tĭv)   also called *manic depressive psychosis*; major psychosis having periods of elation and profound depression. Lithium and other drugs are used to treat it.

bulimia nervosa (bū-lĭm-ē-ă nĕr-vō-să)   an eating disorder; occurs in both men and women, usually of normal weight. Symptoms include binging on high-fat or sweet junk foods and secretly purging by self-induced vomiting or ingestion of laxatives or diuretics. Unlike anorexics, bulimics are aware of their abnormal behavior.

catatonic (kăt-ă-tŏn-ĭk)   does not talk, move, or react; observed in schizophrenia.

delirium (dĕ-lĭr-ē-ŭm)   mental confusion or excitement.

delusion (dē-lū-zhŭn)   false belief, such as megalo **ma** nia.

depression (dē-prĕsh-ŭn)   all bodily functions slowed down; lack of hope; symptoms include irritability, exhaustion, overeating or weight loss, low self-esteem, difficulty concentrating or making decisions, and/or anxiety. Antidepressant drugs or, in severe depression, electroconvulsive (shock) therapy (ECT), may be helpful.

eating disorders   emotional and psychological disorders related to eating behavior as a way of coping with stress, low self-esteem, helplessness, depression, or anxiety. Include anorexia nervosa, bulimia nervosa, and binge eating; one or more disorders may occur simultaneously.

echolalia (ĕk-ō-lā-lē-ă)   repetition of anything that is said instead of answering.

hallucination (hă-lū-sĭ-nā-shŭn)   auditory or visual; hearing or seeing things not really present.

hypochondria (hī-pō-kŏn-drē-ă)   preoccupation with body; imaginary illnesses.

hysteria (hĭs-tĕ-rē-ă)   extreme emotional state; also hysterical blindness, and so on.

illusion (ĭl-lū-zhŭn)   a false interpretation of something seen or heard.

involutional melancholia (ĭn-vō-lū-shŭn-ăl mĕl-ăn-kō-lē-ă)   mental illness in menopause; depression.

malingering (mă-lĭng-ĕr-ĭng)   making believe; pretending (to be ill, for example).

megalomania (mĕg-ă-lō-mā-nē-ă)   delusions of being someone important.

narcissistic (năr-sĭs-sĭst-ĭk)   grandiose feeling and preoccupation with self, arrogance, and self-importance, excluding others and lacking empathy.

nervous breakdown   layperson's term for mental illness. Nerves are not actually involved.

neurasthenia (nū-răs-thē-nē-ă)   ill-defined weakness; weak, tired feeling that rest does not alleviate.

neurosis (nū-rō-sĭs)   having a feeling of extreme anxiety and sometimes hypochon **dri** asis; person with a neurosis is still in touch with reality.

obsessive-compulsive (ŏb-**sĕs**-ĭv kŏm-**pŭl**-sĭv)   neutralizing or suppressing thoughts, impulses, or actions by engaging in repetitive behaviors (such as hand-washing, compelled spotless cleaning, etc.).

paranoid (**păr**-ă-nŏyd)   having feelings of persecution (paranoia).

phobia (**fō**-bē-ă)   exaggerated fear (for example, inability to leave the house); some medical dictionaries list all phobias.

posttraumatic stress disorder (PTSD) (pōst-trăw-**măt**-ĭk)   recurrent replay of some traumatic event that intrudes via thoughts, images, or dreams; feeling as if trauma is "here and now"; numbing of response to later events, hypervigilance (e.g., increased arousal), shame, despair, sleep difficulty, etc.

psychosis (sī-**kō**-sĭs)   mental illness in which person is out of touch with reality.

schizophrenia (skĭz-ō-**frĕn**-ē-ă)   major mental illness (several types) usually affecting young people; symptoms include delusions, hallucinations, incoherent speech, and/or disorganization. Heavy tranquilizers are used in treatment.

stress   Any real or imagined force that disrupts equilibrium or produces strain, especially in amounts that the system cannot handle—in which case it may produce pathologic changes. Some people react to stress (stressors) in a negative way, others thrive on it.

■ **Note:** The term *functional* when referring to mental illness usually means there is no organic cause for it or there is no apparent brain damage. The term *organic* usually means there *is* brain damage that is causing the symptoms.

You may encounter the following names of **psychological tests:** Bender Visual Motor Gestalt Test, MMPI (Minnesota Multiphasic Personality Inventory), Rorschach Inkblot Test, Stanford-Binet Intelligence Scales, TAT (Thematic Apperception Test), WAIS (Wechsler Adult Intelligence Scale), WISC (Wechsler Intelligence Scale for Children).

Abbreviations

ANS   autonomic nervous system.

CNS   central nervous system.

CVA   cerebrovascular accident.

ECT or EST   electroconvulsive therapy (shock therapy) used in treatment of severe depression.

EEG   electroencephalogram (or echoencephalogram). Do not confuse with ECG or EKG, electrocardiogram.

ICP   intracranial pressure; due to edema secondary to trauma.

LP   lumbar puncture (spinal tap).

MS   multiple sclerosis.

NTD   neural tube defect.

PTSD   posttraumatic stress disorder.

REM   rapid eye movements; eye movement during dreaming.

TIA   transient ischemic attack.

Worksheet

Fill in the blank:

1. The cerebrum is the _____largest_____ part of the _____brain_____

2. The dura mater, arachnoid, and pia mater are _____

   _____

3. The cranial nerves for vision are _____ ; sense of smell _____ ;

   and hearing _____

4. Write the abbreviation for the fourth thoracic spinal nerve: _____ ;

   third cervical _____ ; and first coccygeal _____

5. The bony protection for the brain is the _____

   and for the spinal cord _____ .

   The fluid protection for the brain and cord is _____

6. Neurons are _____ . The encephalon is the _____

7. Name two tumors of the nervous system: _____

8. A weakness on one side of the body is called _____

9. Paralysis on one side of the body is called _____

10. Define:

    gyri _____

    sulci _____

    Write the singular form of both: _____

11. Ventricles in the brain are _____ ;

    if they are distended, the condition resulting is _____

12. A stimulus is followed by a _____ when the nervous system is intact.

13. CSF is obtained by performing a spinal tap, also called a _____ .

    This fluid may be required for examination for _____ purposes.

14. Caudal anesthesia is injected into _____

15. Meningitis is _____

16. The sympathetic and parasympathetic are divisions of the _____ nervous system.

17. Match the words in the left column with those in the right column.

   a. no speech   _____   shock treatment

   b. flaccid   _____   response

   c. Babinski   _____   hyperextension

   d. craniotomy   _____   convulsion

   e. Romberg   _____   paralysis

   f. myelogram   _____   skull incision

   g. palsy   _____   to view cord

   h. seizure   _____   balance

   i. whiplash   _____   flabby

   j. ipsilateral   _____   aphasic

   k. stimulus   _____   same side

   l. ECT   _____   without cause

   m. functional   _____   foot reflex

18. Name and describe briefly two nervous system conditions not mentioned in this worksheet

   _____

   _____

   _____

19. What are the three types of "rhythms" or "waves" mentioned in the EEG report?

   _____

   _____

20. Define "nervous breakdown": _____

   _____

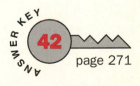

ANSWER KEY 42 page 271

Test Part I p. 353, Part 2 p. 357
Alternate Part I Test p. 355

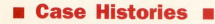

■ Case Histories ■

CASE HISTORY 17

RADIOLOGY REPORT: Skull radiograph

Procedure Skull radiograph. Four views of the skull are obtained. Two burr holes are demonstrated in the left and right frontal parietal regions. Otherwise the bony calvarium is intact. There is no evidence of fracture. No abnormal intracranial calcifications are identified. The sella appears normal.

CASE HISTORY 18

RADIOLOGY REPORT: Cervical spine radiograph

Procedure Cervical spine radiograph. AP, lateral, and oblique views of the cervical spine were obtained. The vertebral bodies and disk spaces appear well maintained. There is no evidence of fracture or dislocation. Minimal degenerative changes are noted.

CASE HISTORY 19

RADIOLOGY REPORT: Myelogram

Procedure Myelogram. Contrast was injected into the lumbar subarachnoid space, and appropriate films were obtained. There was excellent demonstration of the lumbar subarachnoid space. Again evident is the left L4–5 extradural defect, as demonstrated on April 18, 1995, showing no appreciable change. There continues to be slight compression of the L5 nerve rootlet on that side. Impingement into the anterior subarachnoid space is observed on the upright cross-table lateral view. Interpretation: L4–5 extradural defect compatible with a disk bulge is observed, as demonstrated previously, with no significant change.

CASE HISTORY 20

RADIOLOGY REPORT: Brain scan

Procedure Brain scan. Neuroanatomic structures reviewed include cerebellar hemispheres; temporal, frontal, parietal, and occipital lobes; brain stem; ventricles; subarachnoid spaces and cisterns. Bilateral parietal bony defects are noted, and subjacent to the left parietal defect the brain is slightly more dense, although there is no contrast enhancement or mass effect. There is a slight widening of the left sylvian fissure and slight reduction in the left temporal density above that region, again subjacent to bone. Ventricles are normal. Midline is undisplaced with minimal widening of cerebral sulci over the convexities. Impression: Minimal left temporal atrophy. Bilateral bony defects consistent with patient's prior surgical history.

CASE HISTORY 21

EEG REPORT: Electroencephalogram

Electroencephalogram Report Most of this tracing was obtained while the patient was awake, but there are several periods of drowsiness or light sleep. Dominant rhythms include well-formed symmetrical 9–10 cycle per second alpha rhythm and beta activity, which is usually in the 20–30 cycle per second frequency range. Occasional theta waves are present. There are prominent eye blink artifacts. Hyperventilation produced no significant change. There are no spikes, paroxysms, or persistent asymmetries. Conclusion: normal EEG.

■ **Assignment:** Now that you have read these cases, list the words new to you along with their meanings. You may also want to reread Chapter 17 on the musculoskeletal system in which some neuromuscular disorders are presented.

✔ Check Your Progress

Congratulations again! You have nearly made it to the end of Part 2. This is the final Check Your Progress, and at this point you should have a solid foundation and framework in medical terminology. At this point, if you find certain words from Part 2 are still giving you trouble, make and use flash cards and review some of the worksheets that contain the difficult terms.

You may now be given a **review test** for Chapters 22–24, which can be found on page 359 in Appendix F. These three chapters have focused on the male and female reproductive systems and the nervous system. You have learned how to construct words that describe these intricate systems as well as related areas of study such as neonatology, genetics, sexually transmitted diseases, and psychiatry.

You have just about completed the *Medical Terminology* text. The final two chapters in Part 2 contain terminology describing the sense organs and the endocrine system and stress response.

▲ Health Promotion Tip

Symptoms of a CVA, or stroke, are often ignored. Not seeking immediate intervention can result in paralysis or death. By recognizing early warning signs, you can protect yourself.

These warning signs include:

- Numbness or tingling progressing from one specific area to a larger area or an entire side of the body; lasts longer than 1–2 minutes and has no apparent cause.
- Unexpectedly dropping an object held in the hand.
- Inability to communicate (slurred speech, inability to understand words or speak them).
- Vision disturbance (for example, half of visual field disappears, temporary blindness in one eye, blurred or double vision, or partial blindness).
- Vertigo or gait disturbance.
- Intensely painful headache.
- Denial of symptoms.
- Seizure.

Call 911 immediately if stoke is suspected. Time is crucial.

CHAPTER 25

Sense Organs: Eyes, Ears, and Mouth

Anatomy and Physiology of the Eye

Function

The eyes provide receptors for vision.

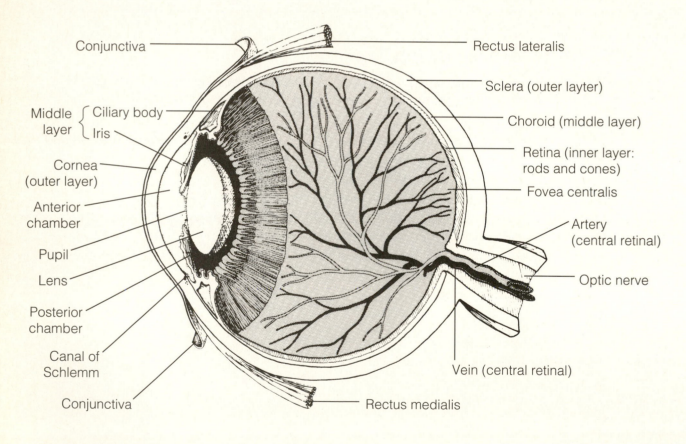

Conjunctiva

Rectus lateralis

Sclera (outer layter)

Middle layer { Ciliary body
Iris

Choroid (middle layer)

Retina (inner layer:
rods and cones)

Cornea
(outer layer)

Fovea centralis

Anterior
chamber

Artery
(central retinal)

Pupil

Lens

Optic nerve

Posterior
chamber

Canal of
Schlemm

Vein (central retinal)

Conjunctiva

Rectus medialis

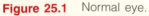

Figure 25.1   Normal eye.

The Eye and Its Parts

See Figure 25.1.

eyes   rest in eye sockets; in orbital cavities of the cranium (eyebrow area).

lacrimal apparatus (lăk-rĭm-ăl ăp-ă-răt-ŭs)   tear ducts and glands.

sclera (sklĕ-ră)   outer covering (rear part is the white of the eye; clear front part is the *cor nea*).

conjunctiva (kŏn-jŭnk-tī-vă)   mucous membrane covering eyeballs and eyelids.

choroid (kō-rŏyd)   dark-brown layer between sclera and retina; it is part of the *u vea* (iris, ciliary body, and choroid) that contains blood vessels for the eye.

iris (ī-rĭs)   colored band of choroid surrounding the pupil and behind the cornea.

pupil (pū-pĭl)   a "hole" in the iris; the iris regulates the size of the pupil.

lens (lĕnz)   transparent, colorless structure encapsulated and held in place behind the pupil by a ligament attached to the ciliary body; refracts (bends) light rays so that they are focused on the retina.

ciliary body (sĭl-ē-ăr-ē)   muscle that changes the shape of the lens by contracting and relaxing.

aqueous humor (ā-kwē-ŭs hū-mŏr)   watery liquid in anterior chamber in front of the lens; it circulates through the anterior and posterior chambers of the eye.

vitreous humor (vĭt-rē-ŭs hū-mŏr)   jellylike transparent substance inside eyeball.

optic nerve (ŏp-tĭk)   transmits images from the retina to the brain.

retina (rĕt-ĭ-nă)   innermost (third) layer of the eye; receives images formed by the lens. Contains sensitive nerve fibers including rods, cones, and fibers connected with optic nerve.

rods   light-sensitive nerve cells that work in dim light and provide black-and-white images.

cones   light-sensitive nerve cells responsible for bright light and color vision.

Muscles attached to the outside of the eyeball provide eye movements.

Pathophysiology of the Eye

Eye Diseases and Disorders

amblyopia (ăm-blē-ō-pē-ă)   weakening, dimness or dullness of vision; "lazy eye"; one eye not being used; treatment is to patch the used eye to force use of the lazy eye; if not treated early (preschool), unused eye will lose visual acuity.

astigmatism (ă-stĭg-mă-tĭzm)   irregularity of the curvature of the eye (cornea and lens); corrected with lenses.

blepharitis (blĕf-ă-rī-tĭs)   inflammation of the eyelids (blephar = eyelids).

blepharoptosis (blĕf-ă-rō-tō-sĭs)   drooping of the upper eyelids.

cataract (kăt-ă-răkt)   progressively blurred, double, or halo vision; opaque lens (instead of clear); most are of the senile type, especially in diabetics; can also be congenital or a result of trauma. Treatment is surgery to extract lens; this may include intraocular lens implant, or person may wear glasses following surgery. Surgical success rate greater than 95%; one of the three leading causes of blindness.

central retinal artery occlusion (sĕn-trăl rĕt-ĭ-năl ăr-tĕr-ē ŏ-klū-zhŭn)   may be due to embolism or thrombus in a sclerotic central artery, cranial arteritis, or fat emboli; produces painless, sudden unilateral blindness; immediate treatment is imperative (reduction of intraocular tension and other measures to reduce the area of retinal ischemia).

central retinal vein occlusion   occurs in elderly arteriosclerotic patients, especially those with glaucoma, covert diabetes mellitus, increased blood viscosity. Blindness may develop in a few hours. Treatment involves destruction of secondary neovascular overgrowth by laser photocoagulation to decrease vitreous hemorrhages. No other treatment available, except anticoagulants if indicated.

chalazion (kă-lā-zē-ŏn) mei **bo** mian cyst on eyelid (enlarged sebaceous gland); may need surgical removal.

color blindness most cases are congenital (in males) but can be caused by injury, disease, or drugs; may be limited to red/green only.

conjunctivitis (kŏn-jŭnk-tĭ-**vī**-tĭs) inflamed conjunctiva (membrane covering the front of the eyeball and lining eyelids); acute type called "pink eye"; other types result from irritation from swimming pools and allergies; see *neonatorum conjunctivitis*.

corneal ulcer (**kŏr**-nē-ăl **ŭl**-sĕr) usually the result of injury or inflammation; contact lenses may also be partial cause.

dacryoadenitis (dăk-rē-ō-ăd-ĕn-**ī**-tĭs) inflammation of the lacrimal (tear) gland.

dacryocystitis (dăk-rē-ō-sĭs-**tī**-tĭs) inflammation and obstruction of lacrimal sac following nasal trauma, deviated septum, nasal polyps (any prolonged obstruction).

dacryolith (**dăk**-rē-ō-lĭth) a "stone" in the lacrimal duct.

detached retina (dē-**tăcht** **rĕt**-ĭ-nă) may be a small detachment or involve almost the entire retina; occurs in myopics frequently; may be the result of injury; treatment is to use laser to "reattach" (see Figure 25.2).

dry eye tear production decreases with age; also associated with a type of arthritis (Sjögren's syndrome). Treatment is with "artificial tears" (an OTC type of eye drops).

esotropia (ĕs-ō-**trō**-pē-ă) a type of strabismus involving one or both eyes turning in.

exotropia (ĕk-sō-**trō**-pē-ă) a type of strabismus involving one or both eyes turning out.

"floaters" (in vitreous) (**flō**-tĕrs) common complaint among older people; bits of protein or cells floating in vitreous fluid that cause visual disturbances; there is no treatment; not considered significant in itself.

foreign bodies in eye if imbedded they may require surgery; chemicals in the eye should be washed out immediately. Safety goggles could prevent many of these types of injuries.

glaucoma (glăw-**kō**-mă) increase in intraocular pressure due to the closing of canal of Schlemm; fluid cannot circulate, and pressure builds up. Usually occurs after age of 40 years and may be asymptomatic; diagnosis is made with ton **om** etry. Treated with miotic drugs (pilo **car** pine); several types of surgery are also possible if needed. One of the three leading causes of blindness.

gonorrheal conjunctivitis of newborn (gŏn-ō-**rē**-ăl kŏn-jŭnk-tĭ-**vī**-tĭs) see *neonatorum conjunctivitis*.

hemorrhages (subconjunctival) (**hĕm**-ĕ-rĭj-ĕz) blood under the membrane as a result of injury; can also occur spontaneously; usually resolves itself.

herpes zoster (ophthalmic) (**hĕr**-pēz **zŏs**-tĕr, ŏf-**thăl**-mĭk) involvement of the fifth cranial nerve (face, eye, and nose) with the herpes virus; a serious form of herpes.

hyperopia (hī-pĕr-ō-pēă) farsightedness; cannot see at close range (to read, for example); see *presbyopia*.

hypertropia (hī-pĕr-**trō**-pē-ă) a type of strabismus involving one eye turning up.

hypotropia (hī-pō-**trō**-pē-ă) a type of strabismus involving one eye turning down.

injuries (**ĭn**-jūr-ēz) foreign body, lacerations, contusions (black eye), and burns.

intraocular pressure (ĭn-tră-**ŏk**-ū-lăr **prĕsh**-ŭr) see *glaucoma*.

iritis (ĭ-**rī**-tĭs) inflammation of the iris; acute or chronic; cause may be unknown but is often associated with rheumatic diseases, diabetes, and trauma; treatment consists of medications and warm compresses.

keratoconus (kĕr-ă-tō-**kō**-nŭs) cone-shaped cornea causing severe myopia; contact lenses may improve vision for a time; corneal transplant is performed when vision deteriorates.

macular degeneration (**măk**-ū-lăr dē-jĕn-ĕr-**ā**-shŭn) damage to macula, in which layers of retina separate due to fluid under the retina; degenerative type of eye condition due to aging wear and tear; central vision lost but peripheral vision may remain.

meibomian cyst (mī-**bō**-mē-ăn) see *chalazion*.

myopia (mī-**ō**-pē-ă) nearsightedness, usually corrected with lens, either in eyeglasses or contact lenses. RK (radial keratotomy) is also being used to treat myopia in some people.

neonatorum conjunctivitis (nē-ō-nă-**tŏr**-ŭm kŏn-jŭnk-tĭ-**vī**-tĭs) purulent conjunctivitis usually due to GC and passed to newborn in the birth canal. Prophylaxis involves treatment with eye drops at birth (silver nitrate, PCN).

nystagmus (nĭs-**tăg**-mŭs) rapid, side-to-side movement of eyeball (usually due to nervous system or inner ear disturbance).

papilledema (păp-ĭl-ĕ-**dē**-mă) swelling of the optic nerve (choked disk); usual cause is intracranial pressure; can be observed with ophthalmoscope.

presbyopia (prĕz-bē-ō-pē-ă) affliction of older-age people; lens loses elasticity (loss of accommodation); treatment is reading glasses or bifocals (presby = old).

retinal detachment see *detached retina.*

retinitis (rĕt-ĭ-**nī**-tĭs) many types, including ac **tin** ic; reti **ni** tis pigmen **to** sa is hereditary; chronic progressive degeneration of retina.

retinoblastoma (rĕt-ĭ-nō-blăs-**tō**-mă) malignant gli **o** ma of retina.

retinopathies (rĕt-ĭn-**ŏp**-ă-thēz) any disorder of retina; arteriosclerotic, hypertensive, diabetic, solar, syphilitic.

strabismus (stră-**bĭz**-mŭs) misaligned (or squinted) eyes; any deviation from normal (convergent or divergent); muscle defect that is correctable by surgery with good results.

stye (hordeolum) (stī, hŏr-**dē**-ō-lŭm) inflammation of sebaceous gland of eyelid.

trachoma (trā-**kō**-mă) chronic infection of conjunctiva and cornea; not common in the United States except in some Native American populations; one of the three leading causes of blindness.

uveitis (ū-vē-ī-tĭs) inflammation of iris and blood vessels.

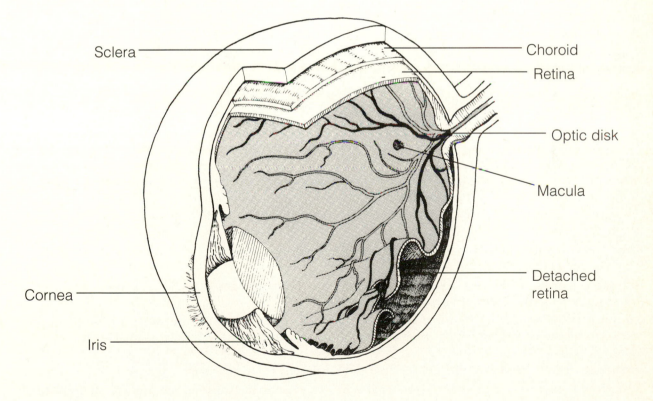

Figure 25.2 Detached retina. (Courtesy of Stanley R. Shorb, M. D., Phoenix, AZ.)

Surgical, Diagnostic, and Treatment Terms

angiography (ăn-jē-ŏg-ră-fē) see *fluorescein*.

cataract extraction (kăt-ă-răkt ĕks-trăk-shŭn) with or without intraocular lens implant, the lens is removed surgically; see *cryoextraction* and *phacoemulsification*.

corneal transplant (kŏr-nē-ăl) surgical procedure with donor cornea used. Treatment for keratoconus and some other corneal abnormalities.

cryoextraction (krī-ō-ĕks-trăk-shŭn) standard cataract removal procedure requiring a rather large incision where cornea meets sclera; uses liquid nitrogen, which forms an ice ball attaching the lens to the probe (cryo = cold).

cryoretinopexy (krī-ō-rĕt-ĭn-ō-pĕk-sē) fixation of detached retina with cold; scar tissue forms and reattaches the retina. Used especially for tears in the outer edges. Retinopexy can also be done with laser (heat).

dacryocystotomy (dăk-rē-ō-sĭs-tŏt-ō-mē) incision of the lacrimal sac.

enucleation (ē-nū-klē-ā-shŭn) surgical removal of eye.

eye muscle surgery shortening and/or lengthening muscles that regulate eye movement for correction of deviation, such as crossed eyes (strabismus).

fluorescein angiography (flū-ō-rĕs-ē-ĭn ăn-jē-ŏg-ră-fē) injection of a dye intravenously to detect retinal blood vessels.

fundoscopy, funduscopy (fŭn-dŏs-kō-pē) examination of the inner eye with ophthalmoscope or funduscope; this examination enables the viewer to see the blood vessels clearly and can aid in early diagnosis of hypertension; if vessels in the eye show damage, it can be assumed other vessels are also suffering damage.

gonioscopy (gō-nē-ō-skō-pē) using a special optical instrument to inspect the angle of the anterior chamber, useful in diagnosing closed-angle glaucoma.

grid test used to detect blind spots or distortions of vision via vertical and horizontal lines on chart.

iridectomy (ĭr-ĭ-dĕk-tō-mē) excision of part of the iris; one type of surgery used in glaucoma to allow fluid to circulate.

iridencleisis (ĭr-ĭ-dĕn-klī-sĭs) similar to iridectomy; used for glaucoma.

keratomileusis (kĕr-ă-tō-mī-lū-sĭs) cornea removed, frozen, ground to a new shape, thawed, and replaced.

keratoplasty (kĕr-ă-tō-plăs-tē) corneal transplant (using donor cornea); surgical success rate about 90%.

keratotomy (RK) (kĕr-ă-tŏt-ō-mē) surgical slits made in the cornea to treat myopia (cosmetic option to contact lenses or eyeglasses).

laser photocoagulation (lā-zĕr fō-tō-kō-ăg-ū-lā-shŭn) laser produces intense heat; used in treatment of retinal detachment and other eye conditions.

phacoemulsification (fă-kō-ē-mŭl-sĭ-fĭ-kā-shŭn) treating cataract by disintegrating it with ultrasound for extraction (phaco = lens).

pterygium surgery (tĕ-rĭj-ē-ŭm) growth of conjunctiva over inner portion of eye (an abnormal growth that can be removed surgically).

slit lamp examination slit lamp is a microscope that illuminates and magnifies structures within the eye. It produces a narrow beam of high-intensity light.

tonometry (tonometer) (tōn-ŏm-ĕ-trē) instrument for measuring pressure within eyeball to diagnose glaucoma before it destroys vision; several types of tonometers are used (Schiötz tonometer is a popular one).

trabeculectomy (tră-bĕk-ū-lĕk-tō-mē) excision of fibrous bands (connective tissue).

ultrasound test (ŭl-tră-sŏwnd) uses sound waves to explore structures in the eye. Echoes from sound waves are reflected back from the retina and are converted into an image that is recorded.

visual field testing test for peripheral vision, in a dark room with spots of light projected for patient to detect.

vitrectomy (vĭ-trĕk-tō-mē) aspiration of vitreous fluid and replacement with saline solution or vitreous to clear opaque vitreous.

YAG laser (yăg) YAG = yttrium, aluminum and garnet. 30% of patients who have extracapsular cataract surgery later have clouding in the membrane behind the lens. This requires that a small opening be made in the membrane; YAG laser is used to do this. Retinal complications reduced if YAG laser is used after surgery instead of during.

Miscellaneous Terms

accommodation (ă-kŏm-ō-**dā**-shŭn)   ability of the eye to adjust to seeing at different distances with ease (near/far).

anesthesia (ăn-ĕs-**thē**-zē-ă)   for eye procedures is usually topical (eye drops); may also be injected locally behind the eye (retrobulbar).

anisocoria (ăn-ī-sō-**kō**-rē-ă)   unequal pupils.

Braille (brāl)   raised alphabet in books for the blind.

canal of Schlemm (kă-**năl** ŭv shlĕm)   opening through which aqueous humor must flow out, or pressure in eye increases.

canthus, canthi (plural) (**kăn**-thŭs, **kăn**-thī)   corner of eye; inner and outer canthi.

cc with correction (lenses).

cryoprobe (**krī**-ō-prōb)   surgical instrument used with liquid nitrogen.

cystotome (**sĭs**-tō-tōm)   instrument for cutting anterior lens capsule. Also spelled *cystitome*.

diopters (dī-**ŏp**-tĕrz)   unit of measure for lenses.

emmetropia (ĕm-ĕ-**trō**-pē-ă)   normal vision.

eye bank   for donor corneas.

eye drops   for treatment of several conditions, especially for reducing intraocular pressure in glaucoma. *Important note:* although eye drops are introduced into the eye, they may have a systemic effect.

fundus (**fŭn**-dŭs)   in the eye, the back part.

fundoscope (**fŭn**-dŭ-skōp)   spelled with *u* or *o* (fundoscope); see *ophthalmoscope*.

guide dogs   formerly called *seeing-eye dogs*; for the blind.

lacrimation (lăk-rĭ-**mā**-shŭn)   production of tears by lacrimal apparatus.

laser (**lā**-zĕr)   acronym for light amplification by stimulated emission of radiation (if you care to know). Produces a highly concentrated beam of light and creates a tiny spot of intense heat. It is very useful in eye surgery of many types.

miotic (myotic) (mī-**ŏt**-ĭk)   (either spelling is correct) drug used to contract pupil; for example, pilocarpine.

mydriatic (mĭd-rē-**ăt**-ĭk)   drug that dilates pupil; for example, atropine or cocaine.

ophthalmologist (ŏf-thăl-**mŏl**-ō-jĭst)   (or oculist) medical doctor who treats eye disorders.

ophthalmometer   device for obtaining prescription of eyeglasses.

ophthalmoscope (ŏf-**thăl**-mō-skōp)   instrument for looking into the eye; same as funduscope.

optometrist (ŏp-**tŏm**-ĕ-trĭst)   (not a medical doctor) fits eyeglasses or contact lenses.

optician (ŏp-**tĭsh**-ăn)   (not a medical doctor) eye product specialist.

peripheral vision (pĕr-**ĭf**-ĕr-ăl **vĭ**-zhŭn)   vision out to the side (at the outer edges).

refractive errors (rē-**frăk**-tĭv **ĕr**-rŏrs)   vision disorders that are correctable with lenses.

Snellen eye chart (**snĕl**-lĕn)   with letters, or "illiterate E," chart for vision screening.

20/20 vision   *not* perfect vision; only means a person can see at 20 feet what most adults see at 20 feet; a screening term meaning the person is not nearsighted.

10/10 vision   *not* perfect vision; only means a child can see at 10 feet what most children (ages 3 to 5 years) can see at 10 feet; a screening term.

Specialists

The ophthalmologist (sometimes called oculist) is the primary person for treating eye disorders. In eye surgery they tend to specialize; one does cornea transplants, one does mostly cataracts or detached retina cases, and so on. The optometrist (not a medical doctor) is qualified to fit glasses or contact lenses. The internist may treat some eye infections, and in some cases a neurologist may be involved.

Abbreviations

OD   right eye (oculus dexter).

OS   left eye (oculus sinister).

OU   both eyes (oculi unitas).

PERLA   pupils equal, react to light and accommodation; neurological screening for quick assessment; **PERRLA:** extra *r* means "round."

sc   without correction (glasses).

VA   visual acuity, clearness, sharpness of vision.

Anatomy and Physiology of the Ear

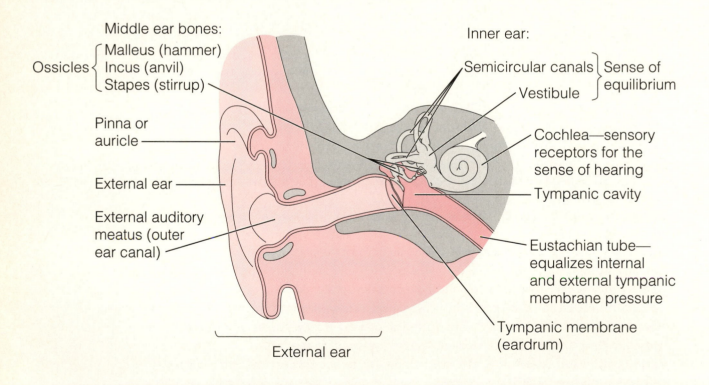

Figure 25.3   Diagram of the internal and external ear. Adapted from Sloane, S.B., *The Medical Word Book* (Philadelphia: W.B. Saunders Company, 1991)

Function

The ears provide receptors for hearing.

Parts of the Ear

external ear   **aur** icle, or pinna, and auditory meatus (mē-**ā**-tŭs) (ear canal).

middle ear   from tympanic membrane, it is lined with mucous membrane; three bones: **mal** leus, **in** cus, **sta** pes (**stā**-pēz).   (Middle ear ends after stapes).

inner ear   **ves** tibule, semi **cir** cular canals, and **coch** lea.

tympanic membrane (eardrum or **myringa)** (tĭm-**pǎn**-ĭk, mĭr-**ĭn**-gǎ)   separates middle ear from external ear.

eustachian tubes (auditory tubes) (ū-**stā**-shŭn)   from middle ear to pharynx (throat); equalize pressure. Horizontal from 0–5 years then gradually tilt vertically thus allowing exudate (such as drainage secondary to inflammation) and nasal material to drain off more efficiently.

Pathophysiology of the Ear

Ear Diseases and Disorders

aerotitis or **barotitis media** (āyr-ō-**tī**-tĭs, bǎr-ō-**tī**-tĭs mē-dē-ǎ)   during a sudden increase in atmospheric pressure, as in airplane descent or deep-sea diving, air must move from the nasopharynx into the middle ear to maintain equal pressure on both sides of the eardrum. Retraction of the eardrum may occur and further complications leading to rupture of the membrane can also result. People with acute upper respiratory infections or allergic reactions should not fly or scuba dive. Scuba diving and flying should be planned 48 hours apart.

deafness (**děf**-nĕs)   *hearing impaired* is the preferred term; hearing loss may be conductive (sound waves cannot be transmitted) or preceptive (nerve damage); causes may include injury, disease, toxic drugs, congenital defects, recurrent otitis media, or scar tissue thickening due to recurrent surgery or a tympanic membrane perforation.

eustachian salpingitis (ū-**stā**-shŭn sǎl-pǐn-**jī**-tĭs)   inflammation of eustachian tube.

foreign body in ear   such as insects, beans, and so on. Insect in ear may be flushed out with oil; in case of beans, peas, and so on, never instill water or fluid that would cause the bean to swell—immediate medical attention should be sought. Also, do not use wax or putty as ear plugs.

impacted cerumen (ĭm-**pǎk**-tĕd sĕ-**rū**-mĕn)   cerumen is normally a soft wax found in the ear canal (auditory meatus), impacted cerumen is hard, dry cerumen that often causes ear discomfort or infection.

labyrinthitis (lǎb-ĭ-rĭn-**thī**-tĭs)   otitis interna; inner ear disturbance.

mastoiditis (mǎs-tŏy-**dī**-tĭs)   inflammation of the mastoid process, which is a process of the temporal bone.

Ménière's disease (mān-ē-**ǎrz**)   or syndrome; cause usually unknown; characterized by tinn **i** tus, dizziness, feeling of pressure in ear; recurrent and progressive.

myringitis (mĭr-ĭn-**jī**-tĭs)   inflammation of the eardrum due to infection or trauma.

otitis externa (ō-**tī**-tĭs ĕks-**tĕr**-nǎ)   bacterial, fungal ear canal infection.

otitis media (ō-**tī**-tĭs mē-dē-ǎ)   middle ear inflammation; common infection in children, usually treated with antibiotics. Characterized by sleep difficulty, ear discomfort, ear drainage, and/or fever.

otosclerosis (ō-tō-sklĕ-**rō**-sĭs)   anky **lo** sis of the stapes (one of the middle ear bones) causing deafness, especially in low tones.

presbycusis (prĕz-bĭ-**kū**-sĭs)   form of nerve deafness in older people.

trauma (**trǎw**-mǎ)   cauliflower ear is a neglected hematoma; trauma can occur to any part of the ear as a result of a blow to the head or from inserting objects into the ear.

Surgical Terms

cochlear implant (kŏk-lē-ăr)   procedure to restore some hearing, still experimental at this time.

fenestration (fĕn-ĕs-**trā**-shŭn)   artificial opening is made to bypass the damaged middle ear, allowing sound waves to pass and reach inner ear (in otosclerosis).

mastoidectomy (măs-tŏy-**dĕk**-tō-mē)   excision of mastoid cells; since the use of antibiotics, this procedure is seldom necessary (ear infections are treated before mastoid is involved).

myringotomy (mĭr-ĭn-**gŏt**-ō-mē)   incision into eardrum; when eardrum is in danger of rupturing spontaneously, this may be done and may include insertion of pressure-equalizing (PE) tube for drainage.

otoplasty (ō-tō-plăs-tē)   surgical repair or plastic surgery on the ear (pinna).

pressure-equalizing (PE) tubes   inserted following a myringotomy to promote drainage from and air flow to the eustachian tube.

stapedectomy (stā-pē-**dĕk**-tō-mē)   excision of stapes (middle ear bone) to restore hearing; an artificial stapes is inserted.

tympanoplasty (tĭm-păn-ō-**plăs**-tē)   plastic surgery on eardrum using a skin graft to refashion a tympanic membrane (corrects large perforations).

tympanotomy (tĭm-păn-**ŏt**-ō-mē)   see *myringotomy*.

Specialists

Ear disorders may be treated by an otolaryngologist, an otologist, and an internist. Surgery is done by an otologist, with the use of microscopes (microsurgery) for better visualization of tiny structures.

Miscellaneous Terms

acoustic meatus (ă-**kū**-stĭk mē-**ā**-tŭs)   opening or passage in the ear.

audiometer (ăw-dē-**ŏm**-ĕ-tĕr)   device for testing hearing.

audiometrist (ăw-dē-**ŏm**-ĕ-trĭst)   person who performs hearing tests.

auditory, acoustic (**ăw**-dĭ-tō-rē, ă-**kū**-stĭk)   pertaining to the ear or hearing.

decibel (**dĕs**-ĭ-bĕl)   unit of measure for sound.

electronystagmography (ē-lĕk-trō-nĭs-tăg-**mŏg**-ră-fē)   method of testing vestibular function by assessing eye motion.

exudate (**ĕks**-ū-dāt)   exit or drainage of cellular debris secondary to inflammation.

hearing aids   types include bone conduction receiver and air conduction receiver.

hearing-ear dogs   dogs trained to respond to sounds and alert the hearing-impaired person.

otic (**ō**-tĭk)   pertaining to ear.

otolaryngologist (ō-tō-lăr-ĭn-**gŏl**-ō-jĭst)   medical doctor specialist of ears and larynx (ear, nose, and throat).

otologist (ō-**tŏl**-ō-jĭst)   medical doctor ear specialist.

otoscope, otoscopy (**ō**-tō-skōp, ō-**tŏs**-kŏ-pē)   instrument and procedure for looking into ear.

sign language   use of hands to communicate.

tinnitus (tĭn-**ī**-tŭs)   "ringing" and other sounds in the ear.

tuning fork   a forklike steel instrument used in testing hearing.

vertigo (**vĕr**-tĭ-gō)   sensation of whirling motion, dizziness.

Abbreviations

AD	right ear	**ENT**	ear, nose, and throat MD specialist (otolaryngologist)
AS	left ear	**PE**	pressure-equalizing tubes inserted postmyringotomy
AU	both ears	**TM**	tympanic membrane

Anatomy and Physiology of the Mouth

Function

The mouth provides a receptor for taste and is a component of the digestive system, housing salivary glands and teeth. Teeth are the organs of mastication (chewing).

Teeth (Organs of Mastication)

For structure, see Figure 25.4 on p. 242.

crown (krŏwn)   made of **enamel**; the portion above the gums.

root (root)   portion embedded in socket (al **ve** olus) of jawbones; include:

  dentin (**dĕn**-tĭn)   hard, ivorylike substance.

  pulp cavity (pŭlp **kăv**-ĭt-ē)   holds vessels, nerve endings.

  cementum (sē-**mĕn**-tŭm)   bony substance that covers the dentin.

  gingiva (plural, **-ae**) (**jĭn**-jĭ-vă)   gum, soft tissue surrounding tooth.

  periodontal membrane (pĕr-ē-ō-**dŏn**-tăl)   surrounds the root and holds tooth in socket.

  root canal (root kă-**năl**)   contains nerves and blood vessels.

  alveolus   the bony socket that holds a tooth.

dentition (dĕn-**tĭ**-shŭn)   eruption of teeth (approximate) (see Figure 25.4).

  deciduous (baby) teeth (dē-**sĭd**-ū-ŭs)   "falling away"; total 20 (see Figure 25.5 on p. 243).

Total teeth	At age
6	1 year
12	1½
16	2
20	2½

  permanent teeth   starting at age 6–7; total of 32 is complete at age 12–13 except for third molars at 17–25 (wisdom teeth).

names of teeth   same, upper and lower.

  incisors (ĭn-**sī**-zŏrz)   front cutting teeth; 4 upper, 4 lower.

  cuspids (canines) (**kŭs**-pĭdz)   anterior teeth (one cusp); 2 and 2.

  bicuspids (bī-**kŭs**-pĭdz)   premolars (two cusps); 4 and 4.

  molars (**mō**-lărs)   posterior grinding teeth; 6 and 6.

tooth surfaces   See Figure 25.4.

  buccal (**bŭk**-l)   refers to cheek side (also called *facial*).

  labial (**lā**-bē-ăl)   refers to lip side (also called *facial*).

  lingual (**lĭng**-gwăl)   refers to tongue side.

  mesial, medial (**mē**-zē-ăl, **mē**-dē-ăl)   middle (between) sides.

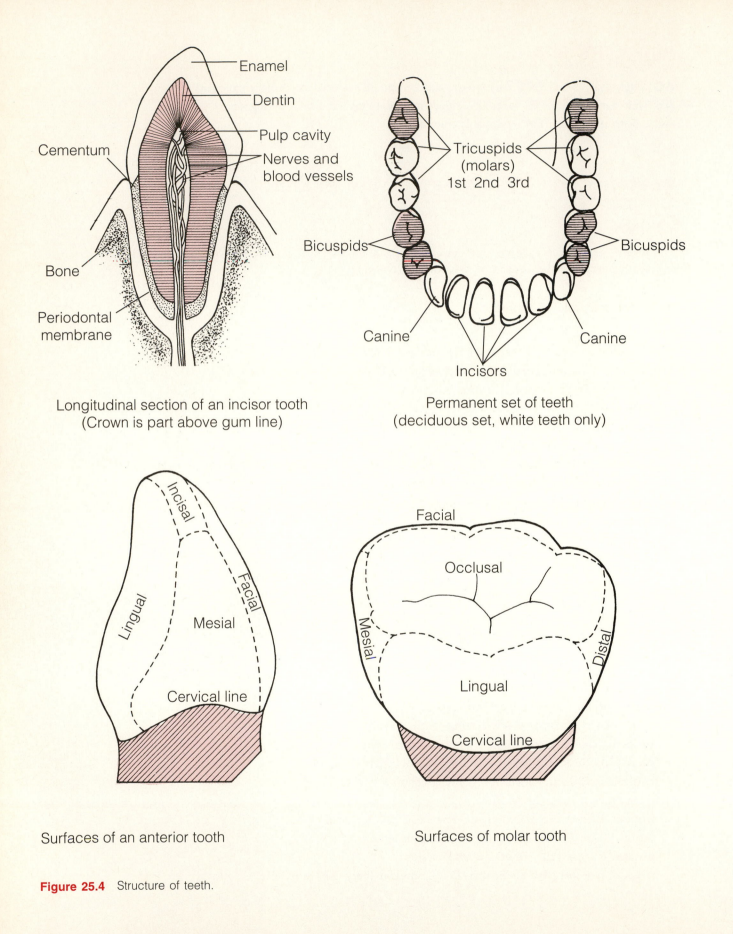

Enamel

Dentin

Pulp cavity

Nerves and blood vessels

Cementum

Bone

Periodontal membrane

Longitudinal section of an incisor tooth
(Crown is part above gum line)

Tricuspids (molars)
1st 2nd 3rd

Bicuspids

Bicuspids

Canine

Canine

Incisors

Permanent set of teeth
(deciduous set, white teeth only)

Incisal

Facial

Lingual

Mesial

Cervical line

Surfaces of an anterior tooth

Facial

Occlusal

Mesial

Distal

Lingual

Cervical line

Surfaces of molar tooth

Figure 25.4 Structure of teeth.

Dental Claim Form

See reverse for instructions

1. ☐ Dentist's pre-treatment estimate ☐ Dentist's statement of actual services Provider ID #	2. ☐ Medicaid Claim ☐ EPSDT Prior Authorization # Patient ID #	3. **Carrier name and address**

PATIENT COVERAGE INFORMATION

4. Patient name first m.i. last	5. Relationship to employee ☐ self ☐ child ☐ spouse ☐ other _____	6. Sex m f	7. Patient birthdate MM DD YYYY	8. If full time student school city

9. Employee/subscriber name and mailing address	10. Employee/subscriber dental plan I.D. number	11. Employee/subscriber birthdate MM DD YYYY	12. Employer (company) name and address	13. Group number

14. Is patient covered by another dental plan yes no If yes, complete 15-a. Is patient covered by a medical plan? yes no	15-a. Name and address of carrier(s)	15-b. Group no.(s)	16. Name and address of other employer(s)

17-a. Employee/subscriber name (if different from patient's)	17-b. Employee/subscriber dental plan I.D. number	17-c. Employee/subscriber birthdate MM DD YYYY	18. Relationship to patient ☐ self ☐ parent ☐ spouse ☐ other _____

19. I have reviewed the following treatment plan and fees. I agree to be responsible for all charges for dental services and materials not paid by my dental benefit plan, unless the treating dentist or dental practice has a contractual agreement with my plan prohibiting all or a portion of such charges. To the extent permitted under applicable law, I authorize release of any information relating to this claim. Signed (Patient* – see reverse) Date	20. I hereby authorize payment of the dental benefits otherwise payable to me directly to the below named dental entity. Signed (Employee/subscriber) Date

BILLING DENTIST

21. Name of Billing Dentist or Dental Entity	30. Is treatment result of occupational illness or injury?	No	Yes	If yes, enter brief description and dates
22. Address where payment should be remitted	31. Is treatment result of auto accident?			
23. City, State, Zip	32. Other accident?			

24. Dentist Soc. Sec. or T.I.N. (see reverse**)	25. Dentist license no.	26. Dentist phone no.	33. If prosthesis, is this initial placement?	(If no, reason for replacement)	34. Date of prior placement

27. First visit date current series	28. Place of treatment Office Hosp. ECF Other	29. Radiographs or models enclosed?	No	Yes	How many?	35. Is treatment for orthodontics?	If service already commenced enter:	Date appliances placed	Mos. treatment remaining

36. Identify missing teeth with "x"	37. Examination and treatment plan – List in order from tooth no. 1 through tooth no. 32 – Using charting system shown.						For administrative use only

		Tooth # or letter	Surface	Description of service (including x-rays, prophylaxis, materials used, etc.)	Date service performed Mo. Day Year	Procedure number	Fee	

38. Remarks for unusual services

39. I hereby certify that the procedures as indicated by date have been completed and that the fees submitted are the actual fees I have charged and intend to collect for those procedures. Signed (Treating Dentist) License Number Date	41. **Total Fee Charged**	
	42. **Payment by other plan**	
40. Address where treatment was performed City State Zip	Max. Allowable	
	Deductible	
	Carrier %	
	Carrier pays	
	Patient pays	

©**American Dental Association, 1994**
J510 (Same as ADA Dental Claim Form - J504, J511, J512)

Figure 25.5 Dental claim form. (Courtesy of The American Dental Association.)

Pathophysiology of the Mouth

Mouth Diseases and Disorders

abscess (ăb-sĕs)   localized pus collection.

anodontia (ăn-ō-dŏn-shē-ă)   without teeth.

bruxism (brŭk-sĭzm)   grinding of teeth, especially at night.

calculus (kăl-kū-lŭs)   hardened plaque deposits at base of teeth (tartar).

Candida albicans (kăn-dĭ-dă ăl-bĭ-kăns)   "thrush," a yeast infection in the mouth.

caries (kār-ēz)   cavities.

edentulous, edentia (ē-dĕnt-ū-lŭs, ē-dĕn-shē-ă)   same as *anodontia*, without teeth.

gingivitis (jĭn-jĭ-vī-tĭs)   inflammation of the gums (gingivae).

impaction (ĭm-păk-shŭn)   tooth embedded in alveolus so that eruption is prevented; requires extraction, usually with anesthesia.

leukoplakia (lū-kō-plā-kē-ă)   white spots or patches on mucous membranes of cheek and/or tongue; may become malignant; leukoplakia buccalis (cheek) or lingualis (tongue).

malocclusion (măl-ŏ-klū-zhŭn)   poor alignment of teeth; may require braces.

neoplasms (nē-ō-plăzms)   malignant growth in oral cavity.

odontalgia, dentalgia (ō-dŏn-tăl-jē-ă, dĕn-tăl-jē-ă)   toothache.

plaque (plăk)   in dentistry, sticky mass of microorganisms that grows on crown of tooth and erodes the gums and bone.

pyorrhea (pī-ŏr-rē-ă)   gum disease with pus pocket formation around tooth; the primary cause of tooth loss.

TMJ (temporomandibular joint) disorder or **dysfunction** (tĕm-pō-rō-măn-dĭb-ū-lăr)   bones of temple and jaw malaligned.

xerostomia (zē-rō-stō-mē-ă)   dry mouth, may aggravate dental problems.

Dental Practice

preventive dentistry   prophylactic care.

regular, periodic dental checkups   including radiographs and fluoride treatments, removal of plaque, examination of oral mucosa, tongue, and cheek for any abnormalities.

> **brushing, flossing, plaque-disclosing agents, limiting sugar intake**
>
> **sealants**   a clear or shaded plastic material that is applied to protect the chewing surfaces of the back teeth (e.g., premolars and molars) from decay.

restorative dentistry

> **fillings**   amalgam, porcelain, gold, silver alloy.
>
> **bonding**   to smooth rough edges, small "chips," or to protect eroded or discolored enamel.
>
> **inlays, crowns, bridgework, caps**
>
> **whitening agents**   cosmetic.
>
> **dentures (prosthodontics)**   partial or full upper, lower.

implantation   setting a tooth into the socket after injury or replacing a lost tooth with an artificial tooth.

dental anesthesia   topical (applied to surface area), local injection, general anesthesia, hypnosis.

Specialists

See the detailed list in Chapter 5, Dental Practitioners and Specialists.

Miscellaneous Terms

alveolectomy (ăl-vē-ŏ-**lĕk**-tō-mē) surgical removal of part of alveolar bone (jaw).

commercial dental laboratory impressions are sent to such a lab instead of being made up in dentist's office.

dental chart teeth are numbered and notation made regarding each tooth condition (see Figure 25.5).

disclosing products exposes areas not being brushed adequately.

exodontia extraction.

extraction surgical procedures to remove tooth.

fissure in dentistry, a groove in tooth enamel.

gingivectomy or gingivoplasty (jĭn-jĭ-**vĕk**-tō-mē, **jĭn**-jĭ-vō-plăs-tē) gum surgery.

impressions molds made by dentist; from these a cast is made in preparation for inlay, crown, and so on.

oral mucosa (ōr-ăl mū-**kō**-să) mucous membranes of mouth including palate, cheek surfaces, tongue.

palate roof of the mouth, hard and soft portions.

rubber dam used by some dentists to cover everything but the tooth on which work is being done.

suction device to keep mouth area dry of saliva during procedures.

sulcus (**sŭl**-kŭs) in dentistry, gum area between teeth.

Current Dental Concerns

Dental personnel need to be concerned with the danger of transmission of AIDS—and, more likely, hepatitis, because hepatitis can be transmitted in saliva. Use of disposable gloves, eyeglasses, and masks is mandatory for dental personnel. Careful sterilization of all nondisposable equipment is essential.

Worksheet

Fill in the blank:

1. Nearsightedness is also called ____myopia____

2. The instrument for measuring pressure within the eyeball is the _____

3. The abbreviation for the right eye is _____; for both or each eye _____; for the left eye _____; for the right ear _____

4. The medical term for a clouded lens is _____

5. Tear glands and ducts are part of the _____ apparatus.

6. Side vision is called _____

7. The specialist who treats refractive errors with glasses (not an MD) is _____

8. Ear wax is also called _____

9. Give two terms meaning "eardrum" _____

10. Inflammation of the middle ear is called _____

11. Tubes from middle ear to pharynx are the _____

12. The machine used to measure hearing ability is the _____

13. _____ is the unit of measure for sound.

14. The nerve to the ear is the _____ nerve.

15. Excision of the mastoid is _____

16. Incision into the eardrum is _____ or _____

17. Plastic surgery on the outer ear is_____

18. People who need reading glasses to see printed material have _____

19. Any disease of the retina is called _____

20. Inflammation of the mucous membrane of the eye is called _____

Identify:

21. ophthalmologist   MD or DO eye specialist_____

22. otologist _____

23. ENT _____

24. lacrimation _____

25. strabismus _____

26. enucleation _____

Define:

27. glaucoma _____

_____

28. accommodation _____

29. PERLA _____

30. otoscope _____

31. papilledema _____

32. conjunctivitis _____

33. amblyopia _____

34. ophthalmoscope _____

35. cerumen _____

36. topical _____

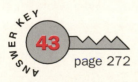
ANSWER KEY 43 page 272

Worksheet

Fill in the blank:

1. Tartar around the base of the teeth is called _plaque_ _____

2. Inflammation of the gums may be called _____ or _____

3. Baby teeth are called _____ because they _____

4. False teeth are called _____

5. TMJ stands for _____

Identify:

6. DDS _Doctor of Dental Surgery_ _____

7. orthodontist _____

8. restorative dentistry _____

9. caries _____

10. malocclusion _____

11. impaction (dental) _____

12. buccal _____

13. incisors _____

14. bruxism _____

15. plaque _____
    _____

16. How many teeth are in a full set (minus the wisdom teeth)? _____

17. How many teeth comprise the baby set? _____

18. Name three dental specialists _____
    _____

19. Good prophylactic dental care includes _____
    _____

20. The crown of a tooth is composed of _____

21. What is the name of the teeth that are also called premolars? _____

22. What do disclosing products do? _____
    _____

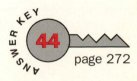

ANSWER KEY 44 page 272

Test Part 1 p. 361, Part 2 p. 363

■ Case Histories ■

CASE HISTORY 22

REPORT OF OPERATION: Cataract extraction

Preoperative dx   cataract, right eye.

Postoperative dx   same.

Operation   cataract extraction, right eye.

Description   The right eye was prepared and draped in the usual sterile fashion for ocular surgery and 10 minutes of ocular massage done to soften the eye. Next, lid drapes and speculum were placed, and the intraocular pressure checked and found to be less than 10 mmHg. A superior rectus fixation suture was placed of 4–0* black silk and a fornix-based conjunctival flap prepared. Next, limbal groove was made with a 64 Beaver blade at the surgical limbus and the anterior chamber entered at 12 o'clock with a Sparta blade. A 180-degree corneal scleral section was then done with scissors and two postplaced 10–0 nylon sutures inserted superiorly and looped out of the way. Peripheral iridectomy was done at 2 o'clock with peripheral iridotomy at 10 o'clock. *Zolyse* was placed into the posterior chamber and irrigated after one minute.

The cataractous lens was extracted with the Amoils cryophake without difficulty or vitreous loss. The two nylon sutures were drawn up and tied and *Miochol* and an air bubble placed in the anterior chamber. Next a total of seven more interrupted 10–0 nylon sutures were used to close the wound. An air bubble and balanced salt solution was placed in the anterior chamber and the wound tested for tightness. Finding it to be so, the rectus suture was removed and the conjunctiva repaired with two wing sutures of 8–0 chromic. Atropine 1% drops were placed on the cornea along with some *Maxitrol* ointment, the eye doubly patched, and the patient returned to the recovery room in good condition. There were no complications.

CASE HISTORY 23

REPORT OF OPERATION: Tympanoplasty

Preoperative dx chronic erythema and edema with pain of the ear canal skin and drum.

Postoperative dx same as above.

Operation   tympanoplasty with resection of canal skin and drum and grafts.

Procedure With appropriate premedication, the patient was taken to the operating room and placed in the supine position and given general endotracheal anesthesia. The left ear was placed uppermost and prepped with Betadine and draped in routine fashion. Inspection disclosed erythema of the handle of the malleus and of the posterior two-thirds of the drum, with marked thickening, perhaps three to four times its normal size. The skin also has raised ridges on the posterior quadrant and bleeding of the posterior canal wall.

A retroauricular incision was made, with deepening to the temporalis fascia, a large segment of which was taken and allowed to dry. The canal skin was elevated from the retroauricular position and then incised at the level of the fibrous annulus and elevated anteriorly. The drum was elevated from the fibrous annulus. The fibrous annulus was allowed to remain intact, and the drum posteriorly was resected to the anterior margin of the handle of the malleus. Care was taken to dissect it cleanly off the malleus by sharp dissection; the lateral process of the malleus was also dissected off. In entry into the mastoid cortex, I found a small black piece of material, which was of undetermined origin, that measured approximately 0.5 cm. It seemed very hard. This may be the foreign body of which he was complaining. It was sent to pathology, and the immediate report was that it was nonspecific material.

The temporalis fascia segment was rehydrated and placed on a bed of Gelfoam and Hydeltrasol and clipped with Wegner's microclips to the anterior tympanic membrane remnant and led out the posterior

---

*The zero is referred to as "aught," so in dictation this is "four aught."

canal wall. The posterior skin was then draped over this, and a parachute dressing of Owen's silk was applied through the canal. The retroauricular incision was closed with 4–0 chromic and 6–0 nylon, continuously locked, with a rubber band drain led off the inferior segment of the wound. A mastoid dressing was applied. He was then awakened and returned to the recovery room in good condition.

CASE HISTORY 24

CONSULTATION: Dental examination

Routine examination. Last dental work completed approximately two years ago. General oral condition good. Apparent gingival irritation in upper right quadrant.

This patient was referred to me for a consultation by her physician. She is a 50-year-old female, divorced, mother of two married daughters. She appears to be in good health. She gives a history of some burning of the mouth and lips ever since a bridge was placed in November, two years ago. The bridge replaced tooth #7, resting on the lingual of a previously constructed ¾ crown on #8. Previous to that time she had worn the ¾ crown on #8 for many years. The burning is most severe late in the day.

Oral examination shows an apparently healthy mouth with no evidence of irritation. The tissue has a healthy pink appearance. The bridge is well constructed. There are seven silver amalgam restorations in the mouth which she says have been in for many years. None of these contact the bridge. Previous treatments have been given by dentists and physicians and they included injections of vitamin B. No relief was obtained.

My immediate reaction to her problem is that it is of systemic origin and unrelated to the dental work. The timing, its occurrence at the time the last bridge was placed, may be coincidental. As a beginning, laboratory tests to determine her hydrochloric acid level are recommended. If the tests are negative, I would suggest the removal of the plastic facing from the bridge first; then removal of the silver amalgam restorations, as they are small and no great expense would be involved. This would give a positive test regarding the electrolytic action.

■ **Assignment:** After reading these cases, list any words new to you. Define them.

▲ Health Promotion Tips

To prevent eye and ear disorders, familiarize yourself with the risk factors and symptomatology. Early assessment and intervention are the keys to optimal health.

Eyes

Glaucoma risk factors:
- Family history of diabetes or glaucoma
- 40 years of age or greater
- Past eye trauma
- Current steroid use
- African ancestry

Cataract risk factors:
- Eye trauma
- Extreme heat exposure
- Radiation exposure
- Heredity
- 60 years of age or greater

Symptoms of glaucoma:
- Impairment or loss of side vision
- Sudden or gradual visual dimness
- No pain (or severe eye pain)
- Colored halos seen around bright objects

Symptoms of cataracts:
- Blurred or double vision
- Need to read closer to book than usual for focus

Ears

Otitis media risk factors:
- Child age 0–5 years (especially)
- History of URI (upper respiratory infection), allergies, or depressed immune response
- Family history of sinusitis or URI
- Group environment (such as child care or school) with more than two children under the age of 5 years
- Smoke exposure

Symptoms of otitis media:
- Ear pain or pressure
- Poor auditory response
- Febrile
- Difficulty sleeping
- Irritability
- Exudate or blood draining from ear (not yellow or tan cerumen)
- There may be no symptoms

CHAPTER 26

Endocrine System and Stress Response

Anatomy and Physiology of the Endocrine System

Function

The endocrine system regulates body activity and, together with the nervous system, helps maintain homeostasis.

Anatomical Terms

All of the organs in the endocrine system are glands (see Figure 26.1). They are called *ductless glands* (or glands of internal secretion) because they have no ducts. (A duct is a narrow tube that carries secretions.) Ductless glands secrete hormones internally, *directly into the bloodstream*, instead of into ducts. Hormones affect many body functions.

Endocrine glands	*Location, Function*
pituitary (pĭ-**tū**-ĭ-tār-ē)　(**hy *poph* ysis**; anterior and posterior)	deep in cranial cavity; called the master gland, as it affects all others.
thyroid (**thī**-rŏyd)　(shaped like a shield)	aside and in front of larynx (neck); alters metabolic rate and secretes thyroxine (high in iodine).
parathyroids (păr-ă-**thī**-rŏydz)　(four)	behind thyroid; regulate calcium and phosphorus content of blood and bones.
adrenals (ă-**drē**-năls)　(cortex, outer; medulla, inner)	one atop each kidney; secrete steroids (corticoids) and catecholamines and help body cope with stress.
pancreas (**păn**-krē-ăs)	behind stomach; controls use of sugar and starch. Islets of Langerhans' beta cells secrete insulin.
sex glands (gonads) (**gō**-năds)	ovaries secrete estrogens and progesterone; testes secrete testosterone.
pineal gland (**pĭn**-ē-ăl)	base of brain; still being researched, produces melatonin, which may affect the body's day/night cycles.
thymus (**thī**-mŭs)	pleural cavity (mediastinum); decreases in size in adult (may have some function in immune responses).

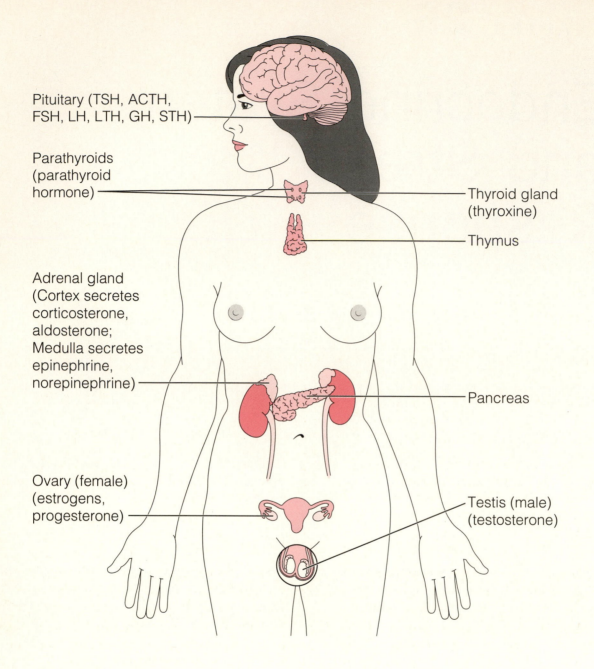

Pituitary (TSH, ACTH, FSH, LH, LTH, GH, STH)

Parathyroids (parathyroid hormone)

Thyroid gland (thyroxine)

Thymus

Adrenal gland (Cortex secretes corticosterone, aldosterone; Medulla secretes epinephrine, norepinephrine)

Pancreas

Ovary (female) (estrogens, progesterone)

Testis (male) (testosterone)

Figure 26.1 Endocrine glands, small but very important ductless glands that secrete hormones directly into the bloodstream. Hormones produced are shown in parentheses. (See abbreviations for each of the pituitary hormones in Appendix H).

Pathophysiology of the Endocrine System

Endocrine System Diseases and Disorders

Endocrine diseases occur when a gland secretes too much or too little hormone, as listed here. Descriptions follow.

Hypersecretion	**Hyposecretion**
Pituitary 　　Acro **meg** aly 　　Gi **gant** ism	Dwarfism (congenital) Simmonds' (adults)
Thyroid 　　Exoph **thal** mic or toxic 　　goiter (Graves' disease)	Goiter (simple) due to lack of iodine **Cre** tinism (children) Myxe **de** ma (adults)
Parathyroids 　　Loss of calcium from bones (increased fragility)	Tetany (low calcium level); neuromuscular 　　hyperexcitability
Adrenals 　　Cushing's (cortex hormone) 　　Pheochromocy **to** ma (medulla)	Addison's disease
Pancreas 　　Hypogly **ce** mia	Dia **be** tes $\genfrac{}{}{0pt}{}{\text{mel } \mathbf{li} \text{ tus}}{\mathbf{mel} \text{ litus}}$ (both pronunciations used)
Ovaries and testes 　　Overdevelopment of sex characteristics	Inability to carry through a pregnancy

acromegaly (ăk-rō-**měg**-ă-lē)   enlarged and distorted extremities and face, especially the jaw; monsterlike appearance; partial hypophy **sec** tomy or radiotherapy are treatments of choice.

Addison's disease (**ād**-dĭs-ŏnz)   weakness, weight loss, jaundice, hypoglycemia; treatment is with cortisone.

cretinism (in children) (**krē**-tĭn-ĭzm)   slow, physically and mentally; treatment is with thy **rox** ine.

Cushing's disease (**kŭsh**-ĭngs)   weak, obese, hypertensive, hyperglycemic, moon facies (moon face, edematous); if caused by tumor, treatment is adrenalectomy.

diabetes mellitus (dī-ă-**bē**-tēz měl-**lī**-tŭs)   poly **dip** sia (thirst), poly **u** ria, weakness, and fatigue are early symptoms; see discussion later in this chapter; treatment is with diet, oral hypoglycemic drugs, insulin.

exophthalmic goiter (ĕks-ŏf-**thăl**-mĭk **gŏy**-tĕr)   (Graves' disease or toxic goiter); swelling of the thyroid gland in neck; tachy **car** dia, weight loss, protruding eyes, diapho **re** sis, shaking, mental symptoms; treatment is with surgery or antithyroid drugs.

goiter (simple) (**gŏy**-tĕr)   swollen thyroid caused by lack of iodine in diet; treatment is with iodine.

hypoglycemia (hī-pō-glī-**sē**-mē-ă)   an abnormally low blood glucose level. Two types: reactive, in response to a meal or drugs; and spontaneous, in the fasting state. Reactive type involves rapid absorption of glucose and a subsequent outpouring of excessive insulin, often seen after gastric resection. Reactive hypoglycemia due to delayed insulin response is seen in some mild Type II (non-insulin-dependent) diabetics and may be the first indication of diabetes mellitus. Functional hypoglycemia, following a carbohydrate load, is also seen, and the cause is unknown.

myxedema (mĭks-ĕ-**dē**-mă)   obesity, sluggishness, dry puffy skin due to mucous accumulations under skin; myx/o means "mucous"; treatment is with thyroxine.

pheochromocytoma (fē-ō-krō-mō-sī-**tō**-mă)   *"pheochromo"* means "dusky color"; a tumor of the adremal medulla, producing hypertension, weight loss, personality changes, diaphor **e** sis, tachy **car** dia; treatment is with surgery and antihypertensive medications.

Simmonds' disease (**sĭm**-mŏnds)   atrophy of the pituitary, causes exhaustion, emaciation, cachexia; treatment is with various hormones whose release is dependent upon pituitary function.

tetany (**tĕt**-ă-nē)   severe muscle and nerve weakness causing spasm, twitching, convulsions; opis **thot** onos (severe arching of back type of spasm); treatment is with calcium.

Tests for Endocrine Function

Blood chemistry tests are done to determine the amount of a particular hormone in a blood sample. Urinalysis (especially 24-hour urine tests) are used in many cases. X-ray examination may be helpful in diagnosing tumors of glands. The most frequently used tests are:

thyroid function studies T_3 and T_4; PBI (protein-bound iodine) and BMR (basal metabolism rate) are older tests (new tests for thyroid function rapidly replace older ones); RAIU (radioactive iodine uptake); thyroid scan; ultrasound (ech **og** raphy); needle biopsy.

pancreatic function studies   GTT (glucose tolerance test), FBS (fasting blood sugar), PP blood (postprandial, after meal), urinalysis.

Specialists

Specialists who deal with the endocrine system are endocrinologists and internists.

Miscellaneous Terms

acidosis (ăs-ĭ-**dō**-sĭs)   disturbance of acid-base balance; accumulation of acids or excessive loss of bicarbonate (diabetic coma).

anorexia (ăn-ō-**rĕk**-sē-ă)   loss of appetite.

cachexia (kă-**kĕks**-ē-ă)   a state of malnutrition and wasting, emaci **a** tion.

cataract (**kăt**-ă-răkt)   clouding of the lens of the eye; surgical extraction is the treatment.

convulsions (kŏn-**vŭl**-zhŭns)   involuntary muscular contractions.

diaphoresis (dī-ă-fō-**rē**-sĭs)   excessive perspiring.

emaciation (ē-mā-sē-**ā**-shŭn)   wasting; extremely thin condition.

gangrene (**găng**-grēn)   death of tissue due to inadequate circulation; amputation is the treatment.

gestational diabetes (jĕs-**tā**-shŭn-ăl)   increased maternal insulin produced due to placental hormones.

gland   any organ that secretes something; glands that are not "endocrine" are "exocrine" (sweat and salivary glands, for example).

hypophysectomy (hī-pŏf-ĭ-**sĕk**-tō-mē)   excision of pituitary gland, partial usually; may be done through sphenoid bone at the base of the frontal lobe (transphenoidal hypophysectomy).

insulin (**ĭn**-sū-lĭn)   first produced for commercial use in 1923; an antidiabetic hormone made from a combination of beef and pork sources. Regular insulin is short-acting; Protamine Zinc & Iletin, NPH Iletin, and Lente are names for longer-acting types. Insulin syringes are special types of syringes, U-40, U-80, U-100, for the different concentrations (units) of insulin. A portable insulin pump has become available and can be worn by the diabetic; it delivers a constant supply of insulin to the patient.

ketosis (kē-**tō**-sĭs)   accumulation of ketone bodies due to incomplete metabolism of fatty acids (consumption of more fat than can be burned completely by the body; the unburned fats produce an acid chemical substance called ketone); excessive ketone produces a form of acidosis in diabetics (vinegary odor to the breath).

neuropathy (nū-rŏp-ă-thē)   any disease of nerves, often observed in diabetes. Examples are loss of Achilles tendon reflex; sensory disorders, such as increased sensation (hyperes **the** sia), peculiar sensations (pares **the** sia), or loss of feeling, especially in lower extremities; footdrop, and so on; **im** potency; postural hypotension.

oral medications (hypoglycemic) (hī-pō-glī-**sē**-mĭk)   medications used by some non-insulin-dependent diabetics; these drugs are not insulin; many physicians feel they are not useful.

Diabetes Mellitus

Diabetes mellitus is the major disease of the endocrine system. There are two major types: Type I (insulin-dependent or IDDM), in which insulin is not produced, and Type II (non-insulin-dependent, or NIDDM), in which not enough insulin is produced or the insulin produced cannot be used by the body. One theory is that interaction between sugar and insulin takes place in cells called insulin receptors. These receptors also attract fat and can only accommodate fat *or* insulin. Fat gets to receptors first, and insulin has nowhere to go.

Long-Term Complications

Diabetes is the leading cause of new cases of blindness (reti **nop** athy and cataract). It is the major cause of kidney disease and neurologic disorders, cardiovascular mortality, peripheral vascular disorders, impotence, nonaccidental amputation, problems in pregnancy, and psychologic damage. In general, diabetes increases susceptibility to infection, so that even minor lesions can lead to gangrene. Elevated blood glucose makes it difficult for diabetics to heal properly.

diet, exercise, and normal weight maintenance   These are important issues in diabetes. This is a chronic, incurable disease; it *can* be controlled in most cases. A "brittle" diabetic is one whose condition is difficult to control (suddenly fluctuates between high and low levels of blood glucose).

drugs   Insulin (many types) must be injected, at least daily, in insulin-dependent patients (more often in some cases). Oral drugs do not replace insulin and can only be used in Type II diabetes. Their use is controversial presently. Some physicians feel that patients who do not require insulin can do just as well with diet and exercise as with the pills.

insulin pump   This is a device worn by the patient (implanted or attached to belt). It dispenses insulin automatically as the body's need arises. It holds about a two-week supply.

urine and blood tests for sugar (used by patients at home)   tablets and dipsticks are occasionally used for urine testing; self-monitoring capillary blood testing is done with an automated spring-loaded lancet to prick finger (such as Glucometer); with both urine and blood tests, visual comparison is made with a color chart (trace, 1-plus up to 4-plus).

Hb A$_{lc}$ test   measures how much sugar attaches to red blood cell's protein during a three-month period. It is important because high blood sugar for a prolonged period may cause damage to blood vessels, thereby increasing risk of complications.

Short-Term Complications

	Diabetic coma (not enough insulin; blood sugar high)	Insulin shock (too much insulin; blood sugar low)
Symptoms	Slow onset, polyuria, thirst, anorexia, nausea, flushed dry skin, deep breathing, abdominal pain, low blood pressure and eyeball tension, air hunger, "sweet" fruity/acetone breath	Sudden onset, double vision, hunger, nervousness, dizziness, moist/cold pale skin, shallow breathing, mental confusion with unusual behavior
Treatment	Insulin	Food, juice, candy
Recovery	Slow	Rapid

Either of the above can proceed to death if not treated in time. Patients who take insulin must learn to recognize early signs and seek necessary treatment.

Stress

stressor   a pressure, force, or strain on a system; may be real or perceived as real.

eustress   "good" stress that increases a person's health or performance.

distress   "excessive" and/or "difficult" stress. Compromises the body's ability to defend itself from all diseases, especially stress that remains unabated for long periods, sometimes longer than required to confront the stressor. Signs of distress may include the following dimensions: mood (irritability, insomnia, feeling uncomfortable, insecure, or worried), visceral (symptoms include chills, nausea, vomiting, diarrhea, vertigo, or tinnitus), musculoskeletal (trembling, muscle tension, twitching of muscles).

stress response   how a body responds to stressors.

target organ   any organ affected by stress; one person may have intestinal disorders such as diarrhea, another may have skin reactions such as hives.

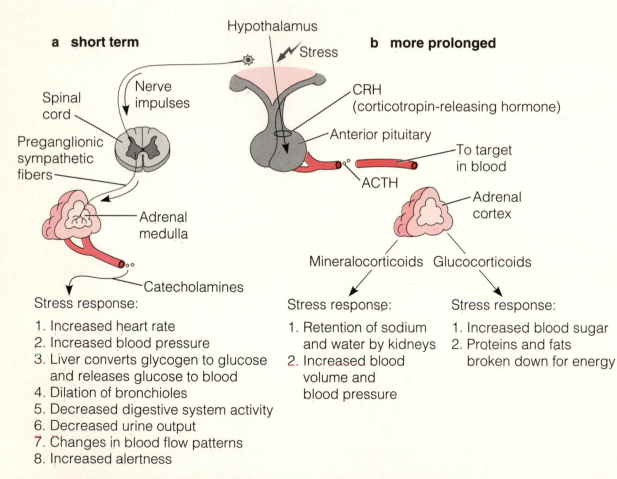

Figure 26.2   Stress and the adrenal gland. Stressful stimuli cause the hypothalamus to activate the adrenal medulla via sympathetic nerve impulses and the adrenal cortex via hormonal signals. (**a**) The medulla mediates short-term responses to stress by secreting catecholamines (epinephrine and norepinephrine). (**b**) The cortex controls more prolonged responses by secreting its steroid hormones.

Worksheet

Fill in the blank:

1. Hormones are secreted only by ___*endocrine*___ glands.

2. Another name for glands of internal secretion or endocrine glands is _____

3. The male hormone is called _____ ;

   and female hormones are _____ and _____

4. Describe the location of the following:

   pituitary gland _____

   _____

   thyroid gland _____

   _____

   Islets of Langerhans _____

   _____

5. Name two tests for thyroid function: _____

   _____

6. Name two tests for glucose (blood tests): _____

   _____

7. _____ is essential for thyroid function.

8. The hormone secreted by pancreas special cells is _____

9. In diabetic coma, the onset is _____

   and the treatment is _____

10. The treatment for insulin shock is _____

11. A goiter is an enlarged _____

12. Sometimes a blood test is done after a meal instead of during fasting. The term for a test done two

    hours after eating is _____

13. In endocrine disorders, the gland is usually producing too much or not enough. The words for this are

    _____ and _____

14. The pancreas is located _____

15. Excision of the pancreas is called _____

16. Another name for the pituitary is _____

17. In acromegaly (pituitary dysfunction), the _____ are enlarged.

18. Some other diseases of the endocrine system not mentioned in this worksheet are _____

    _____ and _____

19. Name the frequent complications in diabetes: _____

20. Define:

a. hypophysectomy   *excision of pituitary* _____

b. neuropathy _____

c. diaphoresis _____

d. goiter _____

e. tachycardia _____

f. cataract _____

g. anorexia _____

h. cachexia _____

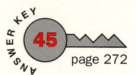

ANSWER KEY **45** page 272

Test p. 365
Alternate test p. 367

■ Case History ■

CASE HISTORY 25

ADMISSION NOTE: Cataract and vitreous hemorrhage

HISTORY AND PHYSICAL

Present Illness Patient is a 79-year-old male who underwent cataract surgery to his left eye in 1985 and had excellent vision results recorded recently. Approximately 1 month ago, he lost the vision in his left eye while straining to dig a ditch from his wheelchair. He saw a large red blob with streaks of black in his visual field followed by flashes of light. Since that time he has no clearing evident in his visual acuity, which is obscured by a diagnosed vitreous hemorrhage. He has poor vision in his right eye due to a dense cataract.

Past History Amputations of both legs due to diabetic small vessel disease. Hernia surgery, fractured hip. Medications: 26 U of NPH insulin daily. Allergies: penicillin. General health: He is an alert, active person considering his advanced years and his disability is coincident with the below-the-knee amputations bilaterally.

Ocular Exam Vision in the right eye is light perception only due to a dense cataract and what was found on B-scan ultrasonography to be a scatter of intermittent echoes, suggesting vitreous hemorrhaging in the right eye. The left eye had vision of hand motion with light projection into all four quadrants. There is a full superior iridectomy, and the left eye shows no evidence of rubeosis. Intraocular pressures are 18 and 14 in the right and left eyes respectively. Fundus examination of the left eye reveals white stalklike emanating tissue from the region of the optic nerve obscuring all fundus view. The ultrasonography of the left eye reveals multiple linear echoes suggestive of vitreous bands and hemorrhage, but there is no evidence of retinal detachment on the B-scan dynamically or in the photographs.

Impression Cataract, right eye, with probable vitreous hemorrhage. Vitreous hemorrhage, left eye. Surgical aphakia, left eye.

The patient is to undergo vitrectomy via the pars plana under general anesthesia February 20. (The pars plana is the thin part of the ciliary body, called the ciliary disk; it connects the choroid and the iris.)

■ **Assignment:** Now that you have read this case, underline and define new words. This case provides good examples of diabetic complications and eye terminology.

▲ **Health Promotion Tip**

As we learned earlier in this chapter, *eustress* is the "good" stress that helps your body gear up for a challenge. Once this challenge is met, however, there is potential for your body to feel *distress*. In order to prevent this potential physical distress, try the following exercises:

- Tell yourself that the stress is over and no longer real.
- Do progressive muscle relaxation exercises.
- Engage in some type of physical activity, such as a brisk 30-minute walk.

For a prolonged stressor, the second and third steps are also helpful.

These cognitive and environmental coping techniques can prevent the activation of target organ distress caused by prolonged stress.

APPENDIX **A**

Answer Keys

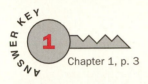

Chapter 1, p. 3

1. a word part, at the beginning of a word (can change the word to opposite meaning). **2.** a word part, at the end of a word. **3.** main part of a word, to which may be added a prefix, a suffix, or another root word. (In medicine, many root words are derived from Latin, Greek, etc.) **4.** two or more root words plus suffix. **5.** root word plus /o used when two or more root words are combined. **6.** before maturity or ahead of time. **7.** excessively active. **8.** study or science of the "mind." **9.** excision of tonsils. **10.** inflammation of the bronchial tubes. **11.** instrument for looking at microscopic objects. **12.** treatment with water. **13.** infection in lungs and bronchial tubes. **14.** pertaining to heart and vessels. **15.** pertaining to stomach and intestines. **16.** "without blood" (low red blood count). **17.** to cut out. **18.** excessive amount of urine. **19.** the study of the structure of the body. **20.** inflammation in sac around heart (peri = around).

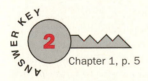

Chapter 1, p. 5

1. excision of the tonsils. **2.** excision of the appendix. **3.** excision of the adenoids. **4.** excision of the thyroid gland. **5.** excision of the spleen. **6.** excision of the

uterus (womb). **7.** excision of the gallbladder. **8.** excision of hemorrhoids (commonly called piles), actually are varicose veins at anal opening. **9.** excision of the gums (dental surgery for diseased gums). **10.** removal of breast. **11.** excision of the adrenal gland. **12.** excision of the pancreas. **13.** excision of the colon (large intestine). **14.** excision of a nerve. **15.** excision of the duodenum (first part of small intestine, follows stomach). **16.** excision of the larynx (watch pronunciation: lărinks). **17.** excision of the ureter (tubes from kidney to the bladder). **18.** excision of the stomach. **19.** excision of the cervix (of the uterus; extends down into vagina). **20.** excision of the eardrum (tympanum). **21.** excision of the ovary. **22.** excision of the urinary bladder or cystic duct of the gallbladder; can also mean excision of a cyst.

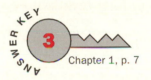

Chapter 1, p. 7

1. tonsillectomy. **2.** adenoidectomy. **3.** thyroidectomy. **4.** adrenalectomy. **SPELL: (5–20) 5.** appendectomy. **6.** hysterectomy. **7.** hemorrhoidectomy. **8.** colectomy. **9.** laryngectomy. **10.** gastrectomy. **11.** cervicectomy.* **12.** tympanectomy. **13.** cholecystectomy. **14.** cystectomy. **15.** mastectomy. **16.** splenectomy. **17.** neurectomy. **18.** duodenectomy. **19.** odontectomy. **20.** pancreatectomy. **21.** cutting out. **22.** cutting into.

---

* The word *cervix* means "neck". The neck of the uterus, or the part that extends down into the vagina, is the cervix. The vertebrae in the neck are also called *cervical* vertebrae.

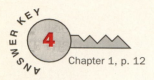

4 Chapter 1, p. 12

SPELL: (1–12) **1.** adenoidectomy: excision of adenoids. **2.** gingivectomy: excision of gum tissue. **3.** splenectomy: excision of spleen. **4.** gastrectomy: excision of stomach. **5.** cholecystectomy: excision of gallbladder. **6.** laryngectomy: excision of larynx. **7.** lobectomy: excision of lobe of lung. **8.** pancreatectomy: excision of pancreas. **9.** duodenectomy: excision of duodenum. **10.** nephrectomy: excision of kidney. **11.** neurectomy: excision of a nerve. **12.** oophorectomy: excision of an ovary. **13.** thyroidectomy. **14.** adrenalectomy. **15.** hysterectomy. **16.** tonsillectomy. **17.** hemorrhoidectomy. **18.** appendectomy. **Extra:** tonsillectomy and adenoidectomy.

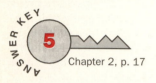

5 Chapter 2, p. 17

1. new permanent opening into the colon. **2.** new permanent opening into the stomach. **3.** new permanent opening into the ileum. **4.** new permanent opening into the trachea. **5.** new permanent opening into the bladder. **6.** new permanent opening into the intestine. **7.** new permanent opening into the jejunum. **8.** incision into the abdomen. **9.** incision into the trachea. **10.** incision into a vein. **11.** incision into the stomach. **12.** incision into the bladder. **13.** incision into a lobe. **14.** herniorrhaphy, nephrorrhaphy, and so on. **15.** nephropexy, salpingopexy, and so on. **16.** rhinoplasty, arthroplasty, and so on. **17.** lithotripsy, neurotripsy, and so on. **18.** abdominocentesis, thoracocentesis, and so on.

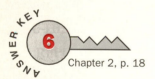

6 Chapter 2, p. 18

1. gastrectomy. **2.** tracheostomy. **3.** cystotomy. **4.** arthroplasty. **5.** nephropexy. **6.** oophorectomy. **7.** neurotripsy. **8.** ileostomy. **9.** colostomy. **10.** cholecystectomy. **11.** thoracocentesis (or thoracentesis). **12.** herniorrhaphy. **13.** arthrocentesis. **SPELL: (14–23)** **14.** appendectomy: excision of appendix. **15.** gastrotomy: incision into stomach. **16.** abdominocentesis: "tapping" of abdomen to remove fluid. **17.** salpingectomy: excision of fallopian tube. **18.** tracheotomy: incision into trachea. **19.** nephropexy: fixation of kidney. **20.** splenectomy: excision of spleen. **21.** gastroduodenostomy:

new permanent opening between stomach and duodenum. **22.** herniorrhaphy: repair of a hernia. **23.** hysterectomy: excision of uterus.

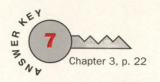

7 Chapter 3, p. 22

1. psychosis. **2.** appendicitis. **3.** neuralgia. **4.** cystocele. **5.** adenopathy. **6.** neurosis. **7.** menorrhagia. **8.** dermatitis. **9.** dentalgia. **10.** acidosis. **SPELL: (11–24)**. **11.** hysteropathy: any disease of the uterus. **12.** rectocele: hernia of rectum. **13.** myalgia: pain in muscles. **14.** nephrosis: condition of kidneys. **15.** hepatitis: inflammation of the liver. **16.** sclerosis: condition of "hardening." **17.** hemorrhage: heavy, uncontrollable bleeding. **18.** myodynia: pain in a muscle. **19.** otitis: inflammation of the ear. **20.** nephropathy: any disease of the kidney. **21.** peritonitis: inflammation of peritoneum. **22.** spondylopathy: any disease of vertebrae. **23.** dentodynia: pain in a tooth. **24.** atelectasis: incomplete dilatation of lung (collapse). **25.** redness, heat, swelling, pain.

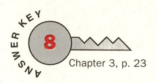

8 Chapter 3, p. 23

1. aseptic: "without sepsis," or in other words, sterile. (Aseptic technique is used in surgery.) **2.** afebrile: "without fever," or normal temperature. **3.** anemic: "without blood," condition in which there are not enough red blood cells. **4.** anesthesia: without feeling (local, regional or general anesthesia). **5.** arrhythmic: "without rhythm," such as the normal rhythm of the heartbeat. **6.** adduction: toward the midline of the body; the opposite of abduction. **7.** adhesion: a growing together of tissues that should not be connected. **8.** abduction: away from the midline of the body. **9.** abnormal: away from the "normal"; deviant in some way. **10.** anteflexion: bending forward or tipped forward (uterus anteflexed, for example). **11.** antibiotic: "against life" of the bacteria; a drug that inhibits or destroys bacterial life. **12.** antiseptic: "against sepsis" or contamination; combats contamination or infection. **13.** anticonvulsive: "against convulsions," a drug used to inhibit convulsions. **14.** antineoplastic: "against" new growths; drug used to treat cancerous growth. **15.** contraindicated: "not indicated," not advisable or recommended. (Certain drugs are contraindicated for diabetics, for example.) **16.** disease: "from ease," or the lack of ease; any abnormal entity. **17.** dysuria: painful urination. **18.** dysmenorrhea: painful menstruation. **19.** dysentery: "painful intestines," severe type of diarrhea.   **20.** dyspnea: difficult, labored breathing.   **21.** hemiplegia: "half paralyzed," one side of body paralyzed.   **22.** hypertension: high blood pressure.   **23.** hypertrophy: excessive growth.   **24.** hypoactive: low activity; sluggishness.   **25.** hypodermic: under dermis (skin) (as in hypodermic needle, for example).   **26.** intercostal: between the ribs (for example, intercostal muscles).   **27.** intramuscular: within a muscle (for example, many medications are injected intramuscularly).   **28.** intravenous: within the vein.   **29.** intrathecal: within spinal canal.   **30.** sepsis: a state of putrefaction (putrid); infected, contaminated, dirty.   **31.** bladder: any hollow sac, usually holds fluid.   **32.** hernia: a rupture or swelling; projection of an organ or a part from normal place.

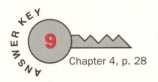

ANSWER KEY 9 Chapter 4, p. 28

1. otoscope, otoscopy.*   **2.** gastroscope, gastroscopy.   **3.** sigmoidoscope, sigmoidoscopy.   **4.** bronchoscope, bronchoscopy.   **5.** ophthalmoscope, ophthalmoscopy.   **6.** rectoscope, proctoscope, proctoscopy.   **7.** anoscope, anoscopy.   **8.** laparoscope, laparoscopy.   **9.** adenectomy.   **10.** appendicitis.   **11.** cardialgia.   **12.** cystocele.   **13.** hysteropathy.   **14.** arthroscope.   **15.** dermatome.   **16.** neurosis.   **17.** cholecystitis.   **18.** electrocardiograph.   **19.** myelogram.   **20.** thyroidectomy.   **21.** mammography.   **22.** nephritis.   **23.** cephalalgia.   **24.** electroencephalogram.   **25.** electromyogram.   **26.** colostomy.   **27.** pyelogram.   **28.** gastrectomy (partial or total).   **SPELL: (29–38)   29.** hemorrhage: uncontrolled bleeding.   **30.** angiogram: X-ray film of vessels (after dye is injected).   **31.** arthroscopy: looking into a joint with a lighted instrument.   **32.** electrocardiography: procedure of taking electrocardiogram.   **33.** echocardiogram: picture of heart action produced by using ultrasound.   **34.** ileostomy: new permanent opening into the ileum.   **35.** ophthalmoscope: instrument for looking into eye.   **36.** bronchoscopy: procedure using a bronchoscope.   **37.** stethoscope: instrument for listening.   **38.** hemiplegia: one side paralyzed.   **39.** instrument for dilating the opening of a cavity so that it can be seen. (Since there is no light attached to it, a flashlight or overhead lamp is used.) Examples are the *vaginal speculum,* used for pelvic exam, and the *nasal speculum,* used for examining interior of nostrils.

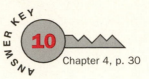

ANSWER KEY 10 Chapter 4, p. 30

1. thermometer.   **2.** adenitis.   **3.** neuralgia.   **4.** tonsillectomy.   **5.** ileostomy.   **6.** bronchoscopy.   **7.** electroencephalograph.   **8.** gastrectomy.   **9.** arthritis.   **10.** electrocardiogram.   **11.** speculum.   **12.** hysterectomy.   **13.** cholecystitis.   **14.** laparotomy.   **15.** nephrosis.   **16.** T.   **17.** F (for looking into the ear).   **18.** F (of the brain).   **19.** T.   **20.** T.   **21.** T.   **22.** F (may be external or internal bleeding).   **23.** T.   **24.** T.   **25.** T.   **26.** instrument used to make an opening larger.   **27.** instrument used to dilate a natural body orifice (vagina, anus, ear, nose).   **28.** instrument used to dilate a stricture (a part that has been closed off).   **29.** instrument to be introduced into a cavity or to dilate a stricture (to detect a foreign body).   **Extra:** *-ograph* suffix usually refers to a machine; in this word it means the X-ray picture.

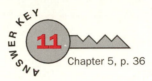

ANSWER KEY 11 Chapter 5, p. 36

1. internist, pediatrician.   **2.** gynecologist, internist.   **3.** urologist, internist, gynecologist (for women).   **4.** orthopedist.   **5.** surgeon.   **6.** allergist, internist, pediatrician.   **7.** dermatologist, internist, pediatrician.   **8.** otologist, otorhinolaryngologist, internist, pediatrician.   **9.** gastroenterologist, internist, pediatrician.   **10.** endocrinologist, internist, psychiatrist; also new specialty for obesity: bariatrics.   **11.** ophthalmologist.   **12.** obstetrician.   **13.** psychiatrist, internist.   **14.** cardiologist, internist.   **15.** internist, orthopedist, gerontologist.   **16.** internist, endocrinologist.   **17.** internist, surgeon, oncologist.   **18.** pediatrician, internist.   **19.** neurologist, internist.   **20.** ophthalmologist, neurologist.   **21.** physician still in training, doing practical work.   **22.** physician who has completed internship, usually getting more experience and may be working toward a specialty.   **23.** "one who practices."   **24.** physician (DO) who attends different kind of medical school than MD student, with more emphasis on the importance of the "skeleton," does some manipulative procedures.   **25.** A radiologist specializes in X-ray treatment and diagnosis.   **26.** An internist often treats children.   **27.** A referral to a medical specialist usually comes from a GP, pediatrician, or other specialist.   **28.** a variety of practitioners ranging from MDs to naturopaths.   **29.** hematologist.   **30.** pathologist.

---

*Accent is always on *os-* in *oscopy.* Pronounce the words in 1–8. Note pronunciations: ō-skōp (oscope), **ŏs**-kŏ-pē (oscopy)

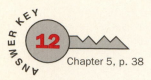

Chapter 5, p. 38

1. optometrist. 2. chiropractor. 3. podiatrist. 4. psychologist. 5. T. 6. T. 7. F. (Although an osteopath does some manipulation, this individual has more education and is qualified to do everything an MD does.) 8. T. 9. T. 10. T. 11. F. (There are "doctors" in every field, such as education and business.) 12. T. Examples * (name any ten). 13. internist, internal medicine: all nonsurgical cases; no obstetrics. 14. orthopedist, orthopedics: skeletal, muscular problems, fractures. 15. obstetrician, obstetrics: prenatal, delivery, postpartum. 16. gynecologist, gynecology: diseases of female reproductive system. 17. urologist, urology: urinary tract, diseases of male reproductive system. 18. cardiologist, cardiology: heart and vessels. 19. endocrinologist, endocrinology: disease of endocrine system; glands. 20. oncologist, oncology: cancerous tumors. 21. pediatrician, pediatrics: children; prevention and treatment of childhood diseases. 22. psychiatrist, psychiatry: mental disorders.

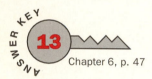

Chapter 6, p. 47

1. vertebrae. 2. ova. 3. diagnoses. 4. thrombi. 5. apices. 6. enemata. 7. cocci. 8. media. 9. nuclei. 10. bursae. 11. bacterium. 12. datum. 13. crisis. 14. prognosis. 15. uterus. 16. speculum. 17. carcinoma. 18. gingiva. 19. focus. 20. appendix. 21. media. 22. appendices. 23. petechiae. 24. diverticulum. 25. protozoa.

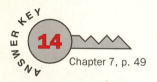

Chapter 7, p. 49

1. without fever (normal temperature). 2. without feeling (local, regional, or general anesthesia). 3. without breathing (periods of no breathing). 4. the rate and extent to which an active drug enters the general circulation. 5. a new field of study related to the ethics of transplants, prolonging life, or ending life (cutting off life support, nourishment, and fluids). 6. slow heart rate. 7. rapid heart rate. 8. remove water or fluid. 9. replace fluid (in dehydrated subject). 10. to happen again; another episode (of an illness). 11. flowing through

---

*There are other possibilities; they should follow this format.

(of feces). 12. increased output of urine. 13. paralysis on one side (although the prefix *hemi-* means "one half," in medicine it always means "one side"). 14. vomiting of blood. 15. substance formed by water combining with various compounds; addition of fluid. 16. high blood pressure (does not mean high tension). 17. excessively active. 18. low blood pressure. 19. under the skin (hypodermic injection). 20. low functioning thyroid gland. 21. a fatty tumor. 22. voiding excessive amount of urine. 23. many cysts. 24. before surgery. 25. before birth. 26. foreknowledge; prediction of outcome of disease. 27. running before; symptom indicative of approaching disease (pertains to initial stage). 28. following surgery. 29. following childbirth.

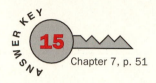

Chapter 7, p. 51

1. without fever (normal temperature). 2. without fever. 3. not typical. (Atypical cells are abnormal cells or cells undergoing some changes.) 4. without a voice; unable to speak. 5. without breathing; periods of no breathing. 6. without development (or wasting away, as with muscles not used). 7. without feeling (a state produced by anesthetics, used for surgical procedures). 8. without pain (analgesic drugs relieve pain). 9. without air (Some bacteria can thrive in anaerobic conditions, without oxygen, such as tetanus.). 10. without rhythm (cardiac arrhythmia). 11. without contamination (sterile). 12. without symptoms. 13. no menstruation (first sign of pregnancy). 14. without oxygen or not enough oxygen. 15. without trauma (injury). 16. "without eating;" unable to swallow. 17. without vessels. 18. without appetite.

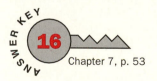

Chapter 7, p. 53

1. T. 2. T. 3. T. 4. F (Dyspnea is difficult breathing; apnea is periods of no breathing.). 5. T. 6. T. 7. antihistamine. 8. hypodermic. 9. tachycardia. 10. prenatal. 11. hemiplegia. 12. anemia. 13. without air (oxygen). 14. "without blood," low red blood count. 15. without growth (wasting away). 16. without pain (pain relieving). 17. the ethics of transplants, life support, right to die, etc. 18. using sensors to train the body to control involuntary functions, such as blood pressure. 19. remove water. 20. high blood pressure. 21. low functioning thyroid. 22. "knowledge before," predicted outcome. 23. after surgery. 24. "much urine," excessive amount of urine. 25. fast heartbeat. 26. the

period before menstrual flow starts.   **27.** running before (early symptoms).   **28.** excessive heat; raising body temperature to destroy cancer cells before radiation; to kill certain types of bacteria.

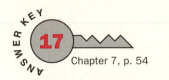

ANSWER KEY 17
Chapter 7, p. 54

1. inflammation of skin of extremities.   **2.** pointed head.   **3.** living in presence of oxygen.   **4.** living without oxygen.   **5.** condition of cells of unequal size.   **6.** difficult labor.   **7.** exaggerated feeling of depression.   **8.** abnormal cell growth.   **9.** an easy labor.   **10.** exaggerated feeling of well-being.   **11.** easy death.   **12.** attraction to those of opposite sex.   **13.** of unlike natures; composed of unlike substances.   **14.** attraction to those of same sex.   **15.** fear of homoxesuality.   **16.** uniform in structure, composition or nature.   **17.** relatively stable state of equilibrium of the internal body.   **18.** condition of cells being equal in size.   **19.** same tension or tone; isotonic solution: one that contains same salt concentratin as body fluids.   **20.** equal temperature.   **21.** ill at ease.   **22.** poorly aligned; not coming together evenly.   **23.** enlarged extremities.   **24.** enlarged heart.   **25.** cessation of menstruation.   **26.** painful menstruation.   **27.** voiding during the night (*not bedwetting*).   **28.** epidemic of great proportions; worldwide.   **29.** evidence of disease; a complaint.   **30.** group of symptoms characteristic of a certain disease; for example, carpal tunnel (wrist), shoulder hand (shoulder).

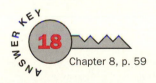

ANSWER KEY 18
Chapter 8, p. 59

The *-oma* words are difficult, as are their definitions; do not concern yourself too much with the exact meanings. Just remember that *-oma* is a new growth or tumor that serves no useful purpose.

1. tumor of a gland (epithelial tissue).   **2.** cancerous tumor.   **3.** tumor of fibrous (connective) tissue.   **4.** tumor of glia cell (nerve cell).   **5.** tumor of liver.   **6.** lymph tissue tumor.   **7.** granulation tissue tumor (at site of injury or ulcer).   **8.** tumor originating in bone marrow (malignant).   **9.** tumor in muscle tissue.   **10.** malignant tumor in connective tissue (cancer).   **11.** blood

tumor (clot).   **12.** increased pressure in eyeball. (Literal meaning is "gray swelling"; this is not really a tumor.)   **13.** difficult or labored breathing.   **14.** no breathing; patients sometimes have short periods of apnea.   **15.** able to breathe only when sitting upright (usually with trunk of body resting on overbed table, and so on).   **16.** rapid breathing.   **17.** slow breathing.

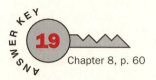

ANSWER KEY 19
Chapter 8, p. 60

1. lipoma.   **2.** hematoma.   **3.** mucoid.   **4.** hypertrophied.   **5.** dyspnea.   **6.** tachypnea.   **7.** hemiplegia.   **8.** paraplegia.   **9.** pyorrhea.   **10.** diarrhea.   **11.** osteomalacia.   **12.** hemolysis.   **13.** carcinoma, sarcoma.   **14.** apneic.   **15.** orthopneic.   **16.** the same throughout; particles dispersed evenly.   **17.** all four limbs paralyzed.   **18.** resembling fat.   **19.** unit of heredity.   **20.** one-sided weakness.   **21.** organs of reproduction.   **22.** tumor of gland.   **23.** inflammation of the lungs.   **24.** overgrowth of cells.   **25.** disease producing.   **26.** yes.   **27.** in position; not spread to surrounding tissue.   **28.** metastatic cancer spread from another site.   **29.** new growth; tumor.   **30.** destruction of fat.

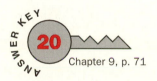

ANSWER KEY 20
Chapter 9, p. 71

1. e **ryth** rocyte.   **2.** cya **no** sis.   **3.** mela **no** ma.   **4.** leu **ke** mia.   **5.** carci **no** ma.   **6.** hydro **ther** apy.   **7.** li **po** ma.   **8.** throm **bo** sis.   **9.** pa **thol** ogy.   **10.** staphylo **co** cci.   **11.** strepto **co** cci.   **12.** ba **cil** li.   **13.** woman having her first child.   **14.** injury, physical or emotional.   **15.** hardening of the arteries.   **16.** control of bleeding.   **17.** gallstones (condition of); *-iasis* similar to *-osis*.   **18.** condition of "dead tissue."   **19.** heating through.   **20.** without feeling or sensation.   **21.** study or science dealing with the blood.   **22.** urine in the blood (components of urine in the blood stream, due to kidney malfunction).   **23.** woman who has been pregnant three times, has had two full-term births.   **24.** T.   **25.** T.   **26.** T.   **27.** F (they cause disease).   **28.** F (they do require oxygen).

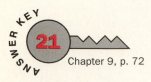

Chapter 9, p. 72

1. white blood cell.   2. condition of "eating cells" (cells that engulf bacteria, and so on).   3. mental illness, "split personality."   4. treatment with water.   5. control of bleeding.   6. paralysis of one side of the body.   7. "without blood," condition in which red blood count is low. 8. urine components in the blood.   9. mania in which person has highly inflated opinion of self.   10. study or science dealing with the blood.   11. cancerous or malignant tumor.   12. nearsightedness.   13. spasm of a nerve.   14. enlarged colon.   15. blood in the urine. **SPELL: (16–32).** prognosis: predicted outcome of a disease.   17. diagnosis: "knowing through," studying symptoms and arriving at decision.   18. hysterorrhexis; rupture of the uterus (breaking open).   19. pathogenic: from which disease arises, disease causing.   20. syndrome: "running together," symptoms that occur together and characterize a certain disease condition.   21. cocci: round bacteria. 22. hemoglobin: a protein in red blood cells; it carries oxygen.   23. nocturia: urinating during the night; *not* bedwetting.   24. multipara: woman who has borne more than one child.   25. thrombosis: condition of clotting (in blood vessels).   26. erythrocyte: red (blood) cell.   27. gravid: pregnant.   28. staphylococcus: round bacteria growing in cluster formatin.   29. virology: study of viruses and viral diseases.   30. cyanosis: bluish color to skin.

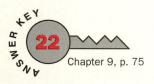

Chapter 9, p. 75

1. diagnosis, symptoms.   2. streptococcus.   3. antibiotic. 4. prognosis.   5. myopia, cannot.   6. hydrotherapy, diathermy, cryotherapy.   7. leukocytes, erythrocytes. 8. WBC, RBC.   9. pathogens, cocci, bacilli. 10. primipara.   11. five pregnancies, two term births. 12. preoperative (preop), anesthetic, postoperative (postop).

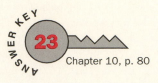

Chapter 10, p. 80

1. movement away from midline (of body); think of kidnapping.   2. movement toward midline.   3. "cutting around" penis (foreskin).   4. not indicated (certain drugs not indicated in pregnancy, for example).   5. arising from outside (body).   6. same as 5.   7. out of place, as a pregnancy outside uterus.   8. secreting externally through a duct. 9. secreting internally directly into bloodstream. 10. arising from within.   11. scope for looking inside body.   12. area over the stomach.   13. outside the uterus (same as ectopic).   14. below the sternum. 15. below normal.   16. on the same side.   17. in the middle of the sternum.   18. suturing of mesentery. 19. spread of cancer cells (change or transformation). 20. tissue change; conversion of food to heat and energy. 21. "beyond ankle" (bones of the foot).   22. "near or beside" medical.   23. similar to typhoid.   24. two like parts paralyzed (lower extremities).   25. around the teeth (gums).   26. around tonsils.   27. around the heart. 28. around the "wastes" (between genitals and rectum). 29. behind the peritoneum.   30. turned backward. 31. through, or by way of, the urethra.   32. through, or by way of, the vagina (normal delivery).

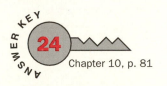

Chapter 10, p. 81

1. standing.   2. bending.   3. lying.   4. straightening. 5. distal; lateral; bilateral.   6. lying.   7. cephalic and superior, caudal and inferior.   8. lithotomy.   9. inside; outside. 10. anteroposterior; posteroanterior, and left lateral of chest (X-ray pictures taken from front to back; from back to front, and from left side).   11. T.   12. T.   13. F (Caudal anesthesia is injected into the tail end of the spinal cavity.)   14. T.   15. T.   16. F (In the peritoneal cavity, not perineum; perineum is area between anus and vulva.) 17. T.   18. T.   19. F. (Hemiplegia is paralysis on one side; paraplegia involves lower half of the body.)   20. T. 21. T.   23. T.   24. T.

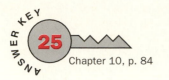

25

Chapter 10, p. 84

1. addicted.   2. abduction.   3. ectogenous.   4. ectopic.
5. retroperitoneal.   6. transurethral.   7. quadrants.
8. ambivalence.   9. tricuspid.   10. lithotomy.
11. bilateral.   12. bilateral.   13. partially in a coma.
14. woman who has borne more than one child.
15. double vision.   16. over the stomach.   17. arising
from within the organism (body).   18. toward the midline.
19. below the sternum.   20. "around the wastes," area
between anus and vulva.   21. on left side, left knee flexed.
22. one side.   23. "around the teeth," gums.   24. bending.   25. coccus, round bacteria found in pairs.   26. OD
27. AP.   28a. vertical body plane; divides body into equal
right and left sides.   28b. vertical body plane; divides body
into front and back.   28c. horizontal plane; divides body
into top and bottom.

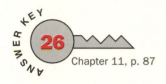

26

Chapter 11, p. 87

1. termination of pregnancy before fetus is viable.
2. area of body from below ribs to pubis.   3. from
below ribs (adjective).   4. localized collection of pus.
5. sudden, severe, usually not long-lasting (disease).
6. growing together (tissues adhering where they should
not).   7. accessory parts of a structure, for example,
adnexa uteri.   8. process of listening for sounds (see no.
43).   9. instrument for sterilizing (steam under pressure).
10. armpit.   11. abnormality.   12. examination of live
tissue.   13. suture material.   14. a tube, usually for withdrawing fluid, such as that for withdrawing urine from the
bladder.   15. pertaining to the neck, for example, cervical
vertebrae (neck area); also, cervix of the uterus.   16. long-
lasting, usually not curable, disease.   17. type of suture
material; chromic catgut.   18. tailbone.   19. present at
birth (born with).   20. process of stretching or opening
up.   21. edema; fluid in body tissues (leaves a "pit" with
pressure); ascites: fluid in peritoneal cavity; anasarca: generalized, severe edema.   22. obstruction of blood vessel,
usually by blood clot.   23. vomiting.   24. introduction of
fluid into rectum (for cleansing purposes, for example).
25. waste matter, elimination.   26. recurrence or flare up
of symptoms after period of remission.   27. connective
tissues (supports and separates muscles).   28. feverish; elevated temperature.   29. quivering type of heartbeat ineffective in pumping blood; restore rhythm (defibrillation).
30. profuse bleeding, internal or external.   31. jaundice:
pigment coloring skin and membranes.   32. preventive
measure to prevent disease.   33. inability to control urination (and bowels).   34. tissue reaction to injury: signs
are redness, heat, swelling, pain (loss of function possible).
35. insufficient supply of blood; for example, ischemic area.
36. yellowing of skin, whites of eyes, membranes, body fluids due to excessive bilirubin (pigment in bile, produced
from hemoglobin) in the blood. It is a symptom, not a
disease. Coombs': test to diagnose hemolytic anemias.
37. spread to other parts of the body, especially cancer
cells. 38. thick, slippery substance secreted by mucous
membranes; mucous (adjective); mucosa = mucous
membrane.   39. fat, excessive overweight.   40. able to
be felt.   41. inablility to move a part (usually caused by
nerve damage).   42. forming the wall of a cavity; for example, parietal pleura.   43. tapping to produce sounds (percussion and auscultation or P and A).   44. area between
anus and genitals.   45. membranous lining of
abdominopelvic cavity (peritoneal cavity).   46. membranous lining of chest cavity (pleural cavity).   47. dropping
down, out of place; for example, prolapsed uterus (dropping
into vagina).   48. preventive measure; for example,
prophylactic dental care—brushing and cleaning, fluoride
treatment.   49. full of pus, producing pus.   50. period
when symptoms disappear temporarily.   51. acute and
chronic condition of sore stiff muscles.   52. having the
nature of serum; membrane that produces serumlike
substance; serum is the yellow fluid part of blood left after
the clot forms.   53. secretion from deep down to
bronchial tubes (not saliva).   54. material used to stitch
up incisions or injuries; also suture lines in cranium.
55. system of sorting patients as to priority of treatment in
emergencies.   56. infectious agent, smaller than bacteria.
57. abdominal organs.   58. to empty bladder; urinate.

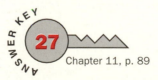

27

Chapter 11, p. 89

1. F (It is an acute disease.)   2. T.   3. F (It is one a person is born with.)   4. T.   5. F (An incontinent person is
one who cannot control voiding.)   6. T.   7. T.   8. T.
9. F (A **bi** opsy is the examination of *live* tissue.)   10. T.
11. emesis.   12. edema, ascites, anasarca.   13. enema.
14. axilla.   15. inflammation. **SPELL: (16–20)** 16. abdominal.   17. sputum.   18. embolism.   19. viscera.
20. immunization.   21. emptied (bladder).   22. pus producing, draining.   23. sagging, dropped down.   24. able
to be felt.   25. prevention.   26. excessive fluid in
peritoneal cavity.   27. severe, generalized edema.

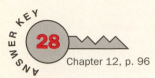

28
Chapter 12, p. 96

1. 600,000 units intramuscularly every eight hours. **2.** 30 milligrams by mouth every four hours, as needed for headache. **3.** grains 1½ at bedtime as needed. **4.** 100 milligrams by mouth, at bedtime. **5.** nothing by mouth after midnight. **6.** 1000 cubic centimeters of 5% glucose in distilled water, intravenously, immediately. **7.** out of bed, twice a day. **8.** give patient plenty to drink, keep record of intake and output. **9.** tid. **10.** gr. **11.** g. **12.** c̄. **13.** s̄. **14.** dc. **15.** H_2O. **16.** O_2. **17.** ac. **18.** BRP (bathroom privileges). **19.** GI. **20.** s̄s̄. **21.** intravenous pyelogram. **22.** 4 times a day. **23.** units. **24.** quantity not sufficient. **25.** suppository. **26.** normal saline. **27.** tender loving care. **28.** intravenously. **29.** electrocardiogram. **30.** temperature, pulse, respirations. **31.** temperature, pulse, respirations, B/P. **32.** computerized (axial) tomography: series of "pictures"; more detailed information than from X-ray films. **33.** cc, +, mg or mgm. **Extra:** see note no. 3, p. 94, see p. 93 for immunizations.

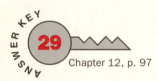

29
Chapter 12, p. 97

1. ER or A & D. **2.** OR, RR, surg. **3.** X-ray. **4.** ER or OPD. **5.** CCU or ICU. **6.** OB, labor, nursery, postpartum unit. **7.** peds. **8.** CS. **9.** lab. **10.** PT. **11.** MR. **12.** morgue. **13.** SS. **14.** NP. **15.** ENT or MOR. **16.** OT or PM & R. **17.** CS.

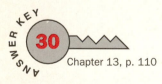

30
Chapter 13, p. 110

1. complete blood count (per cubic millimeter). **2.** white blood count (per cubic millimeter). **3.** red blood count (per cubic millimeter). **4.** hemoglobin (the red coloring in the blood). **5.** hematocrit (volume of red cells in a sample of blood). **6.** fasting blood sugar. **7.** Diff stands for differential, and it means counting each of the different kinds of leukocytes or white blood cells in a blood sample. **8.** neutrophils, eosinophils, basophils, lymphocytes, monocytes. (These leukocytes are names by the kind of dye they "take." Phil means "to love." Eosin is a kind of acid dye. Eosinophils "love" it. Basophils "love" basic dyes. Neutrophils take "neutral" dye. **9.** numbers of cells, size and shape (in other words, how many, how big, and how they look); hematology. **10.** reaction (pH), specific gravity,

test for glucose, albumin, and microscopic findings. **11.** Voided specimen is passed by patient, normally. A catheterized specimen is obtained with a sterile catheter after patient has been washed; so a catheterized specimen is cleaner, less likely to be contaminated, and thus more useful for a test. (This is especially true in the female. Any vaginal discharge will contaminate the specimen, and if the patient is menstruating, it is difficult to get a clean urine specimen.) **12.** serology; STS (serological test for syphilis), VDRL (Veneral Disease Research Laboratories), Kahn. **13.** bacteriology; C&S (culture and sensitivity). **14.** test to detect abnormal (cancer) cells; taken from the cervix of the uterus with a swab or stick; cytology division. **15.** Examination of live tissue; a frozen section. **16.** see pp. 108. **17.** Fasting means not eating; a fasting blood sugar is taken before breakfast, and the patient has been on NPO since midnight. **18.** PMNs, segs. **19.** monos, eos, basos. **20.** enzyme. **21.** 11-16 g/dL.

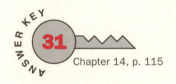

31
Chapter 14, p. 115

1. Physician's Desk Reference: a comprehensive book published yearly, listing all prescription drugs by brand or trade name, generic name (and chemical name) and showing which drug company produces each. Also explains the use of each drug, giving side effects, contraindications, and dosage recommended, among other things. **2.** over the counter: refers to any drug that may be purchased without a prescription. **3.** prescription, recipe; "take." **4a.** increases urinary output. **4b.** relieves pain. **4c.** reduces or relieves nasal congestion. **4d.** a drug that suppresses the immune system's antibody formation to prevent rejection of transplanted organ (renders a patient vulnerable to infection). **5.** Generic refers to the chemistry of the drug; the brand name is one chosen by a drug company for its product that falls in a certain generic class. There are many brand name drugs for every generic drug, and prices vary considerably. The pharmacist may substitute the most reasonable buy for the patient if the physician orders specifically by the generic name, but may *not* substitute a generic for a brand name drug. **6.** A drug sales representative for a certain drug company. **7.** T. **8.** F (All drugs have an expiration date and should be discarded after that date.) **9.** F (Most medical dictionary listings do not contain drugs. The Physician's Desk Reference is the best reference to use.) **10.** T. **11.** T. **12.** You have probably heard of Darvon, Seconal sodium, Premarin, and others. Examples of classifications are anticonvulsives, antineoplastics, cardiovascular preparations, antinauseants, antiinflammatory drugs, hemorrhoid preparations, and so on. You write the examples. **13.** A prescription usually reads as follows: Rx: Darvon Compound, 32 mg, Cap T tid prn, for pain. **14.** Some words that appear frequently are anorexia, nausea, vomiting, diarrhea, alopecia, thrombocytopenia, pruritus, myelosuppression, idiosyncrasies.

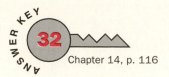

1. Brand and Generic Name Index, pink.   2. Product Category, blue section; acetaminophen, Excedrin, Percocet, Tylenol, etc.   3. This drug is pictured in the Product ID section and the first page number is the picture section. The second page number is the product information.
4. Roche is the manufacturer; diazepam is the generic name; white 2-mg tabs; yellow, 5-mg tabs; blue, 10-mg tabs.
5a. Valium.   5b. Demerol.   5c. Enovid.   5d. Zyloprim.
6a. meprobamate.   6b. norethindrone.
6c. hydrochlorothiazide.   6d. mazindol.   7. Equanil, Fastin.

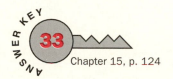

1. peritoneal cavity; thoracic, pleural cavity.   2. cranial cavity.   3. cell.   4. nucleus, cytoplasm or protoplasm, and cell membrane; genes are in the chromosomes (in the nucleus).   5. patent, lumen.   6. perforated.   7. os meatus, orifice.   8. vasoconstriction.   9. stoma.
10. vasodilators.   11. cervix.   12. cardiovascular.
13. musculoskeletal.   14. respiratory.   15. gastrointestinal.   16. musculoskeletal.   17. endocrine.
18. nervous.   19. urinary.   20. reproductive and endocrine.   21. integumentary.   22. reproductive and endocrine.   23. epithelial, connective, muscle, and nervous.   24. group, organs.   25. absorption, storage, and use of foods for growth and repair of tissue; production of energy; elimination of wastes.   26. tissues.   27. muscle.   28. cell division (means of multiplying).   29. legs.
30. striped (voluntary muscle or skeletal muscle).
31. release of a substance.   32. taking in.   33. process of excreting or expelling.   34. study of diseases; diseased state.   35. state of constancy.   36. F (It is one you get because of medical treatment in a medical facility.)   37. T.

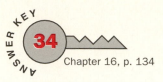

1. dermatologist.   2. protection, receptor, temperature regulator, excretion (any two answers).   3. epidermis.
4. sudoriferous.   5. sebaceous.   6. impetigo, scabies, psoriasis, and so on.   7. corium; blood vessels, nerves, sweat and oil glands.   8. herpes simplex.   9. contact dermatitis, eczema, drug reactions, insect bites or stings (any three.)   10. paronychia.   11. Mantoux: tuberculosis; Dick: susceptibility to scarlet fever; and so on.   12. T.   13. T.
14. T.   15. T.   16. F (A vesicle is a blister.)   17. T.
18. F (It is a loss of pigment and is not infectious.)
19. dermatome.   20. urticaria.   21. nevi; mole.
22. erythema.   23. syphilis, measles (rubeola and rubella), varicella (chickenpox), diabetes mellitus, Hodgkin's disease, Kaposi's, lupus erythematosus (any three).   24. louse.
25. acne vulgaris.   26. papule, macule, bulla, and so on.
27. Kaposi's sarcoma.   28. mammoplasty.   29. bruise, black-and-blue mark.   30. keloid.

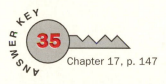

1. cranium, calvaria.   2. sinuses.   3. sutures.
4. fontanels.   5. cervical, thoracic, lumbar, sacral, coccygeal.   6. movement toward the midline.   7. connective fibrous tissue holding one bone to another.
8. connective fibrous tissue holding muscle to bone.
9. small sac filled with fluid, at joints to cushion them.
10. greenstick: bone broken, but not separated; simple: bone broken, not protruding through skin; compound: bone broken and piercing through skin.   11. orthopedist, osteopath, chiropractor.   12. straight; literally, means "straight child," but actually means treatment of bone disorders.   13. another kind of physician who uses all MD methods, but also may use manipulation (more importance placed on "spinal column" alignment).   14. bending; straightening.   15. sternum; vertebral column.
16. inability to move part.   17. wasting away (from disuse).   18. excessive development.   19. knee cartilage: superior aspect of tibia.   20. frontal, occipital, parietal, temporal, and so on (any three).   21. ribs.   22. bones (skeleton).   23. diaphragm.   24. striated, smooth (non-striated), cardiac.   25. osteoarthritis, osteomalacia, rickets.
26. bones.   27. axial, appendicular.   28. larger head proportionately; fontanels in skull; softer bones (cartilage).
29. systemic lupus erythematosus, rheumatoid arthritis, nonsteroidal anti-inflammatory drug.   30. See Fig. 17.3.

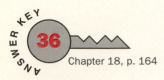

ANSWER KEY 36
Chapter 18, p. 164

1. disease of the heart and/or blood vessels. 2. cerebrovascular accident; rupture or blockage of artery in brain. 3. pulmonary; systemic. 4. pulmonary artery and lungs; left atrium, pulmonary vein. 5. aortic; aorta. 6. tricuspid; mitral. 7. superior vena cava; inferior vena cava. 8. keep blood from backflowing (blood can move in forward direction only). 9. blood vessels. 10. collateral (circulation). 11. oxygen, nutrients, carbon dioxide, wastes. 12. dividing wall between right and left sides of heart. 13. heart ventricles contract; top number in B/P. 14. heart ventricles relax; bottom number in B/P. 15. heart muscle. 16. procedure done before transfusion to be sure of compatibility. 17. study or science of the blood. 18. without oxygen. 19. twisted, tortuous, dilated. 20. arteries that supply heart muscle (myocardium) with blood. 21. A, B, AB, O. 22a. erythrocytes. 22b. leukocytes. 22c. thrombocytes or platelets. 22d. neutrophils, eosinophils, basophils, lymphocytes, monocytes. 23. Rh negative or Rh–. 24. pacemaker. 25. cardiologist; hematologist. 26. coronary occlusion, coronary thrombosis, myocardial infarct or infarction. 27. pericardium; endocardium. 28. electrocardiogram; coronary care unit. 29. exercise or lack of it; eating or fasting; emotions; amount of blood, thickness of blood, condition of arteries. 30. cardio; phlebo; arterio; (hem) angio; thrombo; embolus. 31. type O. 32. prevents antibody production. 33. aneurysm, leukemia, atrial septal defect, transient ischemic attack, and so on. 34a. myocardial infarct. 34b. congestive heart failure. 34c. cerebrovascular accident. 34d. atrial septal defect. 34e. transient ischemic attack. 35. attain normal weight, exercise, cut down on use of salt, stop smoking. 36a. no known cause (disease peculiar to one person). 36b. no cause known. 36c. via, or by way of, an opening (lumen) in a vessel.

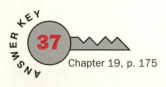

ANSWER KEY 37
Chapter 19, p. 175

1. thoracic, pleural. 2. nares, pharynx, larynx, trachea, bronchi, bronchioles, lungs (alveoli). 3. diaphragm; it moves down; makes more room; during inspiration. 4. epiglottis. 5. pharynx; from pharynx to middle ear; equalize pressure. 6. tiny air sacs in lungs where gaseous exchange takes place. 7. pleurisy. 8. O_2 and CO_2 (oxygen and carbon dioxide). 9. nares; septum. 10. apex; apices; base. 11. sinuses. 12. in front of (It would not be possible to do a tracheotomy if trachea were behind

esophagus.) 13. radiologist or roentgenologist. 14. oto(rhino)laryngologist or ENT specialist. 15. tracheostomy. 16. diaphragm. 17. atelectasis; tuberculosis. 18. amount of air that can be forcibly expelled after deep inspiration. 19. emphysema, asthma, chronic bronchitis (any one). 20. dyspnea. 21. orthopnea. 22. apnea. 23. pharyngitis, sinusitis, tonsillitis, and so on. 24. upper respiratory infection. 25. short of breath. 26. intermittent positive pressure breathing. 27. anteroposterior and side, X-ray. 28. expectorants; aerosols. 29. rales. 30. carcinoma of lung (bronchogenic carcinoma). 31. bronchi. 32. fast breathing. 33. secretions from bronchial tubes. 34. allergic disorder with severe wheezing. 35. cough that produces sputum. 36. machine used to check vital capacity. 37. scope for looking into bronchi. 38. breathing in. 39. tapping chest to remove fluid. 40. both lungs involved. 41. a pneumonia to which AIDS (or immunosuppressed patients) are susceptible; often fatal.

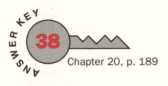

ANSWER KEY 38
Chapter 20, p. 189

1. digestive; peritoneal, abdominopelvic. 2. liver; appendix. 3. teeth, tongue, salivary glands, pancreas, liver, gallbladder. 4. duodenum, jejunum, ileum. 5. esophagus; peristalsis. 6. cecum, ascending colon, tranverse colon, descending colon, sigmoid colon, rectum, anus. 7. anus. 8. feces, stool. 9. upper GI series, lower GI (barium enema), GB series, stool to lab, proctoscopy, biopsy, gastric analysis, gastrocopy, and so on. 10. liver; gallbladder; aids in digestion of fats; cystic, hepatic, common. 11. choledoch; cholecyst; cholangiography or choledochography. 12. introduction of solution into rectum, for cleansing or for X-ray, for example. 13. tiny projections that line small intestine, increase surface area. 14. circular (purse string type) muscle (anal sphincter, for example). 15. instrument for looking into the rectum. 16. fats, carbohydrates, proteins; fats 9, CHO 4, proteins 4. 18. right and left hypochondria, right and left lumbar, right and left inguinal; epigastric, umbilical and suprapubic should be shown in a drawing (see Fig. 20.3). 19. peritoneal; greater, lesser. 20. feeding by tube inserted into stomach. 21. washing out stomach. 22. inflammation of the mouth. 23. inflammation of the tongue. 24. excision of the gallbladder. 25. new permanent opening into colon. 26. inflammation of the liver. 27. condition of gallstones. 28. loss of appetite. 29. small intestine, villi. 30. appendectomy, ileostomy, anastomosis, and so on. 31. peptic or duodenal ulcers, colitis, appendicitis, esophagitis, and so on. 32. surgical repair of the lip (often for cleft lip), eating disorder with periods of binging and vomiting, surgical repair of the outlet from the stomach (pylorus). 33. gallbladder series, X-ray to detect stones;

nothing by mouth, in preparation for procedure or surgery; nasogastric tube, into the stomach through nose, for feeding, to relieve distention, to keep stomach empty; within normal limits, a term often used in histories to describe an organ, system, or lab result.

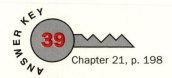

Chapter 21, p. 198

1. kidneys, ureters, bladder, urethra. **2.** unable to control voiding and/or bowels. **3.** obtain a urine specimen (sterile); to relieve distended bladder when person is unable to void. **4.** pyelitis. **5.** any disease of the kidney. **6.** dysuria, anuria, polyuria, hematuria, and so on. **7.** urinalysis, pH, specific gravity, glucose, and so on. **8.** nephrons. **9.** kidneys, ureters, bladder. **10.** to empty bladder. **11.** any substance that increases urinary output. **12.** use of machine to filter blood when kidneys are non-functional (artificial kidney). **13.** "urine in the blood," kidneys not filtering blood, and waste products are in circulating blood. **14.** many urgent trips to the bathroom. **15.** X-ray of KUB using dye introduced through the urethra instead of intravenously. **16.** hematuria. **17.** anuria. **18.** enuresis. **19.** nephrorrhaphy. **20.** cystocele. **21.** nephrolithiasis, nephrosis. **22.** pyelography, pyelitis. **23.** ureterostomy, ureterectomy. **24.** retention catheter (with a balloon to hold it in place in the bladder). **25.** urinary tract infection. **26.** opening of urethra. **27.** using a scope to look into the bladder. **28.** any disease of the renal pelvis. **29.** intravenous pyelogram, an X-ray of kidney after dye has been given IV. **30.** pus in the urine. **31.** X-ray of the bladder. **32.** procedure of crushing stones. **33.** "outside of the body." **34.** See Fig 21.1.

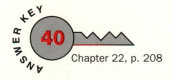

Chapter 22, p. 208

1. ovum, ovary. **2.** cervix, fundus. **3.** fallopian tube. **4.** placenta. **5.** cervix. **6.** tubal ligation or laparoscopic sterilization. **7.** cesarean. **8.** dilation and curettage; dilating cervix and scraping uterus lining. **9.** estimated date of confinement; due date. **10.** fetal heart tones heard by fetoscope. **11.** last menstrual period, used to calculate EDC. **12.** left or right, occiput anterior; normal vertex presentation of infant (back of head toward top) during delivery). **13.** zygote intrafallopian transfer. **14.** delivered 5 live infants; pregnant 7 times. **15.** smear to detect carcinoma, from the cervix. **16.** three-month periods of pregnancy. **17.** ovum leaves ovary. **18.** (usually) buttocks presenting; not the head. **19.** method used to evaluate condition of infant at 1 and 5 minutes after delivery. Top score is 10. **20.** plastic surgery on breasts, postmastectomy or purely cosmetic. **21.** salpingectomy. **22.** hysterectomy. **23.** episiotomy. **24.** pelvimeter. **25.** ectopic.

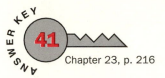

Chapter 23, p. 216

1. sperm, testis. **2.** prostate. **3.** AIDS. **4.** vasectomy. **5.** testis, epididymis. **6.** sexually transmitted disease. **7.** prostate-specific antigen, testing for early prostate cancer. **8.** cryptorchidism. **9.** prostatectomy. **10.** circumcision. **11.** syphilis, gonorrhea, AIDS, chlamydia, etc. **12.** See Table 23.1.

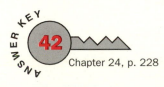

Chapter 24, p. 228

1. largest, brain. **2.** exterior, middle, and interior layers of the meninges (membranes that cover brain and spinal cord). **3.** optic, olfactory, auditory. **4.** T4, C3, Co-1. **5.** cranium, vertebral column; cerebrospinal fluid. **6.** nerve cells; brain. **7.** gliomas, meningiomas. **8.** hemiparesis. **9.** hemiplegia. **10.** convolutions of the brain; deep furrows in brain; gyrus, sulcus (singular form). **11.** cavities through which CSF circulates; hydrocephalus. **12.** response. **13.** lumbar puncture; diagnostic. **14.** the sacrococcygeal area. **15.** inflammation of the meninges (membranes). **16.** autonomic. **17.** l, k, i, h, g, d, f, e, b, a, j, m, c. **18.** For example, parkinsonism affects older people, causing severe tremor and masklike facies; herpes zoster is a viral infection that causes lesions along course of a nerve. **19.** alpha, beta, theta. **20.** lay term for mental illness.

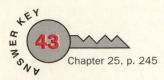

43

1. myopia.   2. tonometer.   3. OD, OU, OS, AD.
4. cataract.   5. lacrimal.   6. peripheral vision.
7. optometrist.   8. cerumen.   9. tympanum, myringa.
10. otitis media.   11. eustachian.   12. audiometer.
13. decibel.   14. auditory.   15. mastoidectomy.
16. tympanotomy, myringotomy.   17. otoplasty.
18. presbyopia.   19. retinopathy.   20. conjunctivitis.
21. MD or DO eye specialist.   22. MD or DO ear
specialist.   23. ear, nose, and throat.   24. excessive tear-
ing of the eyes.   25. "crossed eyes."   26. removal of the
eyeball.   27. increased intraocular pressure, leads to blindness (not a tumor).   28. ability to adjust quickly to near
and far vision.   29. pupils equal, react to light and accommodation.   30. lighted instrument for looking into the
ears.   31. edema of optic nerve where it enters eye.
32. inflammation of the conjunctiva.   33. "lazy eye."
34. instrument for looking into eye.   35. ear wax.
36. applied to the surface.

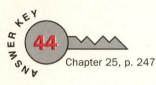

44

1. plaque.   2. pyorrhea or gingivitis.   3. deciduous,
fall out.   4. dentures.   5. temporomandibular joint.
6. Doctor of Dental Surgery.   7. specialist who treats
malocclusion.   8. repair work such as fillings, crowns.
9. cavities.   10. malaligned teeth.   11. tooth cannot
come through the gums.   12. pertaining to the cheek.
13. cutting front teeth.   14. grinding teeth.   15. sticky
mass of microorganisms that grows on teeth; erodes gums
and bone.   16. 28.   17. 20.   18. periodontist,
orthodontist, oral surgeon.   19. brushing, flossing, regular
check-ups.   20. enamel.   21. bicuspids.   22. show
areas that are not being cleaned adequately (red).

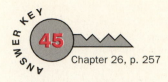

45

1. endocrine.   2. ductless.   3. testosterone; estrogens,
progesterone.   4. in the cranial cavity at base of brain; in
the neck, anterior and aside of larynx; in the pancreas (behind stomach).   5. PBI, protein-bound
iodine; RAU, radioactive iodine uptake; T_3 and T_4; thyroid
scan; ultrasound; needle biopsy.   6. FBS, fasting blood
sugar; GTT, glucose tolerance test; PP blood, postprandial;
urinalysis.   7. iodine.   8. insulin.   9. slow; insulin.
10. food (sugar or juice, for example).   11. thyroid.
12. two-hour postprandial.   13. hyperfunction, hypo-
function.   14. behind the stomach (LUQ).   15. pancreatectomy or pancreectomy.   16. hypophysis.   17. extremities.   18. myxedema, gigantism, exophthalmic goiter,
Cushing's disease, Addison's disease, pheochromocytoma,
Simmonds' disease, cretinism.   19. early arteriosclerosis,
vision and dental problems, gangrene, infection.   20a. excision of pituitary.   20b. any disease of nerves.
20c. excessive perspiring.   20d. enlarged thyroid gland.
20e. rapid heartbeat.   20f. clouded lens of eye.
20g. without appetite.   20h. severe wasting, emaciation.

Disease Report Outline

Your instructor may assign topics or may allow you to choose one that interests you. Reports may be written or given orally, if time permits. Include the following kinds of information, and be concise.

etiology   the cause of the disease (such as bacterial, viral, and degenerative factors). Cause may be unknown, but some theories certainly are prevalent and these can be mentioned.

population affected   factors of age, sex, and race, for example. (Who gets the disease?)

signs and symptoms   What does the patient complain of? What does the physician see (subjective and objective)? Special diagnostic tests necessary for diagnosis can be included here—GB series, GI series, and IVP, for example.

treatment   general kinds of treatment available, for example, surgery, medication, diet, bedrest, radiotherapy, and physical therapy (not too detailed).

prog *no* sis   predicted outcome: Is the prognosis good, fair, guarded, or poor? Are there any sequelae (aftereffects), is complete cure likely, is this a terminal condition, or is it a chronic condition in which the patient may need help to cope with disability?

community resources available   for example, lung associations for emphysema or TB, heart associations for cardiovascular diseases, and special groups such as "ostomy" clubs. (These associations usually have free literature available; see Appendix D.)

bibliography   include at least two current (within last three years) articles or readings from professional sources.

As in any composition, the general outline should also include:

- Introductory paragraph stating the purpose of researching the topic
- Statement of methodology regarding where and how research was done
- Summary or conclusion

APPENDIX C

Using Your Medical Dictionary

Your medical dictionary can be very helpful if you learn how to use it. Look through it to see what it contains. Some dictionaries have a table of contents or index at the front of the book. Some have instructions for use at the front and a table of contents just before the appendix at the back of the book.

All medical dictionaries contain lists of arteries, veins, muscles, and nerves in the appendix. Some also include listings of joints and ligaments and a great variety of other tables, such as weights and measures, signs and symbols, first aid, poisons and antidotes, medical emergencies, phobias, fractures, calorie lists, root words, prefixes, suffixes, plural endings, communicable diseases, immunization schedules, laboratory tests, and normal values.

It is important to learn what your dictionary contains and to become familiar with other medical dictionaries that you may need to use from time to time. Most dictionaries contain some excellent diagrams and illustrations. A picure often tells you more than a definition. In addition to pictures in the text of the book, you may find a section of "plates" showing each of the body systems.

When looking up a word, such as a certain disease, test, or syndrome, you may find it listed under the name of the disease or under "disease"; for instance, it may be listed under "autoimmune disease" or "disease—autoimmune." It will probably be listed in both places.

Dictionaries contain information on body systems. Look under the name of the system. You will learn that some systems have more than one name; for instance, the cardiovascular system is also the circulatory system, and the reproductive system is included in the genitourinary system.

Some abbreviations will be listed alphabetically, and usually there will also be a list of abbreviations in the appendix. There are so many medical abbreviations that you will find separate books of abbreviations used in the medical world.

Before purchasing a particular medical dictionary, look it over carefully. You may find that a large comprehensive dictionary is more confusing than helpful for your purposes. Be sure that the definitions are given in a manner that is understandable to you. There are many medical dictionaries available; it is merely a matter of picking the one that is best suited for you.

Your dictionary, in most cases, will be helpful to you in learning correct pronunctiation. However, pronunciation is best learned by actually practicing saying the words in class and as you work with them in written work.

Your instructor may suggest a dictionary for this class.

Organizations Offering Literature and Information

The location of the office nearest you may be found in the Yellow Pages of the phone directory under "Associations." Sometimes these organizations are listed in the white pages by state or county name, for example, the Arizona Lung Association or the San Mateo County Chapter of the American Heart Association.

AIDS Foundation

Alcoholism Information Center

Alzheimer's Disease and Related Disorders Association

American Cancer Society

American Diabetes Association

American Heart Association

American Red Cross

Arthritis Foundation

Association for Deaf (state)

Asthma and Allergy Foundation

CARES (Epilepsy)

Council of the Blind (state)

Cystic Fibrosis National Research Foundation

Department of Health (state)

Easter Seal Society for Crippled Children and Adults

-ectomy clubs (mastectomy, laryngectomy)

Epi-Hab

Family Planning Council (state)

Foundation for the Blind

Hemophilia Association

Huntington's Chorea

Kidney Foundation (state)

Leukemia Society of America

Lion's Vision Center

Lung Association (state)

March of Dimes

Medical societies (county and state)

Mental health associations (local and state)

Mental retardation associations (local and state)

Multiple Sclerosis Society

Muscular Dystrophy Association of America

Myasthenia Gravis Association

-ostomy clubs (colostomy)

Retired physicians' associations

SIDS Association

United Cerebral Palsy Association

United States Public Health Department—Center for Disease Control

Women's Health Resource Center

Some newspaper medical advice columns, computer programs, and television medical shows are helpful, as they usually provide an understandable explanation of common disorders and diseases. These can be used in class discussions. Keep advised of educational television programs; instructors may remind you to watch them. In some states, public television (PBS) has aired excellent programs on coronary bypass surgery, total hip and knee implants, and many other informative medical/surgical programs.

Support Groups

There are support groups for every imaginable problem area. Some are widely known, such as Alcoholics Anonymous and Child Protection Services. Others are listed here. Some of these may be only local groups and may not be found in small towns but others, such as AA and WeightWatchers, will be found in every locality.

To find a support group:
Check the white pages of the phone directory.
Check under Associations in the Yellow Pages.
Call the local Information and Referral number.
Call the mental health, medical, or nursing associations.
Look for help lines in local newspapers and for news stories on support groups.

Here are some support groups and other services.   The name of the city or state, such as "Arizona" or "Chicago," or "American" or "National," may precede the title of the program.

AIDS Information/Support
AIDS Project
AIDS Referral, Counseling, and
    Education Program
Interfaith AIDS Network
Little Innocent Victims
Shanti Group

Alcoholism Services
Al-Anon Family Group
Alcoholics Anonymous
Adult Children of Alcoholics
Secular Organization for Sobriety

Advocacy
Alliance for the Mentally Ill
Association for Supportive
    Child Care
Community Legal Services

Family Violence Shelters
    (these vary locally)
Autumn House
My Sister's Place
The Shelter

Help Hot Lines
Center Against Sexual Assault
Child Abuse Hot Line

Child Protective Services
Child Crisis Center
Crisis Information and Assistance
Drug Abuse Program
Parents Anonymous
Suicide Prevention
Teens Talking to Teens
Terros

Planned Parenthood
Adoption Services
Pregnancy Counseling

Relief Services
American Red Cross
Goodwill Industries
Salvation Army
St. Vincent de Paul

Support Groups
Alliance for the Mentally Ill
Alzheimer's Disease and Related
    Disorders Association
Alzheimer's Support Group
American Chronic Pain
    Association
Anorexics/Bulimics Anonymous
Bereavement Support Group
Cancer Family Support

Cardiopulmonary Pep Club
Chronic Fatigue Syndrome
    Association
Cocaine Anonymous
Co-Dependent Anonymous
Compassionate Friends
Corneal Transplant Support
    Group
Emotions Anonymous
Grief Support Group
Holistic Support Group
Hospice
Kids Can Cope
La Leche League
Lupus Foundation of America
Make Every Day Count
Mended Hearts
Mothers of Twins
New Horizons Manic Depressive
    and Depressive Support
    Group
Ostomy Association
Overeaters Anonymous
Parents Anonymous
Parents Without Partners
Parkinson's Support Group
United Scleroderma Association
WeightWatchers

Brief Introduction to Diagnostic Microbiology

Steps taken in the laboratory to identify bacteria:

1. Specimen is grown on suitable medium.

2. Colonies grow, organism is isolated, slides are prepared.

3. Gram stain is done. If gram positive, broad-spectrum antibiotics may be started before organism is identified further. If gram negative, different antibiotics are indicated. (If a patient is acutely ill, the antibiotic may be started before full identification has been made. After identification is complete and sensitivity studies have indicated the most effective antibiotic for this organism, the antibiotic may be changed.)

4. Other stains may be done; acid-fast stain, for example.

5. Additional tests:
   - Does the specimen ferment lactose, glucose, mannitol?
   - Does it hemolyze blood?
   - Does it produce acid, indole, gas?
   - Does it liquefy gelatin?

6. Culture and sensitivity are done to find the most effective antibiotic.

Pathogenic Bacteria

Bacteria have been classified, sorted into related groups under Latinized names that can be long and difficult. The following are some pathogenic bacteria.

Pathogen	Action
Borrelia burgdorferi	causes Lyme disease, caused by Ixodes dammini tick.
*Clost **rid** ium tetani*	causes tetanus (it is a spore-forming bacillus).
*Corynebac **ter** ium diphtheriae*	causes diphtheria (a bacillus), effectively controlled with vaccine, DT and DTP.
*Diplo **coc** cus pneumoniae*	commonly known as pneumococcus; causes lobar pneumonia, sinus infections, meningitis, peritonitis, corneal ulceration.
*Esche **rich** ia coli (E. coli)*	a bacillus, normal inhabitant of the GI tract, associated with sporadic outbreaks of diarrhea (named after famous German bacteriologist, Escherich).

He **moph** ilus influenzae	a bacillus, causes meningitis in children, and severe infections of sinuses, middle ear, throat, bronchi, lungs.
He **moph** ilus pertussis	whooping cough, effectively prevented by DTP vaccine.
Mycobac **ter** ium tuberculosis	bacillus that causes tuberculosis.
Neis **ser** ia gonorrhoeae	known as gonococcus (GC), causes gonorrhea. *Gono* means "related to semen or seed."
Neis **ser** ia meningitidis	infection occurs through the nasopharynx into lymphatics and to the blood, producing bacteremia with metastatic lesions—especially in the meninges, but also in lungs, joints, ears, eyes, and skin.
Pseudo **mon** is aeruginosa	a bacillus, causes UTIs, but also eye, ear, intestinal, and skin infections.
Salmo **nel** la typhi	bacillus that causes typhoid fever.
Salmo **nel** la typhimurium	causes salmonellosis (common food poisoning) and other GI illnesses.
Shi **gel** la	bacillus, causes bacillary dysentery.
Staphylo **coc** cus aureus	commonly called "staph" infection; causes boils, cystitis, pyelitis, impetigo, septicemia, endocarditis, meningitis, pneumonia, and puerperal sepsis.
Strepto **coc** cus pyogenes	commonly called "strep" infection; capable of inducing infection in every organ and tissue of the body, including impetigo, cellulitis, erysipelas, tonsillitis, laryngitis, otitis media, pneumonia, scarlet fever, rheumatic fever, pharyngitis (strep throat).

Other Pathogenic Organisms and Parasites

Pathogen	*Action*
Can **did** a albicans	a yeast, causes moniliasis or candidiasis, thrush in infants.
Coccidi **oi** ides immitis	a spore-forming fungus; causes valley fever (coccidioidomycosis).
Enta **moe** iba histolytica	causes ameobiasis (amoebic dysentery).
Giar idia lamblia	a flagellate that causes giardiasis (protozoa).
Peni **cill** ium notatum	a mold; often a culture contaminent but used as an antibiotic.
Peni **cill** ium chrysogenum	a mold; often a culture contaminent but used as an antibiotic.
Plas **mod** ium vivax	cause of malaria.
Pneumo **cyst** is carinii	cause of the deadly lung infection AIDS victims are prone to develop, as are transplant patients, who receive immunosuppressive therapy; an "opportunistic organism."
Ric **kett** siae	transmitted by a tick; causes Rocky Mountain spotted fever.
Tinea	causes ringworm, a communicable fungal infection.
Trepon **em** a pallidum	a spirochete that causes syphilis, which is also called *lues* (pronounced **lū**-ēz).
Trichi **nel** la spiralis	a worm that causes trichinosis.
Tricho **mon** as vaginalis	a flagellate that causes vaginal infections.

Viruses

Viruses have not been rigidly classified. You will hear of the following:

AIDS virus, or HIV (human immunodeficiency virus)

cytomegalovirus

Ebola virus

ECHO virus

Epstein-Barr (EBV) virus (associated with mononucleosis)

herpes virus

polio virus

respiratory syncytial virus (RSV)

retrovirus

rhinovirus

Type I or II flu virus

APPENDIX F

Chapter Tests and Review Exams

Your instructor will decide which tests will be given; some instructors may choose to use their own tests.

Chapter 1	Introduction and Basic Medical Words	281
Chapter 2	Surgical Procedures	283
Chapter 3	Medical Conditions and Diseases	285
Chapter 4	Medical Instruments and Machines	287
Chapter 5	Medical Specialists and Specialties	289
Review Exam 1	Chapters 1–5	291
Chapter 6	Plural Endings	295
Chapter 7	Additional Prefixes	297
Chapter 8	Additional Suffixes and Root Words	299
Chapter 9	Bacteria, Colors, and Review	301
Review Exam 2	Chapters 6–9	303
Chapter 10	Directional, Positional, and Numerical Terms	305
Chapter 11	Additional Terms	307
Chapter 12	General Abbreviations	309
Chapter 13	Diagnostic and Laboratory Abbreviations	311
Chapter 14	Basic Pharmacology	313
Review Exam 3	Chapters 10–14	315
Chapter 15	Structure of the Body	317
Chapter 16	Integumentary System	319
Chapter 16	Alternate Test	321
Chapter 17	Musculoskeletal System	323
Chapter 17	Alternate Test	325
Chapter 18	Cardiovascular System	327
Chapter 18	Alternate Test	329
Chapter 19	Respiratory System	331
Chapter 19	Alternate Test	333

Chapter 20   Gastrointestinal System   335
Chapter 20   Alternate Test   337
Chapter 21   Urinary System   339
Chapter 21   Alternate Test   341
Review Exam 4   Chapters 15–21   343
Chapter 22 and 23   Reproductive Systems   347
Chapter 22 and 23   Alternate Test   351
Chapter 24   Part 1 Nervous System   353
Chapter 24   Part 1 Alternate Test   355
Chapter 24   Part 2 Psychiatric Terms   357
Review Exam 5   Chapters 22–24   359
Chapter 25   Part 1 Sense Organs: Eyes and Ears   361
Chapter 25   Part 2 Sense Organs: Mouth   363
Chapter 26   Endocrine System and Stress Response   365
Chapter 26   Alternate Test   367
Midterm Exam   Chapters 1–14   369
Final Exam   Chapters 1–26   371

Test

points: 100

Do not write on this page until assigned

_____

name

_____

course or section no.

Chapter 1
Introduction and Basic Medical Words

Spell: (4 points each)

1. _____

2. _____

3. _____

4. _____

5. _____

6. _____

7. _____

8. _____

9. _____

10. _____

11. _____

12. _____

Define any eight: (2 points each)

_____

_____

_____

_____

_____

_____

_____

_____

_____

_____

_____

_____

_____

_____

_____

_____

_____

_____

_____

(continued)

Build a word: (6 points each; if correct word but misspelled, only 3 points)

13. Excision of the adenoids _____

14. Excision of the spleen _____

15. Excision of the stomach _____

16. Excision of the pancreas _____

17. Excision of the larynx _____

18. Excision of a nerve _____

Do not write on this page until assigned

_____
name

_____
course or section no.

Chapter 2
Surgical Procedures

Spell: (2 points each)

1. _____

2. _____

3. _____

4. _____

5. _____

6. _____

7. _____

8. _____

9. _____

10. _____

11. _____

12. _____

Define all: (2 points each)

_____

_____

_____

_____

_____

_____

_____

_____

_____

_____

_____

_____

_____

_____

_____

_____

_____

_____

_____

_____

_____

_____

_____

(continued)

13. _____   _____

_____

14. _____   _____

_____

15. _____   _____

_____

Build a word: (4 points each; if correct word but misspelled, only 2 points)

16. Excision of the appendix _____

17. New permanent opening into the stomach _____

18. Crushing of a "stone" (litho) _____

19. Fixation or suturing a fallopian tube _____

20. Incision into the abdomen _____

21. Excision of an ovary _____

22. Surgical repair of a kidney _____

23. Surgical puncture (tapping to remove fluid) of abdomen _____

24. New (emergency) opening into (incision into) trachea _____

25. Excision of the pancreas _____

Do not write on this page until assigned

_____

name

_____

course or section no.

Chapter 3
Medical Conditions and Diseases

Give a word for: (4 points each)

1. Excision of the uterus _____

2. Inflammation of the ear _____

3. A new permanent opening into the colon _____

4. Tapping (puncture) of the chest to remove fluid _____

5. Repair of a hernia _____

6. Any disease of the heart muscle _____

7. Condition of the skin _____

8. "Any disease" of the glands _____

9. Incision into the trachea _____

10. Fixation of a kidney _____

11. Excision of the spleen _____

12. Pain along a nerve _____

13. A hollow sac or organ _____

14. An infected state or condition _____

15. High blood pressure _____

Spell: (2 points each)

16. _____

17. _____

18. _____

19. _____

20. _____

Define: (2 points each)

_____

_____

_____

_____

_____

_____

_____

_____

_____

(continued)

21.

22.

23.

24.

25.

26.

Test

points: 100

_____

name

_____

course or section no.

Chapter 4
Medical Instruments and Machines

1. Name five "scope" instruments used _for looking into_ body parts and name the body part:

Scopes (3 points each)   _Body part_ (2 points each)

_____   _____

_____   _____

_____   _____

_____   _____

_____   _____

2. Name two "scopes" used for _listening_:

Scopes (3 points each)   _Body part_ (2 points each)

_____   _____

                                        _____

_____   _____

                                        _____

Fill in the blank: (2 points each)

3. Electrocardio **og** raphy is a procedure similar to electroencepha **log** raphy, except that the first concerns

   the _____ and the second, the _____

4. An electrocardiogram is placed in the patient's file. It is a _____ of heart action.

   A thermometer records _____

5. There are many kinds of dilators. One that is used to dilate the vaginal orifice is called a _____

   _____ (during pelvic examination).

(continued)

6. List at least 15 *suffixes* you have learned and place them under the proper heading: (1 point each)

cutting or surgical procedure	diseases or conditions	medical instruments and machines and their use

Spell: (2 points each)

7. _____

8. _____

9. _____

10. _____

11. _____

12. _____

13. _____

14. _____

15. _____

16. _____

Define: (2 points each)

_____

_____

_____

_____

_____

_____

_____

_____

_____

_____

_____

_____

_____

_____

_____

_____

_____

_____

_____

_____

Test

points: 101

_____

name

_____

course or section no.

Chapter 5
Medical Specialists and Specialties

Name the medical or osteopathic specialist: Must be spelled correctly. (4 points each)

1. Prenatal care, delivery, and postpartum _____

2. All kinds of nonsurgical conditions _____

3. Children only _____

4. Interpreting and diagnosing by X-ray procedures _____

5. Skin conditions and diseases _____

6. Mental illness _____

7. Eye diseases and eye surgery _____

8. Diseases and injuries, nervous system _____

9. Heart (and blood vessel) diseases _____

10. Hearing disorders _____

True/False: Circle the number of the _true_ statements only. Defend your answers. Explain what is "untrue" in the false statements. (3 points each)

11. Many kinds of different specialists perform surgery; general practitioners also perform surgery.

12. An optometrist treats refractive errors by prescribing glasses.

13. An osteopathic physician has an equal number of years of education as a medical doctor.

14. A psychologist is an MD.

15. Foot disorders can be treated by an MD or a podiatrist.

16. False teeth are called dentures; they are a prosthetic device.

Identify: Spell out. (3 points each)

17. DO _____

18. DDS _____

19. RN _____

20. LPN _____

21. MD _____

(continued)

Fill in the blank: (4 points each)

22. The dental specialist who straightens teeth is the _____

23. The dental specialist who treats gum diseases is the _____

Spell: (2 points each)

Define: (2 points each)

24. _____   _____

    _____

25. _____   _____

    _____

26. _____   _____

    _____

27. _____   _____

    _____

28. _____   _____

    _____

Review Exam 1

points: 113

_____

name

_____

course or section no.

Chapters 1–5 Review

Spell: (2 points each)   **Define:** (2 points each)

1. _____   _____
2. _____   _____
3. _____   _____
4. _____   _____
5. _____   _____
6. _____   _____
7. _____   _____
8. _____   _____
9. _____   _____
10. _____   _____

Build a word: (2 points each, 1 if misspelled)

1. The study or science of the ears.   _____
2. A specialist (OD) who treats refractive errors and fits eyeglasses. _____
3. A specialist dealing in root canal work.   _____
4. The procedure of using a lighted instrument to view the joints. _____
5. A condition of the kidney.   _____

Multiple choice: Circle the most appropriate answer for each statement below. (2 points each)

1. Neuralgia is
   a. a fungal infection that invades the nerves
   b. a medication used for its sedative effect
   c. nerve pain
   d. a condition of the nerves
   e. none of the above

2. Menorrhagia is
   a. bursting forth of menses
   b. a condition of irritation in males
   c. a hernia that occurs exclusively in males
   d. b and c only
   e. none of the above

(continued)

3. An anesthetic
   a. puts you to sleep; a sedative
   b. gives the sensation of being without feeling
   c. is a body part
   d. none of the above
   e. all of the above

4. Hyperactivity is
   a. a byproduct of hypertension
   b. the opposite of hypoactivity
   c. a treatment for some glandular disorders
   d. excessive motionful behavior
   e. b and d only

5. Dyspnea is
   a. a Floridian fantasy land
   b. painful diarrhea
   c. partial paralysis
   d. a condition of the knees
   e. difficult or labored breathing

True or False: Circle T if you agree the statement is true or F if you think it is false. (2 points each)

1. Abdominocentesis is a surgical procedure to remove the stomach.   T   F

2. Neurotripsy is the surgical crushing of a nerve.   T   F

3. Oophoritis is inflammation of the eye.   T   F

4. A colostomy is a new permanent opening into the colon.   T   F

5. Adenopathy is any glandular condition or disease.   T   F

Define: (2 points each)

1. afebrile   _____

2. contraindicated   _____

3. myringotomy   _____

4. aseptic   _____

5. dermatosis   _____

Identification: Identify the root word for each of the following. (2 points each)

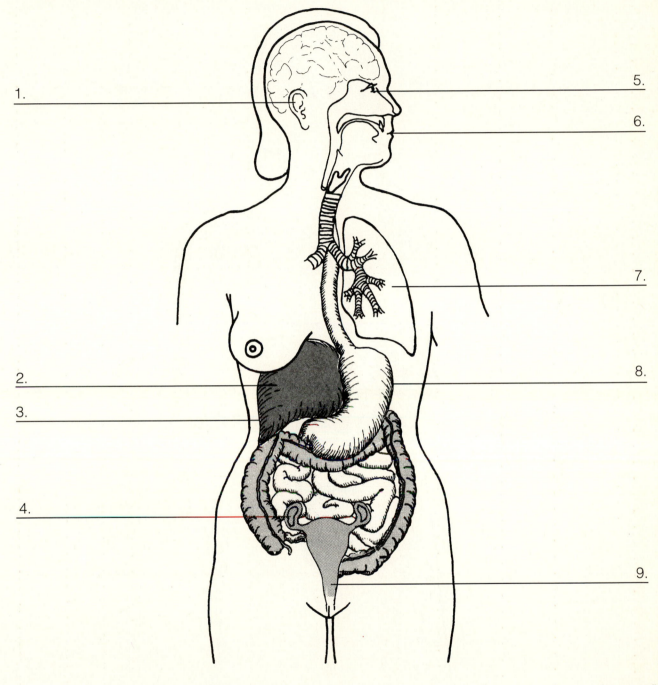

1. _____

2. _____

3. _____

4. _____

5. _____

6. _____

7. _____

8. _____

9. _____

(continued)

Identification: Identify the root word for each of the following. (1 point each)

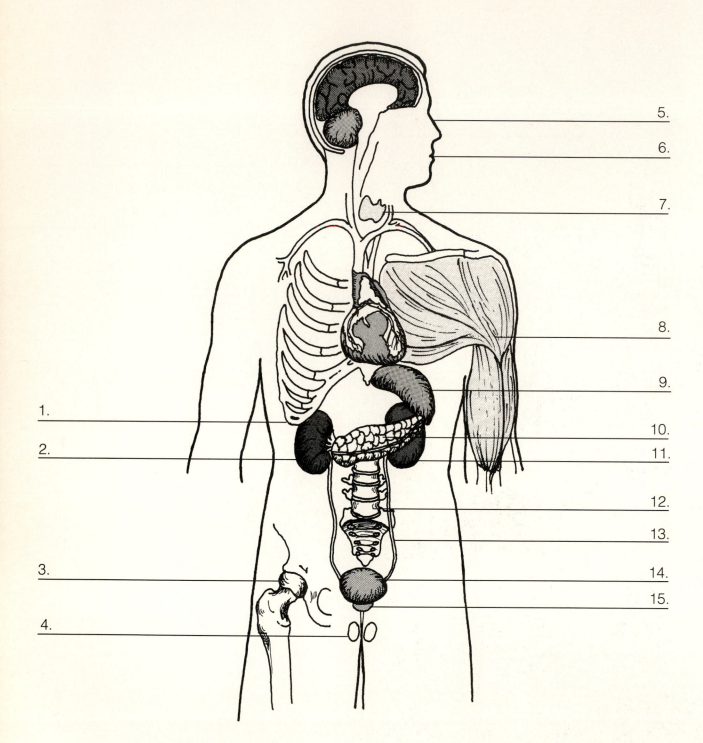

1. _____

2. _____

3. _____

4. _____

5. _____

6. _____

7. _____

8. _____

9. _____

10. _____

11. _____

12. _____

13. _____

14. _____

15. _____

Do not write on this page until assigned

_____

name

_____

course or section no.

**Chapter 6
Plural Endings**

Fill in the blank: (3 points each)

1. The singular form of a female reproductive egg is _____

2. The plural form of the medical term for some blood clots is _____

3. The plural form of the medical term for determining the cause of an illness ("through knowledge") is

    _____

4. The plural form of the medical term for toes is _____

5. The plural form of petechia is _____

Give plural: (3 points each)

6. diagnosis _____

7. apex _____

8. focus _____

9. vertebra _____

10. diverticulum _____

11. lumen _____

Write singular of: (3 points each)

12. data _____

13. bacilli _____

14. crises _____

15. lumina _____

16. enemata _____

Test

points: 100

_____
name

_____
course or section no.

Chapter 7
Additional Prefixes

True/False: Circle the number of the *true* statements only. Defend your answers. Explain what is "untrue" in the false statements. (2 points each)

1. A medication given before surgery is called a postoperative medication.

2. Prognosis is the predicted outcome of a disease.

3. The six-week period following delivery is called postpartum.

4. A patient who cannot void may be said to have polyuria.

5. Dysmenorrhea means painful menstruation.

6. A general anesthetic produces loss of all sensation.

7. An antiseptic helps to prevent infection.

8. Hyperactive people would not be as likely to be overweight as those who are hypoactive.

9. Fear and excitement often cause bradycardia.

10. Bioavailability means the drug is available from the pharmacy.

Spell: (2 points each)

11. _____

12. _____

13. _____

14. _____

15. _____

16. _____

Define: (2 points each)

_____

_____

_____

_____

_____

_____

_____

_____

_____

_____

_____

_____

(continued)

17. _____   _____

                                             _____

18. _____   _____

                                             _____

19. _____   _____

                                             _____

20. _____   _____

                                             _____

Define: (2 points each)

21. ar **rhyth** mia _____

22. dys **u** ria _____

23. hypo **der** mic _____

24. antico **ag** ulant _____

25. he **mol** ysis _____

Fill in the blank: A term will be dictated for the first blank of each sentence below. After supplying the correctly spelled word, fill in the blanks to complete the sentences. (1 point each dictated term for spelling; 2 points each sentence for filling in the blanks)

26. _____ occurs with most illnesses. It means general _____

27. _____ can cause loss of sleep. It means _____

_____

28. _____ is the opposite of _____ (bad feeling).

29. _____ occurs at about age 50. It means _____

30. _____ , when painful, is called _____

31. _____ is disfiguring. A person with this condition has _____

_____

32. _____ means (literally) a condition of _____

33. _____ is best treated by a dentist called an _____

34. _____ means a group of _____ that generally occur together.

35. _____ solutions have an amount of salt equal to that of _____

Test

points: 100

_____
name

_____
course or section no.

Chapter 8
Additional Suffixes and Root Words

Define: (4 points each)

1. anemia   _____

2. thermometer   _____

3. hematology   _____

4. phagocytosis   _____

5. hysterorrhexis _____

6. hemolysis   _____

7. laryngitis   _____

8. sarcoma   _____

9. nocturia   _____

10. in situ   _____

11. pyorrhea   _____

12. orchidoplasty   _____

13. azotemia   _____

14. lipoid   _____

15. paronychia   _____

Fill in the blank: A term will be dictated for the first blank of each sentence below. After supplying the correctly spelled word, fill in the blanks to complete the sentences. (2 points each dictated term for spelling; 2 points each sentence for fill in the blank)

16. _____ is a _____ or _____ tumor.

17. _____ means _____

18. _____ of muscles results from _____

19. _____ is difficult _____

20. _____ is _____ of either _____ of the body.

21. _____ means _____ breathing

(continued)

22. _____ occurs because of dietary deficiency. It means _____ of

_____

23. _____ lesions are producing _____

24. _____ means (literally) _____. It refers to

frequent watery _____

25. _____ is important in surgery. It means _____

Test
points: 90

_____
name

_____
course or section no.

Chapter 9
Bacteria, Colors, and Review

Give a word for: (4 points each)

1. spherically shaped bacteria _____

2. bacteria that need oxygen _____

3. unable to move _____

4. bacterium that grows in clusters _____

5. bacterium that grows in pairs _____

6. poisons _____

7. grown in the laboratory _____

8. liver disease _____

9. disease associated with increase in WBCs _____

10. condition of deficient pigmentation _____

Fill in the blank: A term will be dictated for the first blank of each sentence below. After supplying the correctly spelled word, fill in the blanks to complete the sentences. (2 points each dictated term for spelling; 2 points each sentence for filling in the blanks)

11. _____ is a term for _____ _____ _____

12. _____ is a condition of being _____ in color.

13. _____ is a bacterium that causes illness. It is _____

   in shape and grows in _____

14. _____ is a rod-shaped _____

15. _____ is a term for bacteria that grow in _____ of

   _____

16. _____ organisms cause _____

17. _____ is an illness also known as _____

18. _____ is a characteristic of bacteria that means _____

19. _____ is the study of _____

20. _____ can only be seen with an _____ microscope and

   cannot be successfully treated with _____

(continued)

Draw a picture of staphylococci and a picture of the bacterium referred to in Question 13. (5 points each)

Review Exam 2

points: 100

_____

name

_____

course or section no.

Chapters 6–9 Review

Spell: (2 points each)   **Define:** (2 points each)

1. _____   _____

2. _____   _____

3. _____   _____

4. _____   _____

5. _____   _____

6. _____   _____

7. _____   _____

8. _____   _____

9. _____   _____

10. _____   _____

Build a word: (2 points each, 1 if misspelled)

1. Destruction of red blood cells _____

2. Paralysis of all four limbs _____

3. Inability to eat or swallow _____

4. Malignant growth _____

5. White blood cell _____

Multiple choice: Circle the most appropriate answer for each statement below. (2 points each)

1. Sequelae are
    a. initial signs of a disease
    b. recurrences of a disease
    c. the aftereffects of a disease
    d. b and c only
    e. none of the above

2. Cyanosis is
    a. a condition of sensitivity to light
    b. a type of medicine
    c. a symptom or condition of blueness
    d. a and c only
    e. none of the above

(continued)

3. Multipara means
   a. capable of many pairings
   b. a condition of many illnesses
   c. to bear many children
   d. too much intake
   e. none of the above

4. Syndrome is
   a. a type of symptom
   b. a group of symptoms that occur together in a pattern
   c. a procedure for obtaining thin sections of skin for grafting
   d. an instrument
   e. none of the above

5. Lipoid is
   a. resembling lips
   b. a being from the planet Lip
   c. a condition of lesions on the lips
   d. a condition of fat lips
   e. fat-like

True or False: Circle T if you agree the statement is true or F if you think it is false. (2 points each)

1. It is rare to see one petechiae.   T   F

2. Ova is singular and ovum is plural.   T   F

3. We all have ten phalanx, right?   T   F

4. Hypotension is a clinical term for relaxation.   T   F

5. Cytoplasm is the fluid inside a cell.   T   F

Define: (2 points each)

1. tachycardia _____

2. prodromal _____

3. polyuria _____

4. preoperative _____

5. lithotripsy _____

Identification: Identify the medical root words for the following. (2 points each)

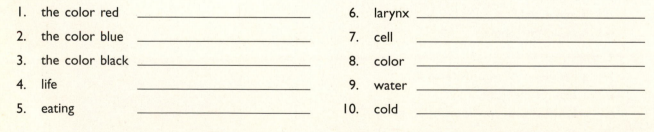

1. the color red _____   6. larynx _____

2. the color blue _____   7. cell _____

3. the color black _____   8. color _____

4. life _____   9. water _____

5. eating _____   10. cold _____

Do not write on this page until assigned

_____
name

_____
course or section no.

Chapter 10
Directional, Positional, and Numerical Terms

Fill in the blanks: (4 points each)

1. The opposite of flexion is _____

2. Distal is the opposite of _____

3. The front surface of the body is _____

4. The back surface of the body is _____

5. The abdomen is divided into four areas called _____

   for describing the area involved.

6. Cephalic means toward the head; _____ means toward the tail (base of the spine).

7. Bedsores are called _____ ulcers because they are caused by lying in bed.

8. Bilateral pneumonia means pneumonia in _____ _____

   (2 words, 4 points total)

9. A person lying face down is in what position? _____

10. Another term for middle is _____

11. Bending is _____

12. A tubal pregnancy is one "out of place" and is called _____

True/False: Circle the number of the _true_ statements only. Defend your answers. Explain what is "untrue" in the false statements. (2 points each)

13. Dorsal recumbent position is lying on back, face up.

14. Epigastric pain is pain over the stomach area.

15. An AP X-ray film of the chest is taken from the back of the patient.

16. Periodontal disease is a gum disease that causes teeth to become loose.

17. The abdomen is divided into four quadrants.

18. Sims' position is lying on the right side.

19. A fever is a temperature over 98.6° F; a temperature below 98.6° F is considered to be a subnormal temperature.

20. Internal hemorrhage is bleeding somewhere inside the body.

21. Rotation means turning.

(continued)

Define: (2 points each)

22. extrauterine _____

23. lithotomy position _____

24. hemiplegia _____

25. abduction _____

Spelling: (2 points each)

26. _____   31. _____

27. _____   32. _____

28. _____   33. _____

29. _____   34. _____

30. _____   35. _____

Describe or draw body planes: (4 points each)

36. midsagittal

37. coronal

38. transverse

Test

points: 91 + 6 bonus

Do not write on this page until assigned

_____

name

_____

course or section no.

Chapter 11
Additional Terms

True/False: Circle the number of the *true* statements only. Defend your answers. Explain what is "untrue" in the false statements. (3 points each)

1. The terms *ascites* and *anasarca* refer to excessive fluid accumulation in the body tissues.

2. Triage is a method of sorting the wounded or ill.

3. Many disease conditions are characterized by periods of remission and exacerbation.

4. If a patient is afebrile, he has a fever.

5. A palpable lesion is one that can be seen.

6. A cadaver is a corpse.

7. Serous drainage is "similar to serum."

8. Adnexa uteri are the ovaries, fallopian tubes, and ligaments.

9. Auscultation has to do with listening to sounds from within the body.

10. Percussion is done along with auscultation. It means tapping or striking to produce sounds.

11. Axillary temperature is taken in the groin.

12. *Anomaly* means some kind of defect or irregularity.

13. A biopsy involves the examination of dead tissue.

Fill in the blank: (4 points for each word)

14. *Abortion* means premature expulsion of a nonviable _____

15. An abscess is a localized accumulation of _____

16. A(n) _____ infection usually starts suddenly and is more severe but shorter in duration than a(n) _____ infection.

17. _____ is a word that means "growing together" of tissues that should not be attached.

Define: (2 points each)

18. incontinent _____

19. voided   _____

20. edema   _____

(continued)

Spell: (1 point each)   **Define:** (1 point each)

21. _____   _____

22. _____   _____

23. _____   _____

24. _____   _____

25. _____   _____

26. _____   _____

27. _____   _____

28. _____   _____

29. _____   _____

30. _____   _____

31. _____   _____

32. _____   _____

33. _____   _____

34. *Underline* words that are incorrectly spelled. (Correct them for a bonus point.)

dilitation _____   pneumocystis _____

coccygeal _____   abdomin _____

sputum _____   recipiant _____

cervicle _____   abdomenal _____

paralyzed _____   fibrilation _____

Chapter 12
General Abbreviations

Give abbreviation or term for the following: (2 points each)

1. Patient is not to have any food or drink _____

2. Patient may get up to go to the bathroom only _____

3. Patient is to be given compassionate nursing care _____

4. Patient is to have a complete blood count _____

5. Patient is to be given a large amount of liquid to drink _____

6. Amount of urine sent to lab for certain test was insufficient _____

7. All fluids patient drinks and voids are to be measured _____

8. Patient is to walk twice a day _____

9. Patient may have aspirin grains ten every four hours as needed _____

Give the abbreviation for: (2 points each)

10. three times a day _____

11. immediately _____

12. with _____

13. without _____

14. water _____

15. oxygen _____

16. grams _____

17. liters _____

18. units _____

19. capsules _____

20. cubic centimeters _____

Identify (spell out): (2 points each)

21. B.E. _____

22. IVP _____

23. GB series _____

24. upper GI series _____

25. ECG (EKG) _____

26. TPR _____

27. EEG _____

(continued)

Spell out and explain: (2 points each)

28. V/S   _____

29. BRP   _____

30. B/P   _____

31. OPV   _____

32. V.S.   _____

33. MMR   _____

34. C̄   _____

Name *ten* hospital departments: Give abbreviations if any. (1 point each)

35. _____   40. _____

36. _____   41. _____

37. _____   42. _____

38. _____   43. _____

39. _____   44. _____

Fill in the blank:

45. Orders for hospitalized patients should include (1 point each) _____

_____

46. Write abbreviations and spell out all combined routine immunizations: (2 points each)

a. _____

b. _____

c. _____

47. Spell out: (2 points each)

DRGs _____

ICD _____

48. Write the Roman numeral for the number: (1 point each)

7 _____

10 _____

4 _____

Five bonus points: Write an Rx for patient to have 50 milligrams of Demerol every four hours as
needed:

_____

_____

Do not write on this page until assigned

_____
name

_____
course or section no.

Chapter 13
Diagnostic and Laboratory Abbreviations

Define: (2 points each)

1. Cardiovascular diagnoses

   CVA _____

   MI _____

   CHF _____

2. Respiratory diagnoses

   URI _____

   COPD or COLD _____

3. Nervous system diagnoses

   CP _____

   MS _____

4. History-taking abbreviations

   PH _____

   PERLA _____

   Dx _____

5. Glucose tests

   FBS _____

   GTT _____

Lab: Name divisions of the medical laboratory and a kind of test performed in each. (2 points each)

Division   _Test_

6. _____   _____

7. _____   _____

8. _____   _____

Fill in the blanks: (2 points each)

9. What is the Pap smear or test used for? _____

_____

(continued)

10. What is meant by cath spec? Spell and explain. _____

_____

_____

11. Name three tests performed in routine urinalysis. _____

_____

_____

Define: (2 points each)

12. erythrocytes _____

13. WBC and diff _____

_____

14. culture and sensitivity (C & S) _____

_____

15. V.A. _____

16. three kinds of leukocytes _____

_____

True/False: Circle the number of the *true* statements only. (2 points each)

17. SMA (SMAC) includes a group of blood chemistry tests.

18. CA is an abbreviation for cancer.

19. Morphology of cells means numbers present.

20. Many kinds of bodily excretions are examined in the laboratory.

Spell: (1 point each)   **Define:** (2 points each)

21. _____   _____

          _____

22. _____   _____

          _____

23. _____   _____

          _____

24. _____   _____

          _____

Define: (2 points each)

25. qd _____

26. q4h _____

Test

points: 70

_____

name

_____

course or section no.

Chapter 14
Basic Pharmacology

Fill in the blank: (5 points each answer)

1. The generic drug name of Bayer aspirin is _____

2. PDR stands for the _____ and lists

   all _____ drugs and information about them.

3. _____ relieve nasal congestion.

4. _____ help prevent rejection in organ transplantation.

5. An _____ tells you when a drug should be discarded.

6. The types of drugs that relieve pain are called _____ drugs.

   These include _____ and _____ such as morphine.

7. A representative of a pharmaceutical company is also known as a _____

Spell out: (2 points each)

8. OTC _____

9. IND _____

10. FDA _____

11. USP _____

12. Rx _____

Explain the difference between generic and trade names for drugs. (10 points)

_____

_____

_____

_____

Review Exam 3

Do not write on this page until assigned

_____
name

_____
course or section no.

Review Chapters 10–14

Spell: (2 points each)

1. _____
2. _____
3. _____
4. _____
5. _____
6. _____
7. _____
8. _____
9. _____
10. _____

Define: (2 points each)

_____
_____
_____
_____
_____
_____
_____
_____
_____
_____

Build a word: (2 points each, 1 if misspelled)

1. Abnormally low temperature _____
2. Movement toward the midline _____
3. On both sides _____
4. On the same side _____
5. On one side _____

Multiple choice: Circle the most appropriate answer for each statement below. (2 points each)

1. Adduction is
   a. to move away from midline
   b. to move toward midline
   c. the term for a type of incision
   d. a and c only
   e. none of the above

2. Superior is
   a. an MD's boss
   b. a term identifying a position
   c. a type of supplement prescribed
   d. above
   e. b and d only

(continued)

3. Epigastric is
   a. a very long stomach
   b. pertaining to a round-shaped stomach
   c. a location above the stomach
   d. a ring on the stomach
   e. none of the above

4. A generic drug is
   a. a "one size fits all" medical placebo
   b. an alternative to a "trade name" substance
   c. a less expensive medication with a nonproprietary name
   d. b and c only
   e. none of the above

5. Acute means
   a. sudden and severe
   b. slowly developing and lasting a long time
   c. chronic
   d. a and b only
   e. none of the above

True or False: Circle T if you agree the statement is true or F if you think it is false. (2 points each)

1. RUQ is identified from the physician's perspective.   T   F
2. Q4h is a physician's order for a medication to be given four times daily (that is, within 24 hours). T   F
3. A UTI is very similar to a URI.   T   F
4. Quadriplegic is paralysis involving all extremities.   T   F
5. Dorsal is the same as anterior.   T   F

Define: (2 points each)

1. prn _____
2. interaction _____
3. abscess _____
4. stat _____
5. tolerance _____

Test

points: 91

Do not write on this page until assigned

_____

name

_____

course or section no.

Chapter 15
Stucture of the Body

Fill in the blank: (3 points each blank)

1. The human body is made up of four structural units. Name them, *in order,* beginning with smallest unit:

    a. _____   c. _____

    b. _____   d. _____

2. Organs that work together are called _____

3. Name three body systems and one organ in each:

    _____

    _____

    _____

4. Give the other name for the thoracic cavity _____ and the abdominopelvic

    cavity _____ (names derived from the *name of the membrane lining cavity*)

5. The dome-shaped muscle that separates the chest and abdominal cavities is the _____

6. The space between lungs where the heart lies is called the _____

7. The chromosomes in the cell nucleus contain the _____,

    which pass hereditary characteristics to offspring.

8. Endocrine glands are also called _____ glands.

9. Cells reproduce by a process called _____

10. GI stands for _____

11. The main parts of a cell (three) are the _____

    _____

True/False: Circle the number of the *true* statements only. Defend your answers. Explain what is "untrue" in the false statements. (2 points each)

12. Congenital diseases are acquired in infancy.

13. The brain and spinal cord lie in the cranial cavity.

14. Metabolism is the sum of all physical and chemical changes that take place in the body.

15. Vascular diseases involve only the heart and brain.

16. The primary tissues (kinds of tissues in the body) are epithelial, smooth, connective, and muscular.

17. People who are immunodeficient are vulnerable to every infection they encounter.

(continued)

Define: (2 points each)

18. colostomy _____

19. cholecystectomy _____

20. stomatitis _____

21. laparotomy _____

Spell: (1 point each)

22. _____

23. _____

24. _____

25. _____

26. _____

27. _____

28. _____

29. _____

30. _____

Define any five: (1 point each)

_____

_____

_____

_____

_____

_____

_____

_____

_____

_____

_____

_____

_____

Test

points: 105

Do not write on this page until assigned

_____
name

_____
course or section no.

Chapter 16
Integumentary System

Fill in the blank: (3 points each blank)

1. The specialist who treats skin disorders is a _____

2. Three functions of the skin are _____

    _____

3. Give three terms used to describe skin lesions and define:

    _____   _____

    _____   _____

    _____   _____

4. Name three skin diseases: _____

    _____

True/False: Circle the number of the _true_ statements only. Defend your answers. Explain what is "untrue" in the false statements. (2 points each)

5. Perspiration serves no useful purpose.

6. Some systemic diseases produce skin symptoms or manifestations.

7. The outer layer of skin is the dermis.

8. Skin cancer should be suspected when a nevus changes in size or appearance, or begins to bleed.

9. Tinea pedis is athlete's foot. One need not be an athlete to get this disease.

10. Sebaceous glands secrete sebum, which keeps the skin pliable.

11. Blood vessels and nerves are present in the epidermal layer.

12. Areola mamma is the halo or ring around the nipple (breast).

13. Contact dermatitis is inflammation of the skin caused by coming in contact with some irritant.

14. Pruritus means inflammation of the breast.

15. The Dick and Schick skin tests may be used to determine susceptibility to scarlet fever and diphtheria respectively.

Write the word that means: (3 points each; only 2 points if misspelled)

16. Process of stretching or opening wider   _____

17. A new permanent opening into the colon   _____

(continued)

18. Plastic surgery on the nose _____

19. Surgical puncture of the abdomen to remove fluid _____

20. Surgical repair of a hernia _____

21. Incision into the trachea _____

Define: (2 points each)

22. Mantoux _____

23. nummular _____

24. biopsy _____

25. erythema _____

26. dermatome _____

Spell: (1 point each)

27. _____

28. _____

29. _____

30. _____

31. _____

32. _____

33. _____

34. _____

Define: (1 point each)

_____

_____

_____

_____

_____

_____

_____

_____

_____

_____

_____

_____

_____

Do not write on this page until assigned

_____
name

_____
course or section no.

Chapter 16
Integumentary System

True/False: Circle the number of the _true_ statements only. Defend your answers. Explain what is "untrue" in the false statements. (2 points each)

1. A dermatologist is a specialist who diagnoses and treats skin disorders.

2. Macules, papules, and vesicles are terms to describe skin lesions.

3. Athlete's foot is an athlete's disease.

4. Oil glands are called sebaceous glands.

5. The breasts are also called the mammae.

6. Some systemic diseases produce skin symptoms.

7. A mole is a nevus; two moles, nevi.

8. A biopsy is an examination of living tissue.

9. Sweat glands are called sudoriferous glands.

Fill in the blank: (2 points each)

10. A blister is called a _____;

    a larger blister is a _____

11. The skin test used to determine susceptibility to diphtheria is the _____

12. The two outermost layers of the skin are the _____ and the _____

13. Herpes simplex is the medical term for _____

14. The halo around the nipple of the breast is called the _____

15. Three functions of the skin are _____

    _____

16. Name three parasitic skin infestations: _____

    _____

17. White patches of skin due to loss of pigment signal the disorder called _____

18. Name and describe three skin diseases:

    _____

    _____

    _____

    _____

    _____

(continued)

Write a word that means: (3 points each)

19. Excision of tonsils _____

20. Fixation of a kidney _____

21. Incision into the abdomen _____

22. New permanent opening into trachea _____

23. Tapping of chest to remove fluid _____

Define: (2 points each)

24. laceration _____

25. benign _____

26. malignant _____

27. sebaceous _____

28. lactation _____

Spell: (1 point each)

29. _____

30. _____

31. _____

32. _____

33. _____

34. _____

35. _____

36. _____

37. _____

38. _____

Define any seven: (1 point each)

_____

_____

_____

_____

_____

_____

_____

_____

_____

_____

_____

_____

_____

_____

name

_____

course or section no.

Chapter 17
Musculoskeletal System

Fill in the blank: (2 points each)

1.   The five sections of the spinal column, *in order*, starting at the neck are (a) _____

   (b) _____   (d) _____

   (c) _____   (e) _____

2.   Two functions of the musculoskeletal system are _____

   and _____

3.   Bones are attached to other bones by fibrous tissue called _____. Muscles are

   attached to bones by _____

4.   Name of fracture: bone broken, protruding through skin _____;

   bone cracked, not separated _____

5.   Flexion and extension mean _____ and _____

6.   Moving the arm out to the side, away from the midline is called _____

Name the bones: (2 points each)

7.   The longest bone in the human body _____

8.   The "shoulder blade" _____   collarbone _____

9.   An individual bone in spinal column _____

10.   Bones of fingers and toes _____

11.   Upper arm bone _____   breastbone _____

True/False: Circle the number of the *true* statements only. Defend your answers. Explain what is "untrue" in the false statements. (2 points each)

12.   Bursae are small sacs that serve to cushion joints.

13.   The extremities are part of the axial skeleton.

14.   The muscles between the ribs are intercostals.

15.   Rickets is a disease caused by bacteria.

16.   Sinuses are cavities or air spaces in the skull.

17.   An osteopath is an MD specialist who treats fractures.

18.   Skeletal muscle is also called involuntary muscle.

19.   Frontal, occipital, temporal, and peritoneal are all names of skull bones.

(continued)

Fill in the blank: (2 points each)

20. Name two kinds of arthritis and age groups affected:

_____

_____

21 Three terms used to describe (in bones) "hollow places" or indentations, parts that project outward, and "holes" in bones _____

_____

22. Tibia and fibula are bones of the _____

Spell out: (1 point each)

23. NSAID _____

24. SLE _____

Define: (2 points each)

25. atrophy _____

26. sutures (in skull) _____

27. orthopedist _____

_____

Spell: (1 point each)　　　　　　　　　**Define:** (1 point each)

28. _____　　_____

_____

29. _____　　_____

_____

30. _____　　_____

_____

31. _____　　_____

_____

32. _____　　_____

_____

33. _____　　_____

_____

34. _____　　_____

_____

35. _____　　_____

_____

Alternate Test

points: 100

_____

name

_____

course or section no.

Chapter 17
Musculoskeletal System

Fill in the blank: (2 points each)

1. Four bones of the cranium are _____

   _____

2. Name and describe three fractures:

   _____

   _____

   _____

3. Tendons attach _____ to _____

4. Other terms that mean: bending _____ and straightening _____

5. Name three large bones of upper extremity: _____

   _____

6. Air spaces or cavities in the cranium are called _____

7. Small sacs that serve to cushion joints are _____

8. Seams or articulations between cranial bones are _____

9. Medical specialist who treats bone disorders is an _____

10. Skeletal muscle is also called _____ or _____ muscle

11. Name two main skeletal divisions: _____

12. Name three kinds of muscle: _____

    _____

13. Name three large bones of lower extremity: _____

    _____

14. Abduction means _____

15. A foramen is a _____

16. Rickets is caused by _____

17. What are the soft spots in an infant skull called? _____

18. Name five segments of the vertebral column, _in order, starting from the bottom_ (tail): _____

    _____

(continued)

Give a word for: (2 points each)

19. "Any disease" of the joints _____

20. Wasting away or shrinking of muscle _____

21. Softening of the bones _____

22. Pain in a joint _____

23. Plastic surgery on a joint _____

24. Inflammation of a joint _____

Spell out and explain: (3 points each)

25. HNP _____

26. DJD _____

Name four other bones not mentioned in previous questions: (2 points each)

27. _____

28. _____

29. _____

30. _____

Test

points: 98

_____

name

_____

course or section no.

Chapter 18
Cardiovascular System

Identify: Define or explain. (2 points each)

1. essential hypertension _____

2. myocardium _____

3. atria _____

4. oxygenated blood _____

5. arteriosclerosis _____

6. embolus _____

_____

7. coronary arteries _____

Fill in the blank: (2 points each)

8. Red blood cells are called _____

9. White blood cells are called _____

10. In a white blood count and differential, the different kinds of WBCs are counted. Name the five basic

    kinds: _____

    _____

11. What procedures are done in laboratory to determine compatibility before a transfusion is given?

    _____ and _____

12. Most people have Rh neg/pos blood. (underline one)

13. The top number in the B/P reading is the _____ and the bottom number is

    the _____ pressure.

14. The tiniest blood vessels are called _____

15. In these tiny vessels _____ and _____ (gases) are exchanged.

    Nutrients and _____ are also exchanged.

16. The dividing wall that separates the right and left sides of the heart is called the _____

17. In atherosclerosis, buildup of deposits in arteries may occlude the opening or _____

    of the vessel (word that means "opening in a tube").

(continued)

True/False: Circle the number of the *true* statements only. Defend your answers. Explain what is "untrue" in the false statements. (2 points each)

18. Other names for heart attack are coronary occlusion, coronary thrombosis, and myocardial infarct (infarction).

19. A stroke is the same as a heart attack.

20. Lymph nodes help filter out injurious particles such as bacteria.

21. Everyone has one of four blood types (A, B, AB, O). Everyone also has the Rh factor.

22. Valves in the heart and in the veins keep blood from backflowing.

23. Anemia literally means "without blood." It actually means low red cell count.

24. The pulmonary arteries carry deoxygenated blood.

25. The left ventricle of the heart has a thicker muscle than the right ventricle because it has to pump blood farther.

26. Platelets help to clot blood.

27. Varicose veins are dilated, tortuous veins that occur when valves "break down."

28. CVA stands for cerebrovascular accident or stroke.

29. Angiography is an X-ray procedure to determine condition of blood vessels.

Identify: (1 point each)

30. CCU _____

31. ECG _____

32. Specialist who treats CVD _____

33. Specialist who treats blood diseases _____

34. Trace the circulation from the vessels that bring blood back to the heart to the vessels that carry it out to all parts of the body; name all structures—vessels, chambers, valves, and organs through which it passes, *in sequence*. (13 structures, 1 point each)

a. _____   f. _____   j. _____

b. _____   g. _____   k. _____

c. _____   h. _____   l. _____

d. _____   i. _____   m. _____

e. _____

Spell: (1 point each)

35. _____   40. _____

36. _____   41. _____

37. _____   42. _____

38. _____   43. _____

39. _____

Alternate Test

points: 98

_____

name

_____

course or section no.

Chapter 18
Cardiovascular System

Fill in the blank: (2 points each)

1. Give two other names for heart attack: _____

   and _____

2. Name the four blood types (Landsteiner): (2 points for all 4) _____

3. In a B/P reading, what is the top pressure called? _____

   Bottom pressure? _____

4. An embolus is a _____ that is floating freely in the bloodstream

5. The receiving chambers of the heart are called _____

6. _Which_ ventricle of the heart has the thicker muscle and _why?_ (4 points) _____

   _____

7. What are the vessels that carry blood _away_ from the heart called? _____

   What are the vessels that carry blood _toward_ the heart called? _____

8. The smallest blood vessels are the _____

9. Three layers of the heart are

   (inner)   _____

   (outer)   _____

   (muscular) _____

True/False: Circle the number of the _true_ statements only. Defend your answers. Explain what is "untrue" in the false statements. (2 points each)

10. A CVA is a cerebrovascular accident or stroke.

11. Everyone has the Rh factor.

12. Hypertension is high blood pressure.

13. Platelets are white blood cells.

14. A CBC is a coronary blood center.

15. Hemiplegia means paralyzed from the waist down.

16. The wall that divides the right and left sides of the heart is the septum.

17. Tachycardia means a slow heart rate.

(continued)

18. Give the names of the five basic kinds of leukocytes: (2 points each) _____

_____

19. Define WBC and diff: (2 points) _____

_____

20. Trace the circulation through the heart, starting with the vessels that bring blood back to the heart from the upper and lower parts of the body, naming all chambers, valves, vessels, and organs, *in order,* until the blood leaves the heart to go to all parts of the body. (13 structures, 1 point each)

_____

_____

_____

_____

_____

_____

Define or explain: (2 points each)

21. valves in veins _____

22. coronary arteries _____

23. erythrocytes _____

24. type and x-match _____

_____

25. arteriosclerosis _____

26. hemostasis _____

27. When does the Rh factor present a problem? (4 points) _____

_____

_____

Spell: (1 point each)   **Define:** (1 point each)

28. _____   _____

_____

29. _____   _____

_____

30. _____   _____

_____

31. _____   _____

_____

32. _____   _____

_____

33. _____   _____

_____

Copyright © 1997 by Addison Wesley Longman

Do not write on this page until assigned

_____
name

_____
course or section no.

Chapter 19
Respiratory System

Matching: Match the terms (A–EE) with definitions (1–25), writing the correct corresponding letter in the space provided before each number. Not all of the terms will be used. (2 points each)

1. _____	Air (gas) expired.	A. vital capacity
2. _____	Combination of inspiration and expiration.	B. aerosol
3. _____	Passageway that carries food and gases.	C. base
4. _____	Tube from middle ear to pharynx.	D. URI
5. _____	Organs of respiration.	E. bilateral
6. _____	Air left in lungs after expiration.	F. adenoids
7. _____	Medical name for croup.	G. isoniazid and PAS
8. _____	Diagnostic skin test for TB.	H. asthma, hay fever
9. _____	A cough that produces sputum.	I. sputum
10. _____	Drugs used to treat TB.	J. lobectomy
11. _____	Excision of part of a lung.	K. rales
12. _____	Allergic disorders of respiratory system.	L. bronchitis
13. _____	Secretion from respiratory tract, examined for diagnosis in TB.	M. CO_2
14. _____	Inflammation of air spaces in cranium.	N. pharynx
15. _____	Abnormal lung sounds.	O. laryngotracheobronchitis
16. _____	Medical name for infection in bronchi.	P. eustachian
17. _____	Excision of glandular structures in pharynx.	Q. lungs
18. _____	Abbreviated term used for standard chest X-ray film.	R. valley fever
19. _____	Flap of tissue that covers larynx when food is swallowed.	S. atelectasis
20. _____	Lower (bottom) part of the lungs.	T. residual
21. _____	Referring to both lungs.	U. Mantoux
22. _____	Mist type of medication that helps dilate air passages and loosens secretions.	V. sinusitis
23. _____	Collapse of lung.	W. tonsillectomy
24. _____	Amount of air that can be forcibly expelled after deep inspiration.	X. epiglottis
25. _____	Infection in upper respiratory tract (abbreviation).	Y. IUR
		Z. productive
		AA. respiration
		BB. AP and lat
		CC. spirometer
		DD. intubate
		EE. mucolytic

(continued)

Give a word for: (2 points each; only 1 point if misspelled)

26. Tiny air sacs in which gases exchange in the lungs _____

27. Air (gas) breathed in (and also given as treatment) _____

28. Muscular partition that separates chest and abdominal cavity _____

29. Dividing wall in nose _____

30. Membrane that covers lungs and lines chest cavity _____

31. Windpipe leading to bronchi _____

32. Top (narrower part) of lungs _____

33. Instrument for looking into bronchi _____

34. Difficult or labored breathing _____

35. New permanent opening into trachea _____

36. Incision into trachea _____

37. Procedure of looking into larynx with instrument _____

38. Disease in which alveoli are greatly distended (stretched) _____

39. Cancerous tumor of lung _____

40. Infectious lung disease with tubercle formation _____

41. Inflammation of lungs _____

42. Inflammation of membrane that lines chest cavity _____

43. Surgical puncture of chest (to remove fluid) _____

44. Other words for common cold _____

45. Inflammation that causes loss of voice _____

46. Section of vertebral column that forms back wall of chest _____

47. Can only breathe sitting up _____

48. Rapid breathing _____

49. Temporary periods of no breathing _____

50. ENT specialist _____

(spell out in medical terminology)

Alternate Test

points: 100

_____
name

_____
course or section no.

Chapter 19
Respiratory System

Fill in the blank: (2 points each)

1. The primary gas inspired in breathing is _____; that expired is _____

2. Name the structure in the throat through which both food and gases pass _____

3. The tubes from the middle ear to the pharynx are called _____

4. Examination of the larynx with an instrument for "looking into" is called _____

5. The cavity in which the lungs lie (chest) is also called _____ or _____

6. The seven organs (including passageways) through which inspired air passes, *in order,* are the

    _____

    _____

7. Another word for rapid breathing is _____. Labored breathing

    may also be called _____

8. The dome-shaped muscle that is located below the lungs and contracts during inspiration is the _____

    _____. A hernia of this muscle (opening) is called a _____ hernia.

9. Name four respiratory system diseases or disorders (not mentioned in this test) _____

    _____

10. Two tests for TB are the _____ and the _____

11. Slow breathing is called _____, and a period of no breathing is called _____

12. Atelectasis means _____

13. In emphysema the _____ become distended and inelastic.

14. Rales are _____

15. URI is an abbreviation that means (2 points total) _____

16. Thoracocentesis means _____

17. The plural of alveolus is _____ and of apex _____

18. Expectorants are medications that _____

    _____

19. A spirometer is an instrument used to test _____

    _____

(continued)

Define: (2 points each)

20. tonsillectomy _____

21. tracheostomy _____

22. mucolytic _____

23. carcinoma (lung) _____

24. radiologist _____

_____

Spell out: (3 points each)

25. COPD _____

26. IPPB _____

27. SOB _____

28. T & A _____

29. ENT (and give technical name for physician who treats ENT conditions) _____

_____

Spell: (1 point each)

30. a. _____

    b. _____

    c. _____

    d. _____

    e. _____

Test

points: 100

_____
name

_____
course or section no.

Chapter 20
Gastrointestinal System

Fill in the blank: (2 points each)

1. Two names for the body cavity in which most of the organs of the GI system lie are _____ _____ and _____

2. The stomach lies in the _____ (quadrant); the appendix is attached to the _____ (part of colon), and lies in the _____ (quadrant).

3. Muscular contractions propelling material through GI tract are called _____

4. Bile is important in the digestion of _____ (food). Bile is produced by the liver and stored in the _____

5. The small intestine is lined with tiny projections called _____. These increase the surface area of the intestine, which increases the _____ of nutrients.

6. Write a word that means: excision of the stomach _____; gallstones _____; use of external sound waves to fragment stones _____

7. Name any two surgical procedures performed on GI organs: _____

    _____

8. Name three procedures used in diagnosing GI disorders: _____

    _____

True/False: Circle the numbers of the *true* statements only. Defend your answers. Explain what is "untrue" in the false statements. (2 points each)

9. Choledochitis is inflammation of the common bile duct.

10. Carbohydrates and fats supply the body with heat and energy.

11. The stomach and the abdomen are the same.

12. When the parotid glands are inflamed, the condition is called mumps.

13. Almost all absorption of digested foods occurs in the small intestines.

14. Proteins are essential for growth and repair of tissue.

15. The right and left hypochondriac regions of the abdomen are directly below the right and left lumbar regions.

16. The cardiac and pyloric are sphincter muscles of the stomach.

17. The hepatic and cystic ducts join to make the common bile duct.

(continued)

18. Digestion is both a chemical and a mechanical process.

19. Name three sections of the abdomen (not quadrants and not those already mentioned in question 15)

_____

Write a word for: (2 points each)

20. Inflammation of the tongue _____

21. Inflammation of the colon _____

22. Inflammation of the stomach _____

23. Inflammation of the mouth _____

24. Inflammation of the ileum _____

25. Name, *in order,* the 14 organs of the GI tract through which food passes—from intake to excretion (1 point each; total 14)

_____

_____

_____

_____

26. Name six accessory digestive organs (1 point each) _____

_____

_____

27. Using some of the following words, fill in the blanks: (1 point each) (colostomy, NPO, barium, enema, diagnosis, prognosis, proctoscopic, enemas, upper GI series, symptoms)

The physician reviewed the patient's _____ and wrote a tentative

_____. He told the patient to take _____

after midnight and to take _____ "until clear" in the morning, in prepara-

tion for a _____ (colon X-ray procedure). He also asked him to schedule

another appointment for a _____ exam (looking into rectum with instru-

ment). The physician tried to reassure the patient by telling him the _____

was favorable, but the patient was worried that the outcome might be a _____

(opening into colon).

Alternate Test

points: 101

name _____

course or section no.

Chapter 20
Gastrointestinal System

Fill in the blank: (2 points each)

1. Two other names for the GI tract are _____ and _____

2. The duodenum, jejunum, and ileum are parts of the _____

3. Which cavity holds the GI viscera? _____ or _____

4. The stomach lies in the _____ (quadrant);

    the liver in the _____ (quadrant).

5. The wormlike appendage, attached to the cecum, which serves no known function except to cause trouble, is the _____

6. During digestion foods are changed into soluble form so that they can be readily _____

    into the _____ for use by body cells.

7. An X-ray picture of the lower GI tract is called a _____

    or _____. It is a diagnostic tool.

8. The liver produces _____, which is important for the digestion of _____

    (certain food). This substance that the liver produces is stored in the _____

9. Name the seven large intestine sections (in order): _____

    _____

    _____

10. Name four accessory digestive organs: _____

    _____

11. The mesentery attaches the _____ to the posterior body wall. It is actually

    part of the membrane that lines the entire cavity, called the _____

12. There are many "scopes" for looking into GI organs. Name three: _____

    _____

13. Name three surgical procedures commonly performed on GI organs: _____

    _____

    _____

14. Peristalsis is _____

(continued)

15. What is the common bile duct? _____

   _____

16. _____ _____ and _____ are three

   main food groups. Two other essential elements for proper nutrition are _____

   and _____

17. Diagram and label the nine sections of the abdomen: (1 point each)

Spell: (1 point each)   **Define:** (1 point each)

a. _____   _____

                                            _____

b. _____   _____

                                            _____

c. _____   _____

                                            _____

d. _____   _____

                                            _____

e. _____   _____

                                            _____

Chapter 21
Urinary System

Spell out and explain the following: (4 points each)

1. UA _____
_____

2. I & O _____
_____

3. TUR(P) _____
_____

4. IVP _____
_____

5. UTI _____
_____

6. KUB _____
_____

Fill in the blanks: (3 points each)

7. A catheter is used to _____
or to _____
The names of two kinds of catheters are: _____
and _____

8. A person who cannot control voiding is _____.
One who cannot void is said to have _____

9. Four organs of the urinary system: _____
_____

Define: (2 points each)

10. pyelitis _____

11. diuretic _____
_____

(continued)

12. dialysis _____

_____

13. uremia _____

_____

14. frequency and urgency _____

_____

15. enuresis _____

16. retrograde pyelogram _____

_____

Write a word that means: (3 points each; spelling counts)

17. hernia of the bladder _____

18. fixation of the kidney _____

19. "any condition" of the kidney _____

20. crushing a stone _____

Spell and define: (1 point each for spelling and definition)

21. _____   _____

    _____

22. _____   _____

    _____

23. _____   _____

    _____

24. _____   _____

    _____

25. _____   _____

    _____

26. _____   _____

    _____

27. _____   _____

    _____

28. _____   _____

    _____

29. _____   _____

    _____

Alternate Test

points: 99

_____
name

_____
course or section no.

Chapter 21
Urinary System

Fill in the blanks: (3 points each)

1. Name the procedure of looking into the bladder with an instrument _____

2. The tube used to drain urine from the bladder is called a _____.

    Name two kinds: _____

3. What is the medication used to increase urinary output (general category of drug)? _____

4. IVP stands for _____

5. Two symptoms of UTI are _____ and _____

6. Name and/or describe three tests done in routine UA: _____

    _____

Give the term for: (3 points each; spelling counts)

7. Any disease of the kidneys _____

8. Pus in the urine _____

9. Bedwetting _____

10. Use of the artificial kidney _____

11. Excessive urinary output _____

12. Scant urinary output _____

13. Blood in the urine _____

14. "Urine in the blood" _____

15. No urinary output _____

16. Kidney stones _____

Spell out and explain: (5 points each)

17. UTI _____

    _____

18. KUB _____

    _____

(continued)

19. TUR(P) _____

_____

20. I & O _____

_____

Spell and define: (I point each for spelling and definition)

21. _____   _____

_____

22. _____   _____

_____

23. _____   _____

_____

24. _____   _____

_____

25. _____   _____

_____

26. _____   _____

_____

27. _____   _____

_____

28. _____   _____

_____

Review Exam 4

points: 104

Do not write on this page until assigned

_____
name

_____
course or section no.

Chapters 15–21 Review

Spell: (2 points each)

1. _____
2. _____
3. _____
4. _____
5. _____
6. _____
7. _____
8. _____
9. _____
10. _____

Define: (2 points each)

_____
_____
_____
_____
_____
_____
_____
_____
_____
_____

Build a word: (2 points each, 1 if misspelled)

1. Inflammation of the heart muscle _____

2. Without muscle coordination _____

3. Blood in the urine _____

4. Surgical repair of the kidney _____

5. Painful urination _____

Multiple choice: Circle the most appropriate answer for each statement below. (2 points each)

1. A burst appendix would likely leak into
   a. a pleural cavity
   b. a cranial cavity
   c. a peritoneal cavity
   d. everywhere
   e. none of the above

2. A meatus is
   a. an opening
   b. a muscle
   c. the smallest airway
   d. the smallest blood vessel
   e. none of the above

(continued)

3. The aorta
   a. carries reoxygenated blood to the heart
   b. exchanges oxygen and carbon dioxide
   c. the first vessel in the systemic circulation
   d. is the largest vein
   e. a and d only

4. Atonic is
   a. a type of medication patients find invigorating
   b. without seltzer
   c. pertaining to none
   d. a and b only
   e. no muscular tone

5. Gavage is
   a. a tube feeding
   b. washing out of stomach contents
   c. a prosthesis that operates like a garage door
   d. a surgical procedure
   e. none of the above

True or False: Circle T if you agree the statement is true or F if you think it is false. (2 points each)

1. A macule is a raised spot (such as a wart).   T   F

2. A nodule and cyst are similar.   T   F

3. Impetigo are vesicles.   T   F

4. Ringworm is a parasite infection.   T   F

5. Urticaria = hives.   T   F

Define: (2 points each)

1. vesicle   _____

2. pruritus   _____

3. verruca   _____

4. arthroscopy _____

5. angiogram   _____

Identification: Identify the diagram in blanks provided. (2 points each)

Identify bone fractures

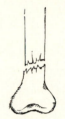

1.   (*Hint:* most common type of fracture; uncomplicated and closed) _____

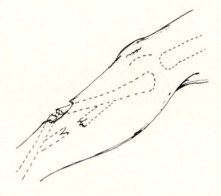

2.   (*Hint:* open fracture with bone protruding through skin) _____

3.   Name and describe any fracture except the two above. _____

_____

_____

(continued)

Identify the following organs: (2 points each)

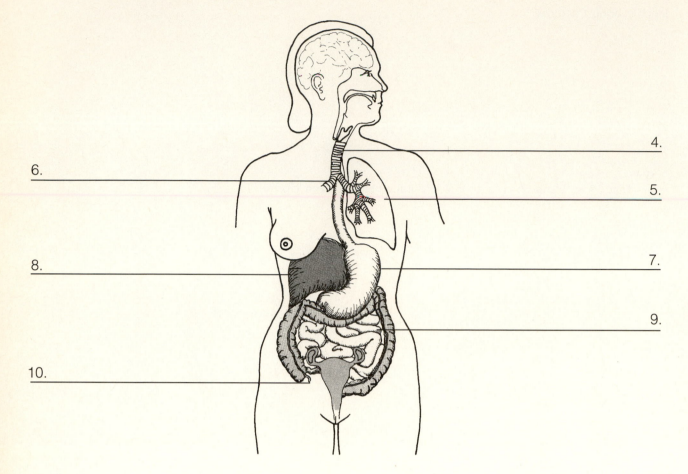

4.

6.

5.

8.

7.

9.

10.

Do not write on this page until assigned

_____
name

_____
course or section no.

**Chapter 22 and 23
Reproductive Systems**

Spell out and explain five: (3 points each)

1. D & C _____

   _____

2. AFP _____

   _____

3. EDC _____

   _____

4. LMP _____

   _____

5. STD _____

   _____

6. Pap smear _____

   _____

   _____

   _____

Fill in the blank: (1 point each)

7. External genitals are called _____ and _____ in men,

   and _____ in women.

8. The sex cell is called _____ in men and _____

   in women.

9. Three organs of reproduction in women are _____

   _____

10. Name three terms used in describing abortions: _____

   _____

True/False: Circle the number of the _true_ statements only. Defend your answers. Explain what is "untrue" in the false statements. (1 point each)

11. An episiotomy is an incision made to facilitate delivery.

12. The vernix caseosa is the afterbirth.

(continued)

13. Menarche is the first menstrual period.

14. ROA and LOA are normal presentations of the infant for delivery.

15. An abortion is a miscarriage.

16. The perineum in the female is the area between the vulva and the anus.

17. Breech always means feet-first delivery of infant.

18. A good Apgar score is 9 to 10 at one minute.

19. An enlarged prostate can block the flow of urine.

Fill in the blank: (2 points each)

20. The three-month periods in pregnancy are called _____

21. Fertilization occurs in the _____

22. The afterbirth is called the _____

23. Plastic surgery on the breast is _____

Give a word that means: (2 points each)

24. Inflammation of the ovaries _____

25. Excision of the prostate _____

26. Surgical fixation of the fallopian tubes _____

27. Pregnancy outside of the uterus _____

Explain or define: (Choose any five; 2 points each)

28. multipara _____

_____

29. episiotomy _____

_____

30. pudendal block _____

_____

31. vasectomy _____

_____

32. PID _____

_____

33. fundus of uterus _____

_____

34. instrument for measuring pelvis _____

_____

Explain this notation on an OB record: (total 4 points)

35. para VII grav IX AB 1, SB 1

_____

Spell and define: (1 point each, spelling, definition)

36. _____
37. _____
38. _____
39. _____
40. _____
41. _____
42. _____
43. _____
44. _____
45. _____
46. _____
47. _____
48. _____
49. _____

Name 3 sexually transmitted diseases: (1 point each)

_____

For one of the STDs listed above, fill in the following information: (10 points)

Disease: _____

Cause: _____

How transmitted: _____

_____

Treatment, if any: _____

Symptoms: _____

_____

Prognosis and/or sequelae: _____

Spell out: (2 points each)

50. GIFT _____

51. CVS _____

(continued)

52. ZIFT _____

53. TSS _____

54. BPH _____

55. PTSD _____

56. FHT _____

57. IVF _____

58. IUD _____

Alternate Test

points: 89

_____

name

_____

course or section no.

Chapter 22 and 23
Reproductive Systems

Fill in the blanks: (2 points each)

1. Name the female sex cell _____ male sex cell _____

2. Procedure for detecting cancer in female cervix _____

3. The score used to determine the infant's condition at 1 and 5 minutes after birth: _____

4. Name three sexually transmitted diseases _____

5. Name the normal vertex presentations of an infant at delivery time (abbreviations) _____
    _____

6. AB is the abbreviation for _____

7. EDC stands for _____

8. The sterilization procedure in men is called _____

    in women it is called _____

9. Where is the perineum (in women)? _____

10. Surgical removal of a breast is called _____

11. Name the external genitals in the male _____

12. Name the sex gland in the female _____; male _____

13. What is the incision made to facilitate childbirth called? _____

14. The first bowel movement of the infant is called _____

Give the term for: (2 points each)

15. Any disease of the uterus   _____

16. Rupture of the uterus   _____

17. Fixation of fallopian tubes   _____

18. Excision of ovaries   _____

19. Inflammation of prostate gland   _____

20. Tapping to remove amniotic fluid   _____

(continued)

Explain or define: (2 points each)

21. gravid _____

22. multipara _____

23. pudendal block _____

24. therapeutic abortion _____

25. spontaneous abortion _____

Fill in the blanks: (2 points each)

26. Name the procedure of opening up the cervix and scraping out the uterus (give abbreviation and spell):

_____

Give two reasons why this is done: _____

and _____

27. Where does fertilization occur? _____

28. Give two complications of pregnancy: _____

and _____

29. An ectopic pregnancy is one that is _____

30. Undescended testes are called "hidden testes." What is another word for this condition?

_____

True/False: Circle the number of the *true* statements only. Defend your answers. Explain what is "untrue" in the false statements. (1 point)

31. The placenta is the afterbirth.

32. A breech delivery is always buttocks first.

33. When delivery is accomplished by an incision into the uterus, the procedure is called cesarean section or C section.

34. The fundus is the neck of the uterus.

35. Dystocia means difficult labor.

36. BPH means high blood pressure.

37. Colporrhaphy is surgical repair of the vagina, sometimes called an A & P repair.

Spell and define: (1 point each)

38. _____   _____

39. _____   _____

40. _____   _____

41. _____   _____

42. _____   _____

Chapter 24 (Part 1 of 2)
Nervous System

(Unless noted otherwise, all answers on this test are 2 points each.)

Fill in the blank:

1. The largest part of the brain is the _____

2. Name four lobes of this part of the brain: _____

   _____

3. The membranes covering the brain and spinal cord are called the _____;

   _____ (outer); _____ (middle); and _____ (inner).

4. Name two cranial nerves: _____ and _____

5. Name two divisions of the autonomic nervous system: _____ and _____

   The autonomic nervous system is also called the _____ nervous system

   because we do not control it.

6. Spinal nerves are designated by abbreviations relating to sections of the spinal column in which they occur;

   C-2 means _____; L-3 _____; T-4 _____

7. The brain and spinal cord are protected by the _____ and _____

   (bony structures) and by _____ (liquid) as well as by membranes.

Define:

8. myelogram _____

9. encephalitis _____

10. subdural hematoma _____

11. EEG (name two) _____

    and _____

12. Name three diseases or disorders of the nervous system not mentioned in this test: _____

    _____

13. Halves or sides of the brain are called _____

14. Glioma and meningioma are kinds of nervous system _____

15. Hemiparesis means _____

(continued)

Write a word that means:

16. inflammation of meninges _____

17. paralysis from the neck down _____

18. deep furrows in the brain _____

19. "water on the brain" _____

20. cavities of the brain _____

21. A spinal tap is also called a _____

22. CSF means _____

23. Injury (damage) to the brain and/or spinal cord generally causes _____

    (loss of motor function).

True/False: Circle the number of the *true* statements only. Defend your answers. Explain what is "untrue" in the false statements.   (1 point each)

24. All of the body's activities are controlled and coordinated by the central nervous system.

25. The occiput is located at the front of the brain.

26. Neurologic diseases are usually disabling, long-term, and require rehabilitative measures.

27. A person who has a "nervous breakdown" has weak nerves.

28. ECG is a record of electrical impulses in the brain.

Matching: (1 point each)

29. _____ ECT   a. LP

    _____ membranes   b. paralysis on one side

    _____ spinal tap   c. convolutions

    _____ functional   d. stimulus

    _____ hemiplegia   e. frontal

    _____ gyrus   f. paralysis waist down

    _____ plexus   g. "tail"

    _____ response   h. shock

    _____ forehead   i. without cause

    _____ paresis   j. meninges

    _____ paraplegia   k. network

    _____ caudal   l. weakness

Spell: (1 point each)

30. _____   33. _____

31. _____   34. _____

32. _____

Do not write on this page until assigned

_____
name

_____
course or section no.

Chapter 24 (Part I Alternate Test)
Nervous System

(All answers in this test are 2 points each.)

True/False: Circle the number of the _true_ statements only. Defend your answers. Explain what is "untrue" in the false statements.

1.   Nerve cells are called neurons.

2.   A lumbar puncture may be done to measure pressure or to obtain a sample of fluid for lab study.

3.   The largest part of the brain is the cerebellum.

4.   Because nervous tissue is very delicate, it is protected with coverings of bone, tough membranes, and CSF.

5.   An ECG is a record of electrical impulses in the brain.

6.   People with weak nerves often have "nervous breakdowns."

Identify: Spell out. Nerves are located by the section of the vertebral column in which they originate.

7.   L-2   _____

8.   T-7   _____

9.   C-5   _____

10.   Co-1   _____

Fill in the blank:

11.   Name the four lobes of the cerebrum: _____

_____

12.   The three membranes that cover the brain and spinal cord are called _____.

Name the external layer:_____; middle layer: _____; and internal

layer:_____

13.   Peripheral means _____. The cranial and spinal _____

are called the peripheral nervous system.

14.   Name the two divisions of the autonomic nervous system: _____

and _____

Which of these aids the body in emergency situations? _____

(continued)

15. The skeletal structures that protect the brain and spinal cord are the _____

    and the _____

16. EEG means _____

    _____

17 Name three diseases or disorders that affect the nervous system _____

    ___ _____

18. The brain is divided into right and left halves; these are called _____

19. The _____ nerve controls vision and the _____ nerve, hearing.

20. The medical specialist who treats diseases of the nervous system is the _____

21. Gyri are convolutions of the _____; sulci are deep _____ in the

    brain.

Define:

22. hemiplegia _____

23. paraplegia _____

24. quadriplegia _____

Fill in the blanks:

25. paresis _____

26. concussion _____

27. myelomeningocele _____

    _____

28. ventricles (in brain) _____

29. cerebral palsy _____

    _____

30. A group of branching and interconnecting nerves is called a _____

31. Inflammation of the brain is called _____

32. Inflammation of the meninges is called _____

33. The encephalon is the _____

34. In which cavity does the brain lie? _____

    The spinal cord? _____

35. What is the term for anesthesia injected into the lower part of the spine? _____

Test
points: 80

_____
name

_____
course or section no.

Chapter 24
Psychiatric Terms (Part 2 of 2)

Spell out and define: (4 points each)

1. PTSD _____

2. REM _____

Define: (4 points each)

3. affect _____

4. aggression _____

5. ambivalence _____

6. anxiety _____

7. autism _____

8. catatonic _____

9. delusion _____

10. depression _____

11. echolalia _____

12. hallucination _____

13. malingering _____

14. manic-depressive _____

15. obsessive-compulsive _____
_____

16. phobia _____
_____

17. psychosis _____
_____

18. schizophrenia _____
_____

19. paranoid _____

20. stressor _____

Review Exam 5

points: 98

_____
name

_____
course or section no.

Chapters 22–24 Review

Spell: (2 points each)

1. _____

2. _____

3. _____

4. _____

5. _____

6. _____

7. _____

8. _____

9. _____

10. _____

Define: (2 points each)

_____

_____

_____

_____

_____

_____

_____

_____

_____

_____

_____

_____

_____

_____

_____

_____

_____

_____

_____

_____

Build a word: (2 points each, I if misspelled)

1. Without speech _____

2. Good feeling (exaggerated) _____

3. Surgical removal of breast _____

4. Viewing of living tissue/cells _____

Multiple choice: Circle the most appropriate answer for each statement below. (2 points each)

1. Tubal ligation is
   a. opening up of a tube
   b. female sterilization
   c. a vascular cleansing
   d. a type of surgical procedure for men
   e. a and b only

2. AFP is
   a. afebrile patient
   b. aneurysm for proxy
   c. after fixed properly
   d. aventricular failing patient
   e. alpha-feto protein *(continued)*

3. GIFT is
   a. an abbreviation for a healthy baby
   b. egg and sperm placed in fallopian tube to fertilize
   c. sperm transfer
   d. something a patient gives
   e. b and c only

4. A stroke is
   a. the position on a clock
   b. a CVA
   c. a heart attack
   d. a TVA
   e. a and d only

5. An EEG is
   a. a type of inflammatory pelvic disease
   b. a cause of sterility
   c. a tuberculin skin test
   d. a and b only
   e. none of the above

True or False: Circle T if you agree the statement is true or F if you think it is false. (2 points each)

1. PTSD may occur post sexual abuse.   T F

2. The parasympathetic system prepares the body for fight or flight.   T F

3. Perceived stress cannot hurt you.   T F

4. "Paranoid" is exactly the same as "phobia."   T F

5. The sympathetic nervous system controls relaxation.   T F

Define: (2 points each)

1. stressor _____

2. TIA _____

3. obsessive-compulsive _____

4. affect _____

5. oophorectomy _____

Identify the five signs or symptoms of a stroke. (4 points each)

1. _____

2. _____

3. _____

4. _____

5. _____

Test

points: 76

_____

name

_____

course or section no.

Chapter 25 (Part 1 of 2)
Sense Organs: Eyes and Ears

Fill in the blank: (2 points each)

1. Sound is measured in units called _____

2. The instrument for looking into the ear is an _____

3. Explain: inflammation OS _____

4. Name the MD specialist who treats eye diseases: _____

5. Give two medical terms for an incision into the eardrum: _____

   or _____

6. A clouded lens is called a _____

7. _____ is a disease in which intraocular pressure is increased.

8. Refractive errors are treated with prescription _____

9. The nerve to the eye is the _____ nerve.

10. The _____ is the machine used for testing hearing.

True/False: Circle the number of the _true_ statements only. Defend your answers. Explain what is "untrue" in the false statements. (2 points each)

11. Astigmatism means "crossed eyes."

12. Good peripheral vision means good vision out to the sides.

13. The lacrimal gland produces tears for crying.

14. All preparations instilled into the eye must be ophthalmic preparations.

15. Presbyopia means inability of the eye to accommodate quickly to near and far vision.

16. The orbit is the bony cavity of the cranium in which the eye rests.

17. The eustachian tubes connect the inner ear with the pharynx.

18. Some forms of hearing loss can be aided with a hearing aid.

19. After cataract extraction, lens implant is one option (the preferred one).

20. Laser is not used in any eye surgery.

21. Corneal transplant requires a donor cornea.

22. Blepharoptosis is drooping of the eyelids.

(continued)

Define: Choose *any* 10 out of 12. (2 points each)

23. tonometer _____

_____

24. conjunctivitis _____

_____

25. inner canthus of eye _____

_____

26. otitis media _____

_____

27. cerumen _____

_____

28. otoplasty _____

_____

29. radial keratotomy _____

_____

30. diopters _____

_____

31. 20/20 vision _____

_____

32. myopia _____

_____

33. amblyopia _____

_____

34. PE tubes _____

_____

Identify the following.   (2 points each)

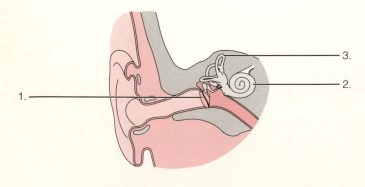

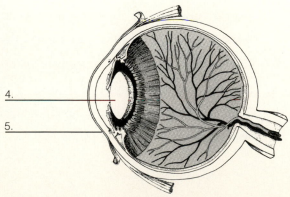

Test

points: 48

Chapter 25 (Part 2 of 2)
Sense Organs: Mouth

Fill in the blanks: (2 points)

1.   Baby teeth are called _____ because they _____

2.   Inflammation of the gums is called _____

3.   The dental specialist who treats gum disease is _____

4.   Permanent first molars usually emerge at about age _____

5.   Dental care that provides devices to replace teeth is called _____ care.

6.   Prophylactic dental care includes: _____ and

     _____

7.   Tartar formation, hardened plaque deposits around teeth at the gumline, is called _____

True/False: Circle the number of _true_ statements only. Defend your answers. Explain what is "untrue" in the false statements. (2 points)

8.   _Buccal_ pertains to the lip.

9.   Most people have the full set of 28 teeth at about age 12–14 (not including wisdom teeth).

10.   The primary cause of tooth loss is caries.

11.   Xerostomia means "dry mouth."

12.   A topical anesthetic (in dentistry) is applied to the gums.

Write a word that means: (2 points each)

13.   Excision of gum tissue   _____

14.   Poorly aligned teeth   _____

15.   Front cutting teeth   _____

16.   Without teeth (toothless)   _____

17.   Toothache   _____

18.   "Grinding" of teeth, usually at night _____

(continued)

Spell and define: (1 point each)

19. _____   _____

    _____

20. _____   _____

    _____

21. _____   _____

    _____

22. _____   _____

    _____

Test

points: 100

_____

name

_____

course or section no.

Chapter 26
Endocrine System and Stress Response

Fill in the blank: (2 points each)

1. Endocrine glands are also called _____ glands because their secretions
   go directly into the bloodstream instead of passing through _____

2. All secretions of endocrine glands are called _____

3. The pituitary glands are located deep in the _____ cavity.

4. The endocrine glands located in the neck, around the larynx, are the _____
   and the _____

5. Estrogen and progesterone are _____ secreted by the _____

6. The endocrine glands located at the top of each kidney are the _____

7. Excision of the pancreas is called _____

8. All of the organs of the endocrine system are called _____

9. The pituitary is called the _____ gland because it regulates all of the other endocrine glands.

10. Hypoglycemia means (three words, 2 points total) _____

11. Diabetes mellitus is a disease caused by dysfunction of the _____.
    Treatment usually involves special diet and an injection of _____ daily.

12. Calcium is the treatment for severe muscle and nerve weakness, called _____

13. RAIU means (2 points) _____
    It is a test of _____ function.

True/False: Circle the number of the *true* statements only. Defend your answers. Explain what is "untrue" in the false statements. (2 points each)

14. The parotid glands are part of the endocrine system.

15. Testosterone is a hormone secreted by the testes.

16. A duct never carries hormones.

17. A goiter is an enlarged adrenal gland.

18. FBS and GTT are tests used to detect diabetes mellitus.

19. The pancreas is located in the LUQ.

20. The islets of Langerhans are cells in the adrenals.

21. Iodine is essential for thyroid function.

(continued)

22. Acromegaly means enlarged extremities and is caused by pituitary dysfunction.

23. Postprandial means "after a meal."

24. Insulin is a hormone secreted by the pancreas.

25. The pancreas functions in two systems, GI and endocrine.

26. Name three disorders of the endocrine system (excluding diabetes):

    _____

    _____

27. People who have diabetes are more susceptible to complications; name three:

    _____

    _____

28. Give the type of onset, symptoms, and emergency treatment for the following: (4 points each; 8 points total)

    Diabetic coma _____

    _____

    Insulin shock _____

    _____

Spell: (1 point each)

29. _____

30. _____

31. _____

32. _____

33. _____

34. _____

35. _____

36. _____

37. _____

38. _____

39. _____

40. _____

Define eight: (1 point each)

_____

_____

_____

_____

_____

_____

_____

_____

_____

_____

_____

_____

_____

_____

_____

_____

Do not write on this page until assigned

_____
name

_____
course or section no.

Chapter 26
Endocrine System and Stress Response

Fill in the blank: (3 points each)

1. Glands of internal secretion are called _____ or _____
    glands.

2. The islets of Langerhans are cells in the _____, which secrete a _____
    called _____

3. The hormone testosterone is secreted by the _____ (organ).

4. Describe the location of the following glands:

    a. hypophysis   _____

    b. suprarenals   _____

    c. thyroid   _____

    d. parathyroids   _____

5. Where is the pancreas located? _____

6. The gonads in the female are the _____

7. Spell out:

    a. FBS   _____

    b. GTT   _____

    c. What are they used for? _____
    _____

8. Name two tests for thyroid function: _____
    _____

9. The master gland is the _____

10. Treatment for diabetic coma is primarily _____

11. Treatment for insulin shock is primarily _____

12. Which endocrine gland lies in the cranial cavity? _____

13. Name three kinds of complications diabetics are susceptible to: _____
    _____

(continued)

Define: (2 points each)

14. acute _____

15. hyperfunction _____

16. edematous _____

Spell: (1 point each)   **Define:** (1 point each)

17. _____   _____

18. _____   _____

19. _____   _____

20. _____   _____

21. _____   _____

22. _____   _____

23. _____   _____

24. _____   _____

25. _____   _____

26. _____   _____

27. _____   _____

28. _____   _____

29. _____   _____

30. _____   _____

Midterm Exam

points: 105

Do not write on this page until assigned

_____

name

_____

course or section no.

Chapters 1–14
Medical Terminology

Define: (2 points)

1. colostomy _____
2. tracheotomy _____
3. arthroplasty _____
4. lithotripsy _____
5. thoracentesis _____
6. neuralgia _____
7. cystocele _____
8. aseptic _____
9. abduction _____
10. hypertension _____
11. hypodermic _____
12. proctoscope _____
13. pelvimeter _____
14. hydrophobia _____
15. prognosis _____
16. orthopedist _____
17. midsagittal _____
18. dysphagia _____

Correct misspelled words and define all words: (1 point each)

19. hemoplegia _____
20. tackycardia _____
21. ophthalmoscope _____
22. erticaria _____
23. vertabra _____

(continued)

24. clavicle _____

25. diaphragm _____

_____

Spell: (1 point each)   **Define:** (1 point each)

26. _____   _____

27. _____   _____

28. _____   _____

29. _____   _____

30. _____   _____

31. _____   _____

32. _____   _____

33. _____   _____

34. _____   _____

35. _____   _____

36. _____   _____

37. _____   _____

38. _____   _____

39. _____   _____

40. _____   _____

41. _____   _____

42. _____   _____

43. _____   _____

44. _____   _____

45. _____   _____

46. _____   _____

47. _____   _____

48. _____   _____

49. _____   _____

50. _____   _____

51. _____   _____

52. _____   _____

53. _____   _____

54. _____   _____

55. _____   _____

56. _____   _____

Final Exam

points: 219

_____

name

_____

course or section no.

Chapters 1–26
Medical Terminology

(Each answer in test is 1 point.)

Name the medical specialist:

1. Children only _____

2. Internal disorders _____

3. Eye diseases _____

4. Mental illness _____

5. Disorders of skeletal system _____

6. Interprets X-ray films _____

Identify:

7. DO _____

   _____

8. podiatrist _____

   _____

9. optometrist _____

   _____

10. Name the two largest body cavities: (two names for each)

    _____ or _____

    _____ or _____

Mark with a check the routine immunizations available and recommended for all with few exceptions. Identify where indicated by blanks:

11. _____   DTP _____   _____   _____

12. _____   varicella

13. _____   parotitis _____

14. _____   influenza

15. _____   rubella _____

16. _____   scarlet fever

(continued)

17. _____ impetigo

18. _____ syphilis

19. _____ poliomyelitis

20. _____ rubeola _____

Write a word that means:

21. Before birth _____

22. Condition of blueness _____

23. Any disease of glands _____

24. Inflammation of kidney _____

25. Excision of ovaries _____

26. Fixation of fallopian tubes _____

27. Enlarged heart _____

28. Malignant tumor _____

29. Fast heartbeat _____

30. High B/P _____

31. Wasting away (muscles) _____

32. Between ribs _____

33. Under the skin _____

34. Treatment with water _____

35. Without rhythm (heart) _____

36. Instrument for cutting thin section of skin _____

37. Instrument for looking into ear _____

38. Excision of gallbladder _____

39. Incision into trachea _____

40. New permanent opening into colon _____

41. Repair of hernia _____

True/False: Circle the number of the *true* statements only. Defend your answers. Explain what is "untrue" in the false statements.

42. Three layers of the heart are endocardium, myocardium, and pericardium.

43. Everyone has the Rh factor (in blood).

44. An isotonic solution has the same salt concentration as that of body fluids.

45. "Diff" in WBC means counting the number of each kind of leukocyte.

46. C & S is a lab procedure done on bacteria to isolate the bacteria causing disease and to determine to which antibiotic the organism is sensitive or resistant (S or R).

47. The words *cervix* and *cervical* pertain to the uterus only.

48. Ligaments, tendons, and fasciae are all kinds of connective tissue.

49. A proctoscope is used for looking into the vagina.

50. During inspiration the diaphragm moves upward.

51. The midsagittal plane divides the body into equal right and left sides.

52. Oxygen and carbon dioxide are exchanged in the alveoli (lungs).

Define:

53. capillaries _____

_____

54. vertebrae _____

55. intravenous _____

56. dehydrated _____

57. etiology _____

58. postpartum _____

59. sinuses _____

60. hypertrophy _____

61. speculum _____

62. osteotome _____

63. aseptic _____

64. gastroscopy _____

65. lipoma _____

66. pyogenic _____

67. arthroplasty _____

68. bradycardia _____

69. prognosis _____

70. neuralgia _____

71. laparotomy _____

72. hysterectomy _____

73. thoracocentesis _____

74. sclerosis _____

75. cystocele _____

76. stomatitis _____

77. lithotripsy _____

(continued)

Matching:

78. _____ AIDS
79. _____ EEG
80. _____ Dick
81. _____ WBC
82. _____ C-2
83. _____ lungs
84. _____ A, B, O
85. _____ Kahn
86. _____ cranium
87. _____ CBC
88. _____ FBS
89. _____ CO$_2$
90. _____ septum
91. _____ voice box

a. pulmonary
b. larynx
c. skull
d. blood types
e. electroencephalogram
f. pneumocystis
g. hematology
h. serological test
i. second cervical vertebra
j. "sugar" test
k. dividing partition or wall
l. scarlet fever
m. carbon dioxide
n. leukocytes

Fill in the blank:

92. Prone means face _____ Supination of the hand means palm _____

93. The proximal end of the femur is near the (pelvis, knee). (Underline the correct word.)

94. The distal end of the humerus is nearer the (shoulder, elbow). (Underline the correct word.)

95. Psoriasis, eczema, and verrucae are disorders of the _____ system.

96. Name the five sections of the vertebral column (in order): _____

    _____

97. Paralysis on one side of the body is _____

    From the waist down _____

    From the neck down _____

98. Flexion and extension mean (in order) _____ and _____

99. Toward the midline: _____

    Away from the midline: _____

100. Name three of the five basic kinds of leukocytes:

    _____

    _____

101. Name any four bones of the extremities: _____

    _____

102. The largest vein in the body is the _____

    The largest artery is the _____

103. Name any two valves of the heart: _____ and _____

_____

104. The two numbers in a blood pressure reading are called _____ (top number)

and _____ (bottom)

105. Name two important pathogenic bacteria: (cluster form) _____

(chain) _____

106. Painful urination is _____ Excessive urination is _____

Urination during night is _____

107. Difficult or labored breathing is called _____

Periods of no breathing is called _____

108. Name four signs of inflammation: _____

109. Rheumatoid arthritis, bursitis, and fractures are disorders of the _____ system.

110. The pulmonary _____ is the vessel that carries deoxygenated blood

from the right ventricle to the lungs.

111. The _____ ventricle of the heart has a thicker muscular wall than the

_____ ventricle because it must pump blood farther.

112. Medical term for heart attack _____

for stroke _____

Give the meaning of:

113. prn _____   117. qid _____

114. stat _____   118. NPO _____

115. URI _____   119. COPD _____

116. CVA _____   120. MI _____

Spell: **Define 121–134:**

121. _____   _____

_____

122. _____   _____

_____

123. _____   _____

_____

124. _____   _____

_____

125. _____   _____

_____

(continued)

126. _____   _____

127. _____   _____

128. _____   _____

129. _____   _____

130. _____   _____

131. _____   _____

132. _____   _____

133. _____   _____

134. _____   _____

135. _____   _____

136. _____

137. _____

138. _____

139. _____

140. _____

141. _____

142. _____

143. _____

144. _____

145. _____

146. _____

147. _____

148. _____

149. _____

150. _____

151. _____

152. _____

153. _____

154. _____

155. _____

Medications

generic name	brand name	major use
acetaminophen	(Tylenol, Actifed, Excedrin, Darvocet-N, Sinutab)	analgesic, antipyretic
acetaminophen with codeine	(Tylenol with Codeine, Phenaphen, Percocet)	analgesic
acetohexamide		oral antidiabetic
acetylcysteine	(Mucosil)	mucolytic
acetylsalicylic acid (aspirin)	(Empirin, Fiorinal, Anacin, Bayer, Ecotrin, Excedrin)*	analgesic, antipyretic
acetylsalicylic acid with codeine	(Percodan)	analgesic
acyclovir ointment	(Zovirax)	herpes infections
albuterol	(Ventolin, Proventil)	bronchodilator
alendronate	(Fosamax)	osteoporosis (after menopause)
alfentanil HCl	(Alfenta)	analgesic; adjunct with anesthesia
allopurinol	(Zyloprim)	reduces uric acid (gout)
alprazolam	(Xanax)	anxiolytic
alteplase (IV)	(Activase)	acute MI; lysis of thrombi
amantadine	(Symmetrel)	antiviral
amiloride	(Moduretic)	diuretic, antihypertensive without excessive potassium loss
aminophylline	(Aminophylline, Mudrane)	bronchodilator, mucolytic
amitriptyline	(Elavil, Triavil, Etrafon, Endep)	antidepressant
amoxapine	(Asendin)	antidepressant
amoxicillin	(Amoxil, Augmentin, Wymox)	semisynthetic penicillin
amphotericin B	(Fungizone)	antifungal, valley fever
ampicillin	(Omnipen)	semisynthetic penicillin
A_1 PI, alpha$_1$-proteinase inhibitor	(Prolastin)	protects against enzymes that destroy lung tissue in inherited emphysema
astemizole	(Hismanal)	antihistamine (nondrowsy)
atenolol	(Tenormin)	angina, hypertension
atropine sulfate		reduces salivation and secretions

---

*Most of these drugs contain another ingredient besides aspirin.

generic name	brand name	major use
attapulgite	(Donnagel, Rheaban, Diasorb)	antispasmodic (GI)
azathioprine	(Imuran)	immunosuppressive; antirejection
azidothymidine (AZT) (see *zidovudine*)		
azithromycin	(Zithromax)	antibiotic
aztreonam	(Azactam)	antibiotic
bacampicillin	(Spectrobid)	semisynthetic penicillin
belladonna	(Donnatal)	antispasmodic
benztropine mesylate	(Cogentin)	parkinsonism
bethanechol	(Urecholine)	urinary retention, postop
bisacodyl	(Dulcolax)	cathartic
bleomycin sulfate	(Blenoxane)	antineoplastic antibiotic
bretylium tosylate		ventricular arrhythmias
bromocriptine mesylate	(Parlodel)	prevents lactation
brompheniramine maleate	(Bromfed, Dallergy, Dimetane, Dimetapp, Lodrane, Respahist)	antihistamine
buspirone HCl	(BuSpar)	anxiolytic
busulfan	(Myleran)	antineoplastic
butalbital-aspirin-caffeine	(Fiorinal)	anxiolytic, muscle relaxant, and analgesic
butorphanol tartrate	(Stadol)	narcotic analgesic
calcitonin-salmon	(Calcimar, Miacalcin)	Paget's disease of the bone
calcitriol	(Rocaltrol)	synthetic vitamin D
captopril	(Capoten)	antihypertensive
carbamazepine	(Tegretol)	anticonvulsant
carbenicillin	(Geocillin)	semisynthetic penicillin
carbidopa/levodopa	(Sinemet)	parkinsonism
carisoprodol	(Soma)	acute musculoskeletal conditions
CDP (see *chlordiazepoxide*)		
cefaclor	(Ceclor)	antibiotic—respiratory/ear infections
cefadroxil monohydrate	(Duricef)	antibiotic
cefamandole nafate	(Mandol)	antibiotic—lower respiratory
cefazolin sodium	(Kefzol, Ancef)	antibiotic
cefotaxime sodium	(Claforan)	antibiotic
cefoxitin	(Mefoxin)	broad-spectrum antibiotic
ceftriaxone	(Rocephin)	penicillin-resistant (gonococcus)
cefuroxime axetil	(Ceftin)	broad-spectrum antibiotic
cephalexin	(Keflex)	broad-spectrum antibiotic
cephalothin sodium		broad-spectrum antibiotic
chlorambucil	(Leukeran)	antineoplastic
chlordiazepoxide	(Libritabs)	tranquilizer
chlordiazepoxide with amitriptyline	(Limbitrol)	depression; anxiety
chlorothiazide	(Diuril, Aldoclor)	diuretic

generic name	brand name	major use
chlorpheniramine maleate	(Codimal, Extendryl, Ornade)	antihistamine
chlorpromazine hydrochloride	(Thorazine)	tranquilizer, antiemetic
chlorpropamide	(Diabinese)	oral hypoglycemic adult-onset diabetes
chlorthalidone	(Hygroton)	diuretic
chlorzoxazone and acetaminophen	(Parafon Forte)	muscle relaxant, analgesic
cimetidine	(Tagamet)	inhibits gastric acid (ulcers)
ciprofloxacin	(Cipro)	broad-spectrum antibiotic
clindamycin	(Cleocin)	antibiotic
clocortolone pivalate		topical steroid
clofazimine	(Lamprene)	antileprosy
clofibrate	(Atromid-S)	lowers cholesterol
clomipramine	(Anafranil)	antidepressant
clonazepam	(Klonopin)	seizure disorders; also used in depression
clonidine hydrochloride	(Catapres)	antihypertensive
clorazepate dipotassium	(Tranxene)	antianxiety
clotrimazole	(Lotrimin)	topical antifungal (tinea)
cloxacillin sodium		synthetic penicillin
codeine	(Empirin with Codeine)	narcotic analgesic
colchicine	(ColBENEMID)	gout
cortisone acetate	(Cortone)	corticosteroid used in many disorders
cromolyn	(Intal)	bronchial asthma
cyclacillin		semisynthetic penicillin
cyclobenzaprine HCl	(Flexeril)	relieves muscle spasm
cyclophosphamide	(Cytoxan)	antineoplastic
cyclosporine	(Sandimmune)	transplant rejection
cyproheptadine HCl	(Periactin)	antihistamine
cytarabine	(Cytosar-U)	antineoplastic
danazol	(Danocrine)	suppresses ovarian function
daunorubicin	(Cerubidine)	antibiotic (cancer)
desipramine	(Norpramin)	antidepression in "crack" users
dexamethasone	(Decadron)	corticosteroid
dexbrompheniramine and pseudoephedrine sulfate	(Drixoral)	antihistamine, decongestant
dexchlorpheniramine		allergic rhinitis
dextroamphetamine sulfate	(Dexedrine)	cerebral stimulation (narcolepsy, obesity)
dextromethorphan	(Anatuss DM)	antitussive
diazepam	(Valium)	tranquilizer
diclofenac	(Voltaren)	NSAID*; arthritis

---

*Nonsteroidal anti-inflammatory drug; many different drugs used in the treatment of arthritis-type illnesses to provide palliation and reduce inflammation. (Pronounced ĕn-sĕd.)

generic name	brand name	major use
dicyclomine hydrochloride	(Bentyl)	GI muscle spasm
dideoxyinosine (ddl)		as yet unapproved experimental AIDS drug in controlled trials
diethylpropion hydrochloride	(Tenuate)	anorectic
diflunisal	(Dolobid)	NSAID*
digoxin	(Lanoxin)	increases strength and force of heartbeat
digoxin immune FAB	(Digibind)	digoxin intoxication
dihydroergotamine mesylate	(D.H.E. 45)	aborts vascular headache
diltiazem	(Cardizem)	angina
diphenhydramine		antihistamine, antitussive
diphenhydramine hydrochloride	(Benadryl, Actifed)	antihistamine
diphenoxylate hydrochloride	(Lomotil)	antispasmodic (diarrhea)
dipyridamole	(Persantine)	angina; post-MI anticoagulant
disopyramide phosphate	(Norpace)	antiarrhythmic
dobutamine hydrochloride	(Dobutrex)	strengthens heart muscle
docusate sodium	(Colace, Dialose, Modane Soft)	stool softener
doxepin hydrochloride	(Sinequan)	treatment of depression or anxiety
doxorubicin hydrochloride	(Adriamycin)	antineoplastic antibiotic
doxycycline monohydrate	(Vibramycin, Monodox)	bacteriostatic
doxylamine succinate	(Unisom)	antiemetic
droperidol	(Inapsine)	analgesic tranquilizer
enalapril	(Vasotec)	angiotensin-converting enzyme inhibitor, antihypertensive
encainide HCl		arrhythmias, V-tach
ephedrine sulfate	(Marax)	relaxes bronchioles
epinephrine (adrenaline)	(Epi-Pen)	respiratory distress and hyper-sensitivity reactions
ergoloid mesylate	(Hydergine)	decline in mental capacity
ergot alkaloids		mental deterioration in elderly
ergotamine tartrate	(Cafergot, Ergomar, Wigraine)	migraine
erythromycin	(Benzamycin, Ilotycin, Theramycin)	antibiotic
esmolol HCl	(Brevibloc)	V-tach with atrial fibrillation
estrogens, conjugated	(Premarin)	menopausal symptoms
estropipate	(Ogen)	menopausal symptoms
ethambutol	(Myambutol)	anti-tuberculosis with isoniazid
ethosuximide	(Zarontin)	anticonvulsant
etretinate	(Tegison)	severe recalcitrant psoriasis
famotidine	(Pepcid)	duodenal ulcers, esophageal reflux
fenoprofen calcium	(Nalfon)	NSAID*

---

*Nonsteroidal anti-inflammatory drug; many different drugs used in the treatment of arthritis-type illnesses to provide palliation and reduce inflammation. (Pronounced ĕn-sĕd.)

generic name	brand name	major use
fentanyl	(Duragesic)	analgesic tranquilizer
ferrous sulfate	(Feosol, Iberet, Fero-Folic-500)	iron deficiency
fluocinolone acetonide	(Synalar)	topical steroid
fluocinonide	(Lidex, Dermacin)	anti-inflammatory, antipruritic
fluorouracil	(Efudex, Fluoroplex)	antineoplastic
fluoxetine	(Prozac)	antidepressant
fluphenazine hydrochloride	(Prolixin)	psychoses
flurandrenolide	(Cordran)	anti-inflammatory, antipruritic corticosteroid (topical)
flurazepam hydrochloride	(Dalmane)	vasoconstriction, hypnotic
flutamide	(Eulexin)	metastatic prostatic cancer
flurbiprofen	(Ansaid)	NSAID*
fluvastatin	(Lescol)	lowers cholesterol
folic acid	(Folvite)	some anemias
furosemide	(Lasix)	diuretic
gemfibrozil	(Lopid)	lowers triglycerides
gentamicin sulfate	(Garamycin)	antibiotic
glipizide	(Glucotrol)	reduces blood glucose
glutethimide	(Doriden)	hypnotic
glyburide	(Diabeta, Micronase)	reduces blood glucose
guaifenesin	(Anatuss, Cheracol, Sudafed Cough, Triaminic)	expectorant
guanabenz	(Wytensin)	antihypertensive
guanethidine sulfate	(Ismelin)	antihypertensive
guanfacine HCl	(Tenex)	hypertension
HCTZ (see *hydrochlorothiazide*)		
heparin sodium	(Hep-Lock)	anticoagulant
hepatitis B vaccine	(Engerix-B, Recombivax HB)	prevention of hepatitis B in high-risk population
H.R.H.	(Ser-Ap-Es)	combination, antihypertensive and diuretic
hydralazine hydrochloride	(Apresoline, Ser-Aps-Es)	antihypertensive
hydrochlorothiazide (HCTZ)	(Esidrix, HydroDIURIL, Oretic, Ser-Ap-Es)	diuretic
hydrocodone	(Vicodin, Lortab)	narcotic analgesic
hydrocortisone	(Cortisporin)	steroid
hydroflumethiazide	(Salutensin)	hypertension
hydromorphone hydrochloride	(Dilaudid)	narcotic
hydroxyzine hydrochloride	(Atarax, Vistaril)	tranquilizer, muscle relaxant
hyoscyamine sulfate, atropine sulfate, phenobarbital	(Donnatal, Arco-Lase, Anaspaz, Cystospaz)	relaxant (GI spasm)
ibuprofen	(Motrin, Advil, Nuprin)	NSAID*

---

*Nonsteroidal anti-inflammatory drug; many different drugs used in the treatment of arthritis-type illnesses to provide palliation and reduce inflammation. (Pronounced ĕn-sĕd.)

generic name	brand name	major use
imipenem-cilastatin	(Primaxin)	antibiotic
imipramine hydrochloride	(Tofranil)	antidepressant
indomethacin	(Indocin)	NSAID*
insulin	(NPH Iletin, Lente, Humulin, Novolin, Velosulin)	injectable in diabetes
interferon, a alfa-2a and 2b recombinant	(Roferon-A, Intron A)	hairy cell leukemia (over age 18)
interferon beta-1b	(Betaseron)	multiple sclerosis
ipecac		emetic
ipratropium bromide	(Atrovent)	bronchodilator, COPD
iron dextran	(INFeD)	iron deficiency
isocarboxazid		monoamine oxidase inhibitor (MAO) in depression
isoetharine	(Bronkosol)	bronchodilator
isoniazid	(Nydrazid, Rifamate, Rifater)	anti-infective (tuberculosis)
isoproterenol solution	(Isuprel Mistometer)	bronchodilator
isosorbide dinitrate	(Dilatrate-SR, Isordil, Sorbide)	vasodilator
isoxsuprine hydrochloride		vasodilator
kanamycin sulfate		antibiotic
kaolin		antispasmodic (GI)
KCl (see *potassium chloride*)		
ketoconazole	(Nizoral)	antifungal, valley fever
ketoprofen	(Orudis)	NSAID*, arthritis
lactulose	(Cholac, Constilac, Constulose, Enulose)	acidifies colon (hepatic coma)
levocarnitine (L-carnitine)	(Carnitor)	carnitine deficiency associated with hypoglycemia, myasthenia
levodopa, Cdopa/Ldopa	(Larodopa, Sinement)	parkinsonism
levothyroxine (L-thyroxine)	(Synthroid)	hypothyroid condition
lidocaine	(Xylocaine)	antirrhythmic, anesthetic
lincomycin hydrochloride	(Lincocin)	antibiotic
lindane (gamma benzene hexa-chloride)	(Kwell)	scabies and lice
liotrix	(Thyrolar)	thyroid hormones
lisinopril	(Prinivil, Zestril)	hypertension
lithium carbonate	(Eskalith)	manic-depression (mania)
lomustine	(CeeNU)	antineoplastic
loperamide hydrochloride	(Imodium)	inhibits peristalsis (acute diarrhea)
lorazepam	(Ativan)	anxiety disorders
lovastatin	(Mevacor)	lowers cholesterol, total and LDL
L-thyroxine (see *levothyroxin*)		

---

*Nonsteroidal anti-inflammatory drug; many different drugs used in the treatment of arthritis-type illnesses to provide palliation and reduce inflammation. (Pronounced ĕn-sĕd.)

generic name	brand name	major use
maprotiline hydrochloride	(Ludiomil)	tetracyclic antidepressant
measles virus vaccine	(Attenuvax)	measles vaccine
mechlorethamine hydrochloride	(Mustargen)	antineoplastic
meclizine hydrochloride	(Antivert)	antihistamine (nausea, vomiting)
meclocycline sulfosalicylate		antibiotic cream
meclofenamate sodium		NSAID*
medroxyprogesterone acetate	(Amen, Provera, Cycrin, Curretab)	secondary amenorrhea and other hormonal imbalances
mefenamic acid	(Ponstel)	analgesic, dysmenorrhea
megestrol	(Megace)	antineoplastic, advanced CA breast and endometrium
melphalan	(Alkeran)	antineoplastic
meperidine	(Demerol)	narcotic analgesic
mephenytoin	(Mesantoin)	anticonvulsant
meprobamate	(Equagesic, Equanil, Miltown)	tranquilizer
mercaptopurine	(Purinethol)	antimetabolite (leukemias)
mesalamine (rectal suspension enema)	(ROWASA)	ulcerative colitis
methenamine mandelate	(Uroqid)	antibacterial (UTI)
methocarbamol	(Robaxin)	musculoskeletal pain
methotrexate	(Rheumatrex)	antimetabolite
methyclothiazide	(Aquatensen, Enduron, Diutensen)	diuretic, antihypertensive
methyldopa	(Aldomet, Aldoril)	antihypertensive
methylphenidate hydrochloride	(Ritalin)	CNS stimulation
methylprednisolone	(Depo-Medrol, Medrol)	steroid, anti-inflammatory immunosuppressive
methysergide maleate	(Sansert)	vascular headache
metoclopramide hydrochloride	(Reglan)	stimulates upper GI motility
metolazone	(Mykrox, Zaroxolyn)	diuretic
metoprolol tartrate	(Lopressor)	hypertension
metronidazole	(Flagyl)	trichomonal and amebicidal action; anaerobic bacterial infections
metyrosine	(Demser)	pheochromocytoma
miconazole nitrate	(Monistat)	fungicidal (moniliasis)
minoxidil	(Loniten)	peripheral vasodilator (antihypertensive)
minoxidil 2% topical	(Rogaine)	treatment for baldness
misoprostal	(Cytotec)	gastric ulcer prevention; used with NSAID* drugs
mitoxantrone HCl inj.	(Novantrone)	antineoplastic in acute nonlymphocytic leukemia

---

*Nonsteroidal anti-inflammatory drug; many different drugs used in the treatment of arthritis-type illnesses to provide palliation and reduce inflammation. (Pronounced ĕn-sĕd.)

generic name	brand name	major use
morphine (inj. and tabs)	(Astramorph, Duramorph, Roxanol)	narcotic analgesic
mumps virus vaccine	(Mumpsvax)	mumps vaccine
muromonab CD-3	(Orthoclone OKT3)	acute allograft rejection (renal transplant)
nadolol		angina, hypertension
naftifine hydrochloride	(Naftin)	fungi and yeast infection (topical)
nalbuphine hydrochloride	(Nubain)	analgesic (synthetic narcotic)
nalidixic acid	(NegGram)	UTI (gram negative)
naloxone hydrochloride	(Narcan)	narcotic antagonist
naproxen	(Naprosyn)	NSAID*
nicardipine	(Cardene)	angina, hypertension
nifedipine	(Procardia, Adalat)	angina, coronary artery spasm
nitrofurantoin	(Macrodantin)	bactericidal (UTI)
nitroglycerin	(Nitro-Bid, Nitrostat, Nitrol)	vasodilator (in angina)
nitroglycerin patch	(Nitrodur-2, Nitrodisc, Nitropatch)	vasodilator (angina)
nizatidine	(Axid)	duodenal ulcer
norepinephrine bitartrate	(Levophed)	peripheral vasoconstictor
norfloxacin	(Noroxin)	broad spectrum antibiotic
nylidrin		vasodilator
nystatin	(Mytrex, Cream, Mycostatin)	antibiotic (fungal); vaginal infections
orphenadrine citrate-aspirin-caffeine	(Norgesic)	analgesic (musculoskeletal)
oxamniquine		*Schistosoma mansoni* infection (blood flukes)
oxazepam	(Serax)	anticonvulsant, antianxiety
oxtriphylline	(Choledyl)	bronchodilator
oxycodone	(Percodan)	narcotic analgesic
oxytocin	(Syntocinon)	uterine stimulant
pancuronium bromide	(Pavulon)	muscle relaxant
papaverine hydrochloride		relieves arterial spasm
penicillin G	(Bicillin, Pfizerpen-G)	antibiotic
penicillin V	(Pen-Vee K)	antibiotic
pentaerythritol		angina
pentamidine	(Pentam)	treatment for PCP in AIDS patients
pentazocine hydrochloride	(Talwin)	analgesic
pentobarbital sodium	(Nembutal)	barbiturate (short acting)
permethrin	(Nix)	pediculosis (lice)
perphenazine-amitriptyline	(Etrafon)	anxiety, agitation

---

*Nonsteroidal anti-inflammatory drug; many different drugs used in the treatment of arthritis-type illnesses to provide palliation and reduce inflammation. (Pronounced ĕn-sĕd.)

generic name	brand name	major use
phenazopyridine hydrochloride	(Azo Gantanol, Pyridium, Azo Gantrisin, Urobiotic)	relief of pain in UTI
phenelzine sulfate	(Nardil)	MAO inhibitor (in depression)
phenobarbital	(Arco-Lase Plus, Bellatal, Donnatal, Quadrinal)	sedative, antispasmodic
phenoxybenzamine hydrochloride	(Dibenzyline)	vasospastic disorders (Raynaud's)
phentermine resin	(Ionamin)	anorexic
phenylbutazone		NSAID*
phenylpropanolamine		decongestant
phenylpropanolamine-phenylephrine-chlorpheniramine	(Atrohist)	antihistamine, decongestant
phenytoin sodium	(Dilantin)	anticonvulsant
phytonadione	(AquaMEPHYTON, Konakion)	synthetic vitamin K
pilocarpine hydrochloride	(Salagen)	antiglaucoma
piroxicam	(Feldene)	NSAID*, arthritis
polymyxin B- and neomycin bacitracin or gramicidin	(Neosporin)	topical antibiotic
plus hydrocortisone	(Cortisporin)	topical antibiotic
potassium chloride	(K-Lor, K-Lyte, Kaon-Cl, Slow K, Micro K, Klotrix)	potassium depletion
povidone-iodine	(Betadine)	germicide
pravastatin	(Pravachol)	lowers lipids
prazosin hydrochloride	(Minipress)	antihypertensive
prednisone	(Sterapred, Deltasone, Prednicen-M)	steroid, anti-inflammatory immunosuppressive; cortisone drugs used in a wide variety of conditions; varied side effects
primidone	(Mysoline)	anticonvulsant
probenecid	(Benemid, ColBENEMID)	gout
procainamide	(Procan SR)	PVCs, arrhythmias
procarbazine hydrochloride	(Matulane)	antineoplastic (Hodgkin's)
prochlorperazine	(Compazine)	tranquilizer, antinauseant
promethazine hydrochloride	(Phenergan, Prometh, Mepergan)	antihistamine, antiemetic, tranquilizer
propantheline bromide	(Pro-BanthĀne)	inhibits GI motility (in ulcers)
propoxyphene hydrochloride	(Darvon, Wygesic)	analgesic
propranolol hydrochloride	(Inderal, Inderide)	antihypertensive, angina, migraine
protamine sulfate		for overdose of heparin
pseudoephedrine hydrochloride	(Sudafed)	decongestant
pseudoephedrine sulfate	(Claritin-D)	decongestant
pyrazinamide (PZA)	(Rifater)	tuberculosis

---

*Nonsteroidal anti-inflammatory drug; many different drugs used in the treatment of arthritis-type illnesses to provide palliation and reduce inflammation. (Pronounced ĕn-sĕd.)

generic name	brand name	major use
quinidine sulfate	(Quinidex)	cardiac depressant (in arrhythmias)
rabies vaccine		pre- and post-exposure vaccine
ranitidine	(Zantac)	ulcers, gastric and duodenal
rauwolfia serpentina	(Raudixin)	diuretic, antihypertensive
reserpine	(Hydropres, Diupres)	hypertension
ribravirin	(Virazole)	antiviral, severe RSV in infants
ritodrine hydrochloride	(Yutopar)	prolongs gestation
salsalate	(Disalcid)	arthritis
scopolamine	(Donnatal, Bellatal)	antidiarrheal
secobarbital sodium	(Seconal Sodium)	barbiturate
selegiline	(Eldepryl)	parkinsonism (an adjunct to levodopa)
spectinomycin hydrochloride	(Trobicin)	antibiotic (penicillin-resistant GC)
spironolactone	(Aldactone)	diuretic
streptomycin sulfate		antibiotic, used to treat tuberculosis
sulfamethoxazole with trimethoprim	(Bactrim, Septra)	UTI; also GI, ear and chest infections
sulfasalazine	(Azulfidine)	sulfonamide (ulcerative colitis)
sulfisoxazole	(Gantrisin)	sulfonamide (UTI)
sulindac	(Clinoril)	NSAID*
tacrine hydrochloride	(Cognex)	Alzheimer's
tamoxifen citrate	(Nolvadex)	antitumor (breast cancer)
temazepam	(Restoril)	sleep medication
terazosin	(Hytrin)	hypertension
terconazole (supp)	(Terazol)	candidiasis (vagina)
terfenadine	(Seldane)	hay fever, allergic rhinitis
tetracycline hydrochloride	(Achromycin)	antibiotic
theophylline	(Marax, Slo-bid)	bronchodilator
thiethylperazine	(Torecan)	nausea, vomiting
thioridazine	(Mellaril)	major tranquilizer
thryoglobulin	(Proloid)	thyroid
thyroid	(Armour)	hypothyroid conditions
ticarcillin disodium	(Ticar)	antibiotic
ticrynafen		antihypertensive, diuretic
timolol maleate (eye drops)	(Timoptic)	reduces intraocular pressure (glaucoma)
tobramycin sulfate	(Nebcin)	antibiotic (gram negative)
tolazamide		oral hypoglycemic
tolbutamide	(Orinase)	oral hypoglycemic

---

*Nonsteroidal anti-inflammatory drug; many different drugs used in the treatment of arthritis-type illnesses to provide palliation and reduce inflammation. (Pronounced ĕn-sĕd.)

generic name	brand name	major use
tolmetin sodium	(Tolectin)	NSAID*
tranexamic acid	(Cyklokapron)	hemostatic, stops bleeding
tranylcypromine sulfate	(Parnate)	MAO inhibitor (depression)
trazodone hydrochloride	(Desyrel)	antidepression
tretinoin	(Retin-A)	antiacne agent
triamcinolone	(Aristocort)	topical and inhaler cortisone drugs
triamterene (some with HCTZ)	(Dyazide, Maxzide, Dyrenium)	diuretic
triazolam	(Halcion)	hypnotic (sleep)
trifluridine	(Viroptic)	antiviral (eye)
trihexyphenidyl hydrochloride	(Artane)	smooth muscle relaxant (parkinsonism)
trimethobenzamide hydrochloride	(Tigan)	antiemetic
trimethoprim with sulfamethoxazole	(Bactrim, Proloprim, Septra)	in AIDS, for PCP
triprolidine hydrochloride and pseudoephedrine hydrochloride	(Actifed)	antihistamine, decongestant
urofollitropin	(Metrodin)	to induce ovulation
ursodiol	(Actigall)	dissolution of stones
valacyclovir	(Valtrex)	herpes
valproic acid	(Depakene)	some seizure disorders
verapamil	(Calan, Isoptin)	angina
vidarabine	(Vira-A)	antiviral drug
vincristine sulfate	(Oncovin)	antineoplastic
warfarin	(Coumadin)	anticoagulant in venous thrombosis
zidovudine (formerly AZT)	(Retrovir)	antiviral, used to treat AIDS patients
zinc undecylenate and undecylenic acid (powder)	(Desenex)	topical antifungal

---

*Nonsteroidal anti-inflammatory drug; many different drugs used in the treatment of arthritis-type illnesses to provide palliation and reduce inflammation. (Pronounced ĕn-sĕd.)

Abbreviations

Hints: Periods are generally omitted. Some abbreviations are shown in capital letters; some will be seen in either capitals or lowercase letters.

Letter(s)	Often means
A	American, association
A/P	anterior/posterior
D	disease
F	Fellow
L/R	left/right
N	national
P	physicians
S	surgeons, syndrome
U/L	upper/lower

General Abbreviations

A   anterior, accommodation, atrium, artery

AA   Alcoholics Anonymous, Associate of Arts (degree)

a͞a   of each (pharmacy)

AAA   abdominal aortic aneurysm

AAE   active assistive exercise (physical therapy)

A & D   admission and discharge (hospital department)

A & P (or P & A)   auscultation and percussion (listening and tapping)

A & P repair   anterior/posterior repair of perineum

A & W   alive and well

AAR   acute anxiety reaction

AAT   alpha-1 antitrypsin; used in deficiency-related emphysema

ab   abortion (if spontaneous, same as miscarriage)

ABC   airway, breathing, circulation

ABG   arterial blood gases, aspiration biopsy cytology

ABO   Landsteiner blood groups

ABS   acute brain syndrome

AC   air conduction

ac   before meals

ACP   American College of Physicians

ACS   American College of Surgeons

ACTA   type of scanner

ACTH   adrenocorticotropic hormone

AD   right ear (auris dextra)

ADA   American Dietetic (Diabetic, Dental) Association; Americans with Disabilities Act

ADAA   American Dental Assistant Association

ADC   Aid to Dependent Children (also AFDC, "Families with")

ADH   antidiuretic hormone

ADHA   American Dental Hygienist Association

ADHD   attention deficit hyperactivity disorder

ADL   activities of daily living

ad lib   as desired, at will

ADR   Adriamycin (antineoplastic drug)

AE   above elbow (amputation)

AFB   acid-fast bacillus (TB and related organisms)

AFP   alpha-fetoprotein

AGA   approximate gestational age (length of pregnancy)

AgNO³ silver nitrate (instilled in newborn's eyes to prevent GC eye infection)

AHA American Heart (Hospital) Association

AI artificial insemination

AIDS acquired immune deficiency syndrome

AJ ankle jerk (reflex)

AK above knee (amputation)

AL axillary line (right or left)

ALL acute lymphocytic leukemia

ALP alkaline phosphatase (high in Ca of prostate)

ALS amyotrophic lateral sclerosis (Lou Gehrig's disease), antilymphocyte serum

AMA American Medical Association, against medical advice

AMD Actinomycin D (antineoplastic drug)

AMI acute myocardial infarction

AML acute myeloblastic (myelocytic, myelogenous) leukemia

ANA antinuclear antibodies (lab test; presence may indicate autoimmune disease), American Nurses' Association

ANLL acute nonlymphocytic leukemia

ANS autonomic nervous system

AP anterior/posterior

APC aspirin, phenacetin, caffeine (analgesic medication)

Apgar score of newborn's condition (Dr. Apgar)

APL anterior/posterior/lateral

Aq aqueous (water)

ARA-C (Ara-C) cytosine arabinoside (antineoplastic drug)

ARC AIDS-related complex

ARDS acute (adult) respiratory distress syndrome

ARE active resistive exercise

ARRT American Registry of Radiologic Technologists (X-ray tech)

ART accredited records technician, assisted reproductive technologies

AS left ear (auris sinstra), aortic stenosis

ASA acetylsalicylic acid (aspirin)

ASAP as soon as possible

ASCP American Society of Clinical Pathologists (medical lab)

ASCVD arteriosclerotic and cardiovascular (or cerebrovascular) disease

ASD atrial septal defect (congenital heart defect)

ASHD arteriosclerotic heart disease, atrial septal heart defect

ASRT American Society of Radiologic Technologists

as tol as tolerated (diet, and so on)

Au gold (metallic element; salts used in treatment; radioactive gold used in certain Ca cases and liver scan)

AV arteriovenous (shunt), atrioventricular

AVR aortic valve replacement

AZT Aschheim-Zondek test (for pregnancy), drug used in treatment of AIDS (zidovudine)

B bacillus, buccal

B₆ pyridoxine vitamin

Ba barium (opaque substance used in X-ray procedures)

B/A backache

Bab Babinski reflex (neurologic test; normal in infant but abnormal after 6 months)

BaE barium enema (also BE)

baso basophil (white blood cell type)

BBB bundle branch block (heart); L or R; blood-brain barrier

BCG bacille Calmette-Guérin (TB bacillus), used as vaccine

BCP blood chemistry profile

BD birthdate

BE barium enema, below elbow (amputation)

BEAM brain electrical activity mapping in diagnosis of tumors, epilepsy

BEB benign essential blepharospasm

BHA bilateral (or benign) hilar adenopathy

BID, bid twice a day

BK below knee

BM bowel movement

BMR basal metabolic rate

BMT bone marrow transplant

BOW bag of waters (amniotic sac)

BP (B/P) blood pressure

BPH benign prostatic hypertrophy

BRP bathroom privileges

BS bowel sounds, breath sounds, blood sugar

BSA body surface area (important measurement in burn patients)

BSP bromosulphthalein, sulfobromophthalein (lab)

BT bleeding time, brain tumor, body temperature

BU Bodansky units (lab term)

BUN blood urea nitrogen (lab test of kidney function)

BVR Bureau of Vocational Rehabilitation

BW birth weight, body weight

Bx biopsy

C centigrade, celsius, costal (rib), cervical, carbon, cesarean

c cubic, centimeter

c̄ with

C-1, C-2, and so on cervical first, second, and so on vertebra or spinal nerve

CA cancer, carcinoma, chronologic age

Ca calcium, cancer

CABG "cabbage" (coronary artery bypass graft)

CAD coronary artery disease

cal calorie

C & S culture and sensitivity (bacteriology lab)

caps capsules

CAT computerized axial tomography (also CT) (scan); multiple X-rays fed into computer provide cross sections of multiple planes

cath catheterized

CBC complete blood count

CBD common bile duct, closed bladder drainage

CBS chronic brain syndrome

CC chief or current complaint, crippled children, compensation case, cardiac catheterization

cc cubic centimeter (also written cm^3)

CCI chronic coronary insufficiency

CCU coronary care unit

CD communicable disease

CDA certified dental assistant

CDC Centers for Disease Control and Prevention, communicable disease center

CF Christmas factor (in blood, bleeding disorder), cystic fibrosis, complement fixation

CHD coronary heart disease, congenital heart disease

CHF congestive heart failure

CHO carbohydrate

CIN cervical intraepithelium neoplasia

CLL chronic lymphocytic leukemia

cm centimeter (cm^3 = cubic centimeter), costal margin (left or right)

CML chronic myelocytic leukemia

CMT certified medical technologist

CMV cytomegalovirus

CN cranial nerve (also written Cr_I, Cr_{II}, and so on)

CNS central nervous system

CO carbon monoxide

Co cobalt (chemical element, used in Ca treatment)

CO_2 carbon dioxide

COLD see *COPD*

comp compensation

COPD chronic obstructive pulmonary disease (also COLD, chronic obstructive lung disease)

CP cerebral palsy

CPD cephalopelvic disproportion (in birth canal, head too large)

CPK creatinine phosphokinase (enzyme released when heart or muscle is damaged)

CPM cyclophosphamide (antineoplastic drug)

CPR cardiopulmonary resuscitation

CPT current procedural terminology (codes)

CPZ chlorpromazine (drug)

CRF chronic renal failure, corticotropin-releasing factor

crit hematocrit (blood test)

CRP (A) C-reactive protein (antiserum)

CS central service (supply), coronary sinus

C section cesarean section (caesarean)

CSF cerebrospinal fluid

CT see *CAT*

Cu copper (metal; small quantities used by body)

cu cubic

cu cm cubic centimeter (cm^3)

cu mm cubic millimeter (mm^3)

CV cardiovascular, cerebrovascular

CVA cerebrovascular accident (stroke); cardiovascular accident

cva costovertebral angle (area over the kidney)

CVD cardiovascular (cerebrovascular) disease

CVP central venous pressure; Cytoxan, vincristine, prednisone (combination of drugs used in cancer treatment)

CVS chorionic villus sampling of placenta (for fetal defects)

CW crutch walking

CXR chest X-ray (procedure)

cysto cystoscopy

D dorsal, diopter, disease, divorced

d deceased, dead, distal, dorsal

D & C dilatation and curettage (uterus)

D & D diagnosis and disposition

D-1, D-2, and so on first, second, and so on dorsal (thoracic) vertebra, spinal nerve, or rib

DAT diet as tolerated

db decibel (unit of sound)

DC (D/C) discontinue, discharged, Doctor of Chiropractic

DD differential diagnosis, dry dressing

DDP Division of Disease Prevention

DDS Doctor of Dental Surgery

DDT insecticide

DES diethylstilbestrol (hormone)

DHS Department of Health Services

DI diagnostic imaging, diabetes insipidus

DIC disseminated intravascular clotting

diff differential (count of each type of WBC)

DIP distal interphalangeal (joint)—joint near tip of finger

DJD degenerative joint disease

DK diet kitchen

DLE disseminated lupus erythematosus

DM diastolic murmur, diabetes mellitus

DMD Doctor of Medical Dentistry

DMSO dimethyl sulfoxide (controversial drug)

DNA deoxyribonucleic acid (present in chromosomes of nuclei cells, carries genetic information)

DNR dorsal nerve root

DNS did not show (for appointment)

D/ns (D/s) dextrose in normal saline (IV solution)

DO Doctor of Osteopathy or Optometry

DOA dead on arrival

DOB date of birth

dorsi dorsiflexion (of foot, turned to posterior aspect of body as in "pointing toes")

DOU definitive observation unit (just below intensive care)

DPT diphtheria, pertussis, tetanus (immunization); also DTP, DT

DR dorsal root, doctor, dressing

DRG diagnostic-related groupings

DSD dry sterile dressing

DTP same as DPT

DTR a deep tendon reflex

DTs delirium tremens (in alcoholism)

DVR Department of Vocational Rehabilitation

DVT deep vein thrombosis

D/W dextrose in water (DW = distilled water)

Dx diagnosis

E enema, eye, extremity

EA educational age

E & H environment and heredity

EBV Epstein-Barr virus

ECF extended care facility, extracellular fluid

ECG electrocardiogram

ECHO virus (enterocytopathogenic human orphan virus)

echo sound

ECM erythema chronicum migrans (skin lesion in Lyme disease)

E. coli *Escherichia coli* (bacterium)

ECT electroconvulsive therapy (shock treatment)

ED emergency department

EDC estimated date of confinement (due date for delivery)

EEG electroencephalogram (brain wave recording)

EFP (R) effective filtration pressure (rate)

EGD esophagogastroduodenoscopy

EIA/ELISA enzyme immunosorbent assay or enzyme-linked immunosorbent assay: screening tests on blood samples to detect presence of HIV antibodies

EKG electrocardiogram

EM electron microscope

EMG electromyogram (muscle)

EMI type of scanner

EMT emergency medical technician

ENG electronystagmography (to test vestibular function by assessing eye motion)

ENT ear, nose, and throat

EOM extraocular movements

eos, eosin eosinophil (type of white blood cell)

ER emergency room, external rotation

ERCP endoscopic retrograde cholangiopancreatography

ERT estrogen replacement therapy

ERV expiratory residual volume (pulmonary function test)

ES emergency service

ESP extrasensory perception

ESR erythrocyte sedimentation rate (blood test)

ESRD esophageal reflux disease

EST electroshock therapy (same as ECT)

ETOH ethynol, ethyl alcohol

EUA examination under anesthesia

ext external

F Fahrenheit, female, Fellow, frequency

FACP, FACS Fellow of American College of Physicians, Surgeons

FANA fluorescent antinuclear antibodies

FAS fetal alcohol syndrome

FB, Fb fingerbreadth, foreign body

FBS fasting blood sugar

FDA Food and Drug Administration

Fe iron

FeSO$_4$ ferrous sulfate

FEV forced expiratory volume

FF force fluids

FH family history

FHT fetal heart tones

F-N finger to nose (coordination)

FOB fiber-optic bronchoscopy, foot of bed

FP flat plate (X-ray procedure)

Fr French (catheter)

FROM full range of motion (of joint)

FS frozen section

FSH follicle-stimulating hormone

FTA fluorescent treponemal antibody (syphilis test)

FTND full-term normal delivery

FU, 5-FU fluorouracil (cancer drug)

FUO fever of undetermined origin

Fx fracture

G glucose, gingival, specific gravity

g (Gm, gm) gram (unit of weight); 29 g in 1 oz

GA gestational age, gastric analysis

Ga gallium (rare metal, used in scans)

GAS general adaptation syndrome, group A streptococcal infection

GB gallbladder

GBS gallbladder series (X-ray film)

GC gonorrhea (sexually transmitted disease)

GE gastroenteritis

GFR glomerular filtration rate (kidney test)

GG gamma globulin (protein in blood, used therapeutically for passive temporary immunity)

GH growth hormone

GI, GIS gastrointestinal, series (X-ray film)

GIFT gamete intrafallopian transfer

GP general practitioner, gram positive

gr grain, gravida, gravity

gram cystogram (X-ray film of bladder), unit of weight

Grav I, II, and so on   gravida I, II, and so on (number of pregnancies)

GT, GTT glucose tolerance (test)

gtt drop

GU genitourinary

GV gentian violet (dye used in lab and as topical medication)

GVHD graft versus host disease

gyn gynecology

H hydrogen, hypo

H⁺ hydrogen ion

h hour

H₂O water

Hb, Hgb hemoglobin (iron-containing pigment in RBCs, carries oxygen to tissues)

HBO hyperbaric oxygen therapy

HBP high blood pressure (hypertension)

HCl hydrochloric acid (normal in the stomach)

HCO₃ bicarbonate

Hct hematocrit (blood test, low in anemias)

HCTZ hydrochlorothiazide (diuretic)

HD Hodgkin's disease (type of cancer), Hansen's disease (leprosy), Huntington's disease, hip disarticulation

HDL high-density lipoprotein ("good" cholesterol)

HEENT head, eyes, ears, nose, throat

HEW Health, Education, and Welfare; see HHS

HF high frequency (sounds)

Hg mercury (metallic element)

Hgb hemoglobin

HGH human growth hormone

HH hard of hearing

HHS Health and Human Services; replaced HEW

HID headache, insomnia, depression (syndrome)

HIV human immunodeficiency virus

HLA homologous (human) leukocytic antibodies

HMD hyaline membrane disease (of newborn babies)

HMO Health Maintenance Organization

HNP herniated nucleus pulposus (hernia of intervertebral disk)

h/o history of

HOH hard of hearing

HP high-power field (microscope); hemipelvectomy

HS heart sounds, head sling

hs bedtime

HSG hysterosalpingography (-gram)

HSO hysterosalpingoooophorectomy

HSV herpes simplex virus (causes cold sores, genital herpes)

HTLV human T-lymphotropic virus type III

HVD hypertensive vascular disease

hypo injection, hypoglycemic diet

Hx history

I iodine (nonmetallic element, used as medication and in diagnosis of thyroid disorders)

¹³¹I radioactive isotope of iodine

I & D incision and drainage

I & O intake and output

IBS irritable bowel syndrome

IC intensive care, intercostal

ICA internal carotid artery

ICD International Classification of Diseases

ICF intracellular fluid

ICM intercostal margin

ICN intensive care nursery

ICP intracranial pressure

ICS intercostal space

ICSI intracytoplasmic sperm injection

ICT insulin coma therapy

ICU intensive care unit

IDDM insulin-dependent diabetes mellitus

IgA immunoglobulin A

IH infectious hepatitis

IHD ischemic heart disease

IHSS idiopathic hypertrophic subaortic stenosis

IM intramuscular (injection)

IND investigational new drug

INH isoniazid (TB drug)

in situ in position or original place (not metastasized)

IOP intraocular pressure

IPPB intermittent positive pressure breathing (treatment)

IQ intelligence quotient

ITP idiopathic thrombocytopenic purpura

IU international units

IUD intrauterine device (for contraception)

IV intravenous (into vein)

IVC intravenous cholangiogram, inferior vena cava

IVD intervertebral disk (between vertebrae)

IVDA IV drug abuser

IVDU IV drug user

IVF in vitro fertilization

IVP intravenous pyelogram (X-ray film of kidney)

J joint, journal, Jewish

JAMA Journal of the American Medical Association

K potassium (mineral)—essential in diet

KAB knowledge, attitudes, and beliefs (or behaviors) survey

KCl potassium chloride (one of the ingredients in Ringer's solution for IV)

KD knee disarticulation

kg kilogram

KJ knee jerk (reflex)

KMnO$_4$ potassium permanganate (antiseptic)

KRP Kolmer Reiter protein (syphilis test)

KS Kaposi's sarcoma

KUB kidneys, ureters, bladder

KVO keep vein open (do not allow IV to run dry)

L liter, left, lower, lumbar

L-1, L-2, and so on first, second, and so on lumbar vertebra or spinal nerve

LI, LII, LIII primary, secondary, tertiary lues (syphilis)

LA left atrium or auricle (of heart)

L & A light and accommodation (eye)

L & D labor and delivery

L & W living and well

laser light amplification by stimulated emission of radiation (has some uses in surgery)

lat lateral

LATS long-acting thyroid stimulator

Lav lymphadenopathy-associated virus

LCM left costal margin

LD Lyme disease

LDH lactic dehydrogenase (enzyme, lab test)

LDL low-density lipoproteins ("bad cholesterol")

LE lupus erythematosus, lower extremity, left eye

LGI lower gastrointestinal (series), same as barium enema

LH luteinizing hormone

LKS/np liver, kidney, spleen (also LSK—liver, spleen, kidney), nonpalpable

LLB lower leg brace

LLL lower left lobe, lower left lid

LLQ lower left quadrant

LMP last menstrual period (to calculate due date)

LN lymph node

LOA, LOP left occiput anterior, posterior (presentation at delivery)

LOC loss of consciousness

LOM limitation of motion

LP lumbar puncture, low power (microscope)

LPN licensed practical nurse (LVN—licensed vocational nurse)

LRQ lower right quadrant

LRS lactated Ringer's solution (for IV)

LS lumbosacral

LSD lysergic acid diethylamide (hallucinogenic drug)

LTB laryngotracheobronchitis (croup)

LTH luteotropic hormone (pituitary hormone, prolactin)

LUL left upper lobe

LUQ left upper quadrant

LV left ventricle

LVH left ventricular hypertrophy

lymph lymphocyte (type of blood cell)

M mean, medium, male, married, medical, morphine, murmur, mortality, mobidity

m murmur, minim, monocyte, meter

M₁ first mitral sound, heart sound at apex

MA mental age, menstrual age, Master of Arts, mentum anterior (presentation at delivery)

M & M morbidity and mortality

MAO monoamine oxidase (inhibitor) (type of medication)

MAST medical antishock trousers

mcg microgram ($1/1000$ of a milligram)

MCH mean corpuscular hemoglobin (blood test), maternal and child health

MCHC mean corpuscular hemoglobin concentration (Hgb in each RBC or per unit of blood)

MCV mean corpuscular volume (measurement of size of individual red cell)

MD Doctor of Medicine, muscular dystrophy

MEG magnetic encephalography

mEq/L milliequivalent per liter (measurement of concentration of a solution)

MF meat free (diet)

MFD minimal fatal dose

MG myasthenia gravis

mg (mgm) milligram

MH mental health, marital history

MI myocardial infarction, mitral insufficiency

mL (ml) milliliter (same as cc)

MM mucous membrane

mm millimeter

mm³ cubic millimeter

mm Hg millimeters of mercury

MMPI Minnesota Multiphasic Personality Inventory (test)

MMR measles, mumps, rubella (combined immunization)

MMWR Morbidity and Mortality Weekly Report (by CDC)

MO mineral oil

MOM milk of magnesia

mono mononucleosis, monocyte (white blood cell)

MOPP nitrogen mustard, Oncovin, prednisone, procarbazine (drugs used in combination for some cancers)

MOR minor operating room

MR may repeat, metabolic rate, mentally retarded, medical records

MRI magnetic resonance imaging (scanner and computer)

MRL medical records librarian

MS multiple sclerosis, mitral stenosis, morphine sulfate, muscle strength, musculoskeletal

MT medical technologist (lab)

MT (ASCP) medical technologist (American Society of Clinical Pathologists)

MTX methotrexate (cancer drug)

MVA motor vehicle accident

MVP mitral valve prolapse (heart valve)

MVR mitral valve replacement

N nitrogen, negative, normal, national

n normal (saline), nasal, nerve

NI, NII, and so on nerves by number

N₂O nitrous oxide (anesthetic gas)

Na sodium

NaCl sodium chloride (salt)

NAD no acute distress

NaHCO₃ sodium bicarbonate

n & t nose and throat

n & v nausea and vomiting

NB newborn

NBM nothing by mouth

NED no evidence of disease

NER no evidence of recurrence

NFTD normal full-term delivery

NG nasogastric (tube)

NGU, NSU nongonorrheal urethritis, nonspecific urethritis

NH₃ ammonia

NIDDM noninsulin-dependent diabetes mellitus

NIH National Institute of Health

nm neuromuscular

NMR nuclear magnetic resonance (gives chemistry of an organ)

NP neuropsychiatric, nasopharyngeal

NPH neutral protamine Hagedorn (insulin)

NPN nonprotein nitrogen (lab test)

NPO nothing by mouth

nr no repeat (no refill of Rx)

ns normal saline (salt solution equal in concentration to that of body fluids)

NSAID nonsteriodal anti-inflammatory drug (pronounced ĕn-sĕd)

NTD neural tube defect

NYD not yet diagnosed

O occiput, oculus, oral, aught (zero), oxygen

O₂ oxygen

OA occiput anterior, old age, osteoarthritis

OAA old age assistance

O & C onset and course

OASI old age and survivor's insurance

OB obstetrics

OB-GYN obstetrics-gynecology

OBS organic brain syndrome

OC oral contraceptive

OCG oral cholangiogram (bile ducts X-ray film)

OD right eye, overdosed, Doctor of Optometry, occupational disease

od every day, once a day

OHS open heart surgery

OI opportunistic infection

OIDS Office of Infectious Disease Services

OJ orange juice

OOB out of bed

OPD outpatient department

OR operating room

ORIF open reduction internal fixation

ORT operating room technician

OS left eye

OSHA Occupational Safety and Health Administration

OT occupational therapy

OTC over the counter (medications)

OTR occupational therapist, registered

OU both eyes, each eye

OV office visit

P phosphorus, pulse, passive, proximal, pupil, para (live births)

p post, pupil (of eye), para, p wave (ECG)

PA posterior/anterior, pulmonary artery, pernicious anemia

PABA para-aminobenzoic acid (sunscreen preparation)

PAD   peripheral arterial disease

PAN   periarteritis nodosa

P & A   percussion and auscultation (tapping and listening)

PaO$_2$ arterial oxygen pressure

PAP   primary atypical pneumonia

Pap   Papanicolaou (smear for cancer detection)

Para I, II, and so on   number of live births, full term

PAT   paroxysmal atrial tachycardia

PBI   protein-bound iodine (thyroid test)

PBZ   Pyribenzamine (antihistamine medication)

pc   after meals

PCA   patient-controlled analgesia

pcn, PCN   penicillin

pCO$_2$ pressure or tension of carbon dioxide

PCP   pneumocystis carinii pneumonia

PCV   packed cell volume

PD   Doctor of Pharmacy

PDA   patent ductus arteriosus (open duct between pulmonary artery and aorta)

PDD   premenstrual dysphoric disorder

PDR   *Physician's Desk Reference* (listing of prescription drugs)

PE   physical examination, pulmonary embolism

Peds   pediatrics

PEEP   positive end-expiratory pressure

PEG   pneumoencephalogram

PELA   percutaneous excimer laser angioplasty

PERRLA   pupils equal, round, react to light and accommodation (eye)

PF   push fluids

pg   pregnant

PGH   pituitary growth hormone

PH   past history, public health

pH   hydrogen ion concentration (measure of acidity/alkalinity)

PICA   posterior inferior cerebellar artery

PID   pelvic inflammatory disease

PIIS   posterior inferior iliac spine

PIP   proximal interphalangeal joint

PKU   phenylketonuria (causes retardation)

PM   physical medicine, postmortem, afternoon

PMI   point of maximum intensity

PMN   polymorphonuclear (leukocyte)

PMS   premenstrual syndrome

PN   peripheral nerve, practical nurse

PND   paroxysmal nocturnal dyspnea, postnasal drip

PNS   peripheral nervous system

PO   phone order, postoperative, per os (orally)

PO$_2$, pO$_2$ pressure of oxygen

PO$_4$ phosphate (important in acid-base balance of blood)

POD   postoperative day

POMP   predisone, Oncovin, methotrexate, 6-mercaptopurine (combination of cancer drugs)

PP   postprandial (after a meal)

PPD   purified protein derivative (TB test), permanent partial disability

PPH   primary pulmonary hypertension

PPLO   pleuropneumonia-like organism (causes atypical pneumonia)

PRE   progressive resistive exercise

prn   as needed

PROM   premature rupture of membranes

PSA   prostate-specific antigen

PSP   phenolsulfonphthalein (renal excretion test)

PSRO   professional standards review organization

PT   physical therapy, prothrombin time

pt   patient

PTA   prior to admission

PTCA   percutaneous transluminal coronary angioplasty (compression of atherosclerotic plaque to increase diameter of lumen)

PTD   permanent total disability

PTH   parathyroid hormone

PTSD   posttraumatic stress disorder

PUD   peptic ulcer disease

PVC/B   premature ventricular contractions/beats

PVD   peripheral vascular disease

pvO$_2$ venous oxygen pressure

PWA   person with AIDS

Px   prognosis

PZA   pyrazinamide (TB drug)

PZI   protamine zinc insulin

q   every

QA   quality assurance

qd   every day

qh, q2h   every hour, every 2 hours

qid   four times a day

qm   every morning

qn   every night

qns   quantity not sufficient (for test ordered)

qod   every other day

QRS   complex (ventricular complex in ECG)

qs   quantity sufficient

R, r   right, rectally, resistant, roentgen, respiration

RA   rheumatoid arthritis, right atrium, residual air

Ra   radium

RAD, rad   radiation absorbed dose (unit of measure for X-rays)

RAI   radioactive iodine

RAIU   radioactive iodine uptake

RATx   radiation therapy

RBC   red blood cell, red blood count

RBD   right border dullness

RBF   renal blood flow

RC   Red Cross, respiratory center, red cell, Roman catheter

RCD   relative cardiac dullness

RCM   right costal margin

RD   retinal detachment (eye), respiratory disease

RDS   respiratory distress syndrome

RE   right eye, readmission

REM   rapid eye movements (during dreams)

rep   repeat

RF   respiratory failure, rheumatic fever, rheumatoid factor

Rh   factor in blood (Rh+ people have the factor)

RHD   rheumatic heart disease

RhoGAM   injection given to Rh-negative women after delivery, miscarriage, or abortion to prevent antibody formation against Rh factor

RLF   retrolental fibroplasia (eye condition that causes blindness)

RLL   right lower lobe

RLQ   right lower quadrant

RML   right middle lobe, right mediolateral (episiotomy)

RMSF   Rocky Mountain spotted fever

RNA   ribonucleic acid

R/O   rule out

ROA   right occiput anterior (presentation at delivery)

ROAD   reversible obstructive airway disease

ROM   range of motion, rupture of membranes

Rom   Romberg (neurologic test for balance)

ROP   right occiput posterior (birth presentation)

ROS   review of systems

RP   retrograde pyelogram

RPR   rapid plasma reagent (syphilis test)

RPT   registered physical therapist

RRA   registered records administrator

RRL   registered records librarian

RRT   registered respiratory therapist

RSB   right sternal border

RSV   respiratory syncytial virus

RT   radiotherapy, recreational therapy, radiologic technologist

RTC   return to clinic

RUE   right upper extremity

RUL   right upper lobe

RUQ   right upper quadrant

RV   right ventricle, residual volume, rubella virus

RVH   right ventricle hypertrophy

RVHD   rheumatic valvular heart disease

Rx   prescription, recipe, treatment, therapy

rx   reaction

S, s sacral, stimulus, sulfur, sinister (left), saline, sensitive, section

s̄ without

S-1, S-2, and so on first, second, and so on sacral spinal nerve or vertebra

SA sinoatrial node (pacemaker in heart), sarcoma

SAD seasonal affective disorder (lack of light)

SAH subarachnoid hemorrhage

SB stillborn, sternal border (right/left, upper/lower)

SBE subacute bacterial endocarditis

SC sickle cell

Sc subcutaneously

scuba self-contained underwater breathing apparatus

SD shoulder disarticulation

sed sedimentation rate (rate at which blood settles)

seg segmented white blood cells (mature forms with segmented nuclei)

SF salt free

sg, sp gr specific gravity (weight as compared to water)

SGOT serum glutamic oxaloacetic transaminase (enzyme, lab test)

SGPT serum glutamic pyruvic transaminase (enzyme, lab test)

SH serum hepatitis (hepatitis B), social history

SHS Sayre head sling

SIADH syndrome of inappropriate antidiuretic hormone

S/ICU surgery/intensive care unit

SIDS sudden infant death syndrome

sig let it be labeled (label on prescription)

SIJ sacroiliac joint

SLB short leg brace

SLC short leg cast

SLE systemic lupus erythematosus (LE)

SMA, SMAC 6, 12, or 18 sequential multiple analysis (series of blood chemistry tests)

SMR submucous resection (nasal surgery)

SNAFU situation normal, all fouled up

SNDO standard nomenclature of diseases and operations

SO₄ sulfate

SOB short of breath, significant other at bedside

SOL space-occupying lesion

soln solution

SOPM stitches out in afternoon

sp gr specific gravity

sq, subq subcutaneously

SR sedimentation rate, systems review, sinus rhythm, stimulus/response

Sr strontium (metallic element)

SS social service, Social Security, soap solution, sterile solution, saline soak, supersaturated, signs and symptoms

s̄s̄ one-half

SSE soapsuds enema

SSKI saturated solution potassium iodide (medication)

stabs nonsegmented white blood cells (immature forms)

staph staphylococcus (bacterium)

stat immediately

STD sexually transmitted disease, skin test dose

STH somatotropin (growth hormone)

strep streptococcus (bacterium)

STS serologic test for syphilis

subq, subcu subcutaneously

SV stroke volume

SVC superior vena cava

SW short wave (diathermy)

Sx signs, symptoms

T, t temperature, thoracic, total, tetanus, tablespoon

T-1, T-2, and so on first, second, and so on thoracic vertebra or spinal nerve

T+1, T+2 increased intraocular tension

T−1, T−2 decreased intraocular tension

T₃, T₄ thyroid function tests

TAB typhoid, paratyphoid A and B (vaccine), therapeutic abortion

tab tablet

TAH total abdominal hysterectomy

T & A tonsillectomy and adenoidectomy, tonsils and adenoids

T & C turn and cough

T & R treated and released

TAT toxin antitoxin, toxoid antitoxin, tetanus antitoxin, Thematic Apperception Test

Tb, Tbc tubercle bacillus, tuberculosis

TBW total body weight

TC tissue culture

TCDB turn, cough, deep breaths

TCNS transcutaneous electrical nerve stimulation (also TENS, TNS)

TED thromboembolus (support hose to prevent emboli)

temp temperature, temporal

TENS transcutaneous electrical nerve stimulation

TF tuning fork

TH thyroid hormone

THA total hip arthroplasty

THI thiamine

THR total hip replacement

TIA transient ischemic attack

tid three times a day

tinc, tr tincture (alcohol preparation)

tiw three times a week

TKA total knee arthroplasty

TKO to keep open (vein)

TKR total knee replacement

TL tubal ligation (sterilization)

TLA translumbar aortogram

TLC total lung capacity, tender loving care

TLCA transluminal coronary angioplasty

TM tympanic membrane, temporomandibular

TMJ temporomandibular joint (jaw)

TNC too numerous to count (lab)

TNM tumor, nodes, metastasis (cancer staging system)

TNS transcutaneous nerve stimulation

TO telephone order

TOF tetralogy of Fallot (congenital heart defect)

TP total protein, testosterone proprionate, *Treponema pallidum*

TPA tissue plasminogen activator

TPC *Treponema pallidum* complement test (syphilis test)

TPI *Treponema pallidum* immobilization test

TPN total parenteral nutrition

TPR temperature, pulse, and respirations

TPUR transperineal urethral resection

Tr trace, tincture, traction

trach trachea, tracheotomy, tracheostomy

TSB total serum bilirubin (lab test)

TSH thyroid-stimulating hormone

TSS toxic shock syndrome

TT tilt table, transfer to

TTD temporary total disability, transverse thoracic diameter

TTH thyrotropic hormone

TUR, TURP transurethral resection of prostate gland

TV tidal volume, total volume, television

TVC timed vital capacity (pulmonary function test)

TW tap water

Tx traction, treatment, tumor cannot be assessed

U unit, upper, uranium

UA (or Ua) urinalysis

U & C urethral and cervical

UC uterine contractions

UCG ultrasound cardiogram

UE upper extremity (arm)

UG urogenital

UGI upper GI series (X-ray film)

ULQ upper left quadrant

UN urea nitrogen (lab test); same as BUN

ung ointment

UNOS United Network Organ Sharing

U/O under observation

UR Utilization Review

URI upper respiratory infection

URQ upper right quadrant

U/S ultrasound

USP US Pharmacopoeia (list of medications)

USPHS US Public Health Service

UTI urinary tract infection

UV ultraviolet

V ventricle, volt, volume, virulence, valve, vein, Roman numeral for number 5

VA Veterans Administration, visual acuity

VBAC vaginal birth after cesarean

VC vital capacity, vocal cord

VCG vector cardiogram

VCR vincristine (cancer drug)

VCU voiding cystourethrogram

VD venereal disease

VDRL Venereal Disease Research Laboratories

Vf ventricular fibrillation, visual field

VR vocational rehabilitation, venous return, ventral root

VS vital signs

VSD ventricular septal defect

VT ventricular tachycardia

VZ virus varicella-zoster (shingles)

W water, week, west, widow, with, watt, weight, width, wife

WAIS Wechsler Adult Intelligence Scale

WB whole blood

WBC white blood count, white blood cell

WBC & diff white blood count and differential (count of each type of WBC)

WC wheelchair

WD well developed, wet dressing

WDWN well developed, well nourished

W/F, wf white female

WHO World Health Organization

WISC Wechsler Intelligence Scale for Children

W/M, wm white male

WN well nourished

WNL within normal limits

WP wet pack, whirlpool

WPW Wolff-Parkinson-White syndrome (disturbance in conduction in Purkinje fibers of heart)

X cross (match), cross section, Roman numeral for 10

X-ray roentgen ray

XU excretory urogram

XX female chromosome

XY male chromosome

Y/O year old

Z zero

ZIFT zygote intrafallopian transfer

Zn zinc

Symbols

♂ male

♀ female

> greater than

< less than

℥ ounce

Ʒ dram

± plus or minus

↑ increased, elevated

↓ decreased, lowered

∥ parallel

Physical Therapy Abbreviations

Kinds of Treatment

E. stim   electrical stimulation

fluido   fluidotherapy

FT$_x$ Fontaine traction

HP   hot pack

HT   Hubbard tank

IC T$_x$ intermittent cervical traction

IP T$_x$ intermittent pelvic traction

MWD   microwave diathermy

parr   paraffin (wax)

PT   physical therapy

ST$_x$ Sayre traction

SWD   shortwave diathermy

TENS   transcutaneous electrical nerve stimulation

US   ultrasound

WP   whirlpool

WT   wading tank

Movement

AAROM   active assistive range of motion

abd   abduction

add   adduction

AROM   active range of motion

elev   elevation

ER   external rotation

ext or /   extension

flex or √   flexion

IR   internal rotation

lat flex   lateral flexion

PROM   passive range of motion

ROM   range of motion

SAQ   short arc quad

SLR   straight leg raise

General

act   active

act assist   active assistive

ADL   activities of daily living

AE amp   above elbow amputee

a g   antigravity

AK amp   above knee amputee

amp   amputation

BE amp   below elbow amputee

BIW   twice a week

BK amp   below knee amputation

FOB   foot of bed

ft   foot or feet

FWB   full weight bearing

LLE   left lower extremity

LUE   left upper extremity

MED   minimal erythemal dosage

NWb   non–weight bearing

‖ bars   parallel bars

pass   passive

PRE   progressive resistive exercise

pt   patient

PWB   partial weight bearing

reed   reeducation

rehab   rehabilitation

RLE   right lower extremity

RUE   right upper extremity

Rx   treatment or therapy

SB   side bending

TIW   three times a week

TO   telephone order

T$_x$ traction

WC   wheelchair

W/cm^2   watts per centimeter squared

WFL   within functional limits

wt   weight

x   times or repetitions

Pulmonary Function Abbreviations

CaO$_2$ concentration of oxygen in arterial blood

CcO$_2$ concentration of oxygen in end capillary blood

C$\bar{v}$O$_2$ concentration of oxygen in mixed venous blood

DL$_{CO}$ diffusing capacity of the lung for carbon monoxide

DL_{O_2} diffusing capacity of the lung for oxygen

ERV   expiratory reserve volume

FE_{CO_2} fraction of carbon dioxide in expired air

$FEF_{25\%-75\%}$ forced midexpiratory flow (between 25% and 75% of FVC)

$FE\ N_2$ fraction of nitrogen in expired air

FEO_2 fraction of oxygen in expired air

FEV_1 forced expiratory volume in 1 second

FEV_3 forced expiratory volume in first 3 seconds

FIN_2 fraction of nitrogen in inspired air

FIO_2 fraction of oxygen in inspired air

FRC   functional residual capacity

FVC   forced vital capacity

IC   inspiratory capacity

IRV   inspiratory reserve volume

MVV   maximum voluntary ventilation

$P\bar{A}_{CO}$ mean partial pressure of carbon monoxide in alveolar gas

PA_{CO_2} partial pressure of carbon dioxide in alveolar gas

$P\bar{A}_{CO_2}$ mean partial pressure of carbon dioxide in alveolar gas

Pa_{CO_2} partial pressure of carbon dioxide in arterial blood

P_{alv} alveolar pressure

PA_{H_2O} partial pressure of water in alveolar gas

Pao   pressure at airway opening

Pa_{O_2} partial pressure of oxygen in arterial blood

PA_{O_2} partial pressure of oxygen in alveolar gas

$P\bar{A}_{O_2}$ mean partial pressure of oxygen in alveolar gas

PB   atmospheric pressure

Pbs   pressure at external suface of chest

P_{CO_2} partial pressure of carbon dioxide

$P\bar{c}_{O_2}$ mean partial pressure of oxygen in capillary blood

$P\bar{E}_{CO_2}$ mean partial pressure of carbon dioxide in mixed expired air

P_L recoil pressure of lung

pN_2 partial pressure of nitrogen

PO_2 partial pressure of oxygen

Ppl   pleural pressure

PRS   recoil pressure of total respiratory system

PW   recoil pressure of chest wall

$\dot{Q}t$ total cardiac output

$\dot{Q}x$ shunt flow

R   respiratory exchange ratio

Raw   resistance of tracheobronchial tree to flow of air into lung

Re   Reynolds number

RQ   respiratory quotient

RUS   resistance of upstream segment of tracheobronchial tree

RV   residual volume

SA_{O_2} percentage saturation of hemoglobin with oxygen in arterial blood

SO_2 percentage saturation of hemoglobin with oxygen

TLC   total lung capacity

$\dot{V}$ gas volume per minute

V_1 inspiratory volume of ventilation per minute

VA   volume of alveolar gas

$\dot{V}A/\dot{Q}c$ ratio of alveolar ventilation to pulmonary blood flow

VC   vital capacity

Vc   volume of blood in pulmonary capillary bed

$\dot{V}_{CO}$ rate of carbon monoxide uptake per minute

$\dot{V}_{CO_2}$ amount of carbon dioxide eliminated per minute

VD   volume of dead space gas

$\dot{V}E$ expiratory volume of ventilation per minute

$\dot{V}_{max}$ maximal rate of airflow during forced expiration

$\dot{V}_{max\ 50}$ rate of airflow at 50% of vital capacity

$\dot{V}_{O_2}$ rate of oxygen uptake per minute (oxygen consumption)

V_T tidal volume (also TV)

Cancer Abbreviations*

This list is presented to acquaint the student with some abbreviations used in cancer cases. The breast is used as an example for the anatomic site of cancer; however, terms dealing with tumor size are generally applicable.

Primary tumor (T)

TX tumor cannot be assessed

TO no evidence of primary tumor

TIS Paget's disease of the nipple with no demonstrable tumor

T1 tumor 2 cm or less in greatest dimension

T1a no fixation to underlying pectoral fascia or muscle

T1b fixation to underlying pectoral fascia and/or muscle

    I tumor—0.5 cm or less

    II tumor—more than 0.5–1.0 cm or less

    III tumor—more than 1.0–2.0 cm or less

T2 tumor more than 2 cm but not more than 5 cm in greatest dimension

T2a no fixation to underlying pectoral fascia or muscle

T2b fixation to underlying pectoral fascia and/or muscle

T3 tumor more than 5 cm in its greatest dimension

T3a no fixation to underlying pectoral fascia or muscle

T3b fixation to underlying pectoral fascia and/or muscle

T4 tumor of any size with direct extension to chest wall or skin (chest wall includes ribs, intercostal muscles, and serratus anterior muscle, but not pectoral muscle)

T4a fixation to chest wall

T4b edema (including peau d'orange), ulceration of the skin of the breast, or satellite skin nodules confined to the same breast

T4c both of the above

Lymph nodes (N) definitions for clinical-diagnostic stage

NX regional lymph nodes cannot be assessed clinically

N0 homolateral axillary lymph nodes not considered to contain growth

N1 movable homolateral axillary nodes considered to contain growth

N2 homolateral axillary nodes considered to contain growth and fixed to one another or to other structures

N3 homolateral supraclavicular or infraclavicular nodes considered to contain growth, or edema of the arm (edema of the arm may be caused by lymphatic obstruction, and lymph nodes may not then be palpable)

Lymph nodes (N) definitions for surgical evaluative and postsurgical treatment—pathologic

NX regional lymph nodes cannot be assessed (not removed for study, or previously removed)

N0 no evidence of homolateral axillary lymph node metastasis

N1 metastasis to movable homolateral axillary nodes not fixed to one another or to other structure; further classified as to number of metastases and size

N2 metastasis to homolateral axillary lymph nodes that are fixed to one another or the other structures

N3 metastasis to homolateral supraclavicular or infraclavicular lymph node(s)

Distant metastases (M) all time periods

MX not assessed

M0 no (known) distant metastasis

M1 distant metastasis present; specify

Tumor size

_____ × _____ × _____ cm
Predominant lesion measured on:
patient
mammogram
pathologic specimen

---

* Adapted from Data Form for Cancer Staging. Used with permission of The American Joint Committee on Cancer. *A.J.C.C. Manual for Staging of Cancer*, Fourth Edition.

Location   (multiple when necessary)

OUQ*

OLQ*

IUQ*

ILQ*

nipple/areola

Performance status of host (H)

Several systems for recording a patient's activity and symptoms are used and are more or less equivalent as follows:

H0   normal activity

H1   symptomatic but ambulatory—cares for self

H2   ambulatory more than 50% of time—occasionally needs assistance

H3   ambulatory 50% or less of time—nursing care needed

H4   bedridden—may need hospitalization

Stage

clinical-diagnostic

surgical evaluative

postsurgical treatment—pathologic

stage TIS: in situ

stage X: cannot stage (unstageable)

stages I–IV (further broken down; too detailed for this text)

---

*Quadrants: outer upper, outer lower, inner upper, inner lower.
**Not otherwise specified.

Histologic type of cancer   check predominant type

Ductal

intraductal (in situ)

invasive with predominant intraductal component

invasive, NOS**

comedo

inflammatory

medullary with lymphocytic infiltrate

mucinous (colloid)

papillary

scirrhous

tubular

other (specify)

Lobular

in situ

invasive with predominant in situ component

invasive

Nipple

Paget's disease, NOS

Paget's disease with intraductal carcinoma

Paget's disease with invasive ductal carcinoma

other (specify)

Histologic grade

G1: well-differentiated

G2: moderately well-differentiated

G3–G4: poorly to very poorly differentiated

Glossary/Index

A

abbreviations: for cancer, 411–412; for cardiovascular disorders, 162–163; diagnostic/laboratory, 99–109; for diet orders, 92; for ears, 241; for eye organ, 238; for gastrointestinal system, 188; for hospital/clinic departments, 94; of immunizations, 93; for insurance, 94–95; for integumentary system, 133; listing of general, 395–408; for musculoskeletal system, 147; for nervous system, 227; for physical therapy, 409; for physician orders, 91–94; for prescriptions, 95–96; for psychiatric terms, 227; for pulmonary functions, 409–410; for respiratory system, 174; for routes of administration, 95; for sexually transmitted diseases, 214, 216; symbols used as, 408; for toileting, 91; for urinary system, 197–198. *See also* medical words

abdomen: front of body between chest and pelvis, 187; illustration showing areas of, 182

abducens, eye muscles that turn eye outward, 220

abduction, away from the midline, 79

abortion, interruption of pregnancy before fetus is viable, 203

abscess: large pustule containing pus, 128; accumulation of pus in lung, 170; of Bartholin's gland, 203; infection in ear/sinuses (brain), 221; inside the mouth, 244; in pleural cavity (empyema), 170

absorption (digestion), takes place in the small intestines, 182

accessory glands, secrete alkaline secretions which (with sperm) make up seminal fluid, 213

accommodation, ability of eye to adjust to seeing different distances, 237

acetabulum, large socket for head of femur, 141

acidosis, disturbance of acid–base balance, 254

acne vulgaris, inflammation of the pilosebaceous glands, 130

acoustic meatus, opening or passage in the ear, 240

acromegaly, enlarged and distorted extremities and face, 253

actinic, pertaining to ultraviolet rays, 132

Addison's disease, weakness, weight loss, jaundice, hypoglycemia, 253

adduction, toward the midline, 79

adenoids, part of the lymphatic system, 169

adhesions, abnormal bands or fibers that bind one organ to another, 183

administrative medicine: administrator of a medical center, 34; concerned with epidemiology and communicable disease, 36

adrenals: atop each kidney, secrete steroids and catecholamines and helps with stress, 251; illustrated, 256

aerobic, needing oxygen, 68

aerosols, medications in spray form for relief of asthma symptoms, 171

aerotitis (barotitis media), sudden increase in atmospheric pressure, air moves from nasopharynx into middle ear/retraction of eardrum may occur as well as further complications, 239

affect, emotional reaction, 226

aggression, hostile attitude, 226

agranulocytes, WBCs produced by spleen and lymph nodes, 156

AIDS, 215, 245, 275–276

albinism, lack of pigment, 132

albuminuria, albumin (protein) in urine, abnormal, 195

alcoholism, addiction to alcohol, leading to malnutrition and liver damage, 183

allergy, acquired hypersensitivity to a substance, 170

alopecia, baldness, 132

alpha-fetoprotein, blood screening test done during pregnancy to measure AFP from fetal circulation to maternal bloodstream, 206

ALS, amyotrophic lateral sclerosis, syndrome marked by muscular weakness and atrophy with spasticity and hyperreflexia, 142, 221

alveolectomy, surgical removal of part of alveolar bone, 245

alveoli (alveolus), tiny air sacs at ends of bronchioles that comprise lung tissue, 168

Alzheimer's disease (presenile dementia), early senility leading to severe deterioration, 221

ambivalence, opposing feelings, 226

amblyopia, weakening, dimness or dullness of vision/"lazy eye," 233

amnesia, loss of memory, 226

amniocentesis, obtaining sample of amniotic fluid to screen for genetic defects, 206

amputation, removal of a limb, 145

anaerobic, growing without oxygen, 68

anasarca, severe, generalized edema, 187

anastomosis (also resection), joining together two parts of intestine or common bile duct when portion has been removed, 186

anemias, groups of diseases characterized by insufficient red blood cells, 158

anencephaly, congenital absence of brain, 221

anesthesia (for eye procedures), usually topical but may be injected locally behind the eye, 237

anesthesia (for OB), regional/general/local types, 204

anesthesiology, anesthesiologist, administers anesthesia during surgery, 34

aneurysm, weak and ballooned area in vessel, 158

angina pectoris, pains in the chest due to spasm of coronary arteries, 158

angiogram (arteriogram) cerebral, radiopaque substance is injected into arteries in neck, then X-ray films are taken, 223

angiography, X-ray examination of vessels, 160, 236

angioplasty, tube or balloon inserted in artery and inflated to open the artery, 160, 223

anisocoria, unequal pupils, 237

ankylosing spondylitis, chronic, progressive inflammation of the vertebrae with spontaneous fusion causing deformity, 142

anodontia, without teeth, 244

anorexia, medical symptom noting that the patient is without appetite, 183, 254

anorexia nervosa, psychological disorder involving a distorted body image and an aversion to food which may result in severe weight loss, malnutrition, and possible death, 183, 226

anoxia, without oxygen, 171

anterior (ventral), toward the front, 76

antibody, protein produced after foreign body invasion, 132

anticoagulant, medication to delay clotting, 160

antigen, any foreign substance that stimulates antibody production, 132

antihistamine, medicine used to treat allergic reactions, 171

antihypertensive drugs, to relax artery walls or neutralize a hormone that causes arterial spasm, 160

anti-rejection drugs, given to try to prevent rejection of transplanted organ, 86

anuria, no urinary output, 195

anus, anal sphincter, 179

anxiety, excessive and long-lasting apprehensive expectation about upcoming life events, 226

aorta, largest heart artery, 154

aortic, between left ventricle and aorta, 153

apgar, numerical expression of condition of newborn infant, 204

aphasia, loss of ability to speak, 225

apnea, temporary periods of not breathing, 171

aponeurosis, flattened tendon, 141

appendectomy, excision of appendix, 186

appendicitis, inflammation of the appendix, ruptured appendix can lead to peritonitis, 183

appendicular, appendages that hang from axial skeleton, 138

aqueous humor, muscle that changes the shape of the lens by contracting and relaxing, 233

arachnoid, middle membrane layer of brain, 218

arrhythmia, irregular heartbeat, often after MI, 158

arteries, always carry blood away from the heart, 154

arteriosclerosis, thickening, hardening, and loss of elasticity of blood vessel walls, 158

arthritis: inflammation of a joint, 142; laboratory tests for, 146

arthrocentesis, puncture into joint to remove liquid, 145

arthroscopy, procedure of looking into joint with scope, 145

arthrotomy, incision into a joint, 145

artificial heart, mechanical heart to sustain a person waiting for a transplant organ, 86

artificial insemination with donor sperm (AID), frozen sperm from donors, screened, and injected into female reproductive tract, 207

ascending colon, large intestine, 179

ascites, edema, collection of fluid in peritoneal cavity, 187

asphyxiation, suffocation due to interference with breathing, 170

assisted hatching, helps embryo hatch from protective membrane to increase chance of implantation, 207

asthma, usually due to allergy/dyspnea and wheezing due to spasm and swelling of airways, 170

astigmatism, irregularity of the curvature of the eye, 233

ataxia, lack of muscle coordination, 142, 225

atelectasis, collapsed lung due to trauma, obstruction, or as complication in lung disease, 170

atherectomy, excision of plaque, 160

atonic, lack of muscle tone, 142

atresias, biliary/absence or closure of normal major bile ducts, 183

atrioventricular node, pacemaker in septum, 153

audiometer, device for testing hearing, 240

audiometrist, person who performs hearing tests, 240

auditory, acoustic, pertaining to the ear or hearing, 240

auditory nerves, hearing and equilibrium, 220

autism, complete withdrawal, unable to communicate, 226

autonomic nervous system (ANA), involuntary functions, 218, 220

axial, skull, thorax, vertebral column, 138

azotemia (uremia), toxic condition/nitrogenous wastes not being excreted, 195

B

Babinski's sign, reflex response/when sole of foot is stroked the big toe turns up instead of down (normal in newborn), 223

bacilli, rod shape bacteria, 68

backache, back pain, 142

ball and socket joint, hip and shoulder joints, 141

bariatrics, bariatrician, treats obesity/science of weight reduction and nutrition, 34

Bartholin's cyst or abscess, inflammation of Bartholin's gland, 203

Bartholin's glands, accessory mucous glands, 203

basophils, WBCs, function unknown, 156

"beating heart" cadaver, body maintained on a respirator in order to "harvest" a usable organ, 86

Bell's palsy, paralysis of one side of face, inflammation of seventh cranial nerve, 222

bibliography, used in disease report, 273

bifurcation, separation into two branches, 171

bilateral, both sides, 76

binge eating disorder, eating large amounts of food when not hungry, eating alone to conceal unusually large portions ingested, 226

biofeedback, training to develop ability to control autonomic nervous system, 225

biopsy, excision of living tissue for examination, 130, 171, 184, 186, 204, 213

bipolar affective disorder, major psychosis having periods of elation and profound depression, 226

bladder distention, full bladder, patient unable to void, 195

blepharitis, inflammation of the eyelids, 233

blood chemistry tests (SMA): abbreviations/terms for, 100; for endocrine functions, 254; listed, 109; sample laboratory report on, 101–106; tests for liver function, 184; for urinary system, 195. *See also* laboratory

blood gases, oxygen and carbon dioxide quantities in laboratory test, 173

blood pressure (B/P), amount of pressure on walls of blood vessels as blood passes through, 157

blood types, 156

blood vessels of the heart (illustrated), 153

bloody show, bloody mucous plug usually passed during late labor, 204

body structure: anatomy and physiology of, 121–123; illustrations of, 9–10, 77–79; integumentary system of, 122, 127–133, 135–136; medical terms for body movements/positions, 78; musculoskeletal system of, 122, 137–147

bone marrow transplant, cells from marrow of matched donor given to patients with leukemia, 160

botulism, caused by toxin in food/GI symptoms, leading to difficulty swallowing and respiratory paralysis, 183, 222

bradycardia, slow heart rate, less than 60 beats per minute, 160

Braille, raised alphabet in books for the blind, 237

brain: illustration of, 219; parts of, 218

brain scan: radioactive element is given and later observed in brain tissue, 223. *See also* scans

brain stem, enlarged extension of spinal cord, 218

breasts: mammary glands, 128; lactation controlled by hormones, 203

bronchi (bronchus), one to each lung/lined with cilia, 168

bronchiectasis, "dilated bronchi" usually secondary to repeated early infections, 170

bronchioles, smaller divisions of bronchi, 168

bronchitis, inflammation of bronchi, 170

bronchodilators, medications to dilate bronchi, 173

bronchoscope, lighted instrument for viewing bronchi, 173

bronchoscopy, use of bronchoscope, 173

bronchospasm, contraction causing bronchi to constrict, 173

bruxism, grinding of teeth, 244

buccal, pertaining to the cheek, 187

bulimia nervosa, eating disorder with binge eating followed by purge vomiting, 183, 226

bulla, large blister, as in burns, 128

bundle of His, conducting fibers, 153

burns, first/second/third degree burns of subcutaneous tissue, 132

burr holes, small openings made with trephine in bone of skull to permit access, 223

bursa(ae), small sacs that cushion joints between tendons and bones, 141

bursitis, inflammation of a bursa, 142

bypass: coronary artery, 160; removal of large portion of small intestine in cases of morbid obesity, 186

C

cachexia, severe malnutrition and wasting, 187, 254

cadaver organ, donor organ from deceased person, 86

Caesarean (C section), delivery by incision into abdomen and uterus, 204

calculus, hardened plaque deposits at base of teeth, 244

calculus (renal), kidney stones, cause blockage with severe pain, 195

callus, localized hyperplasia due to friction, 132

calorie, unit of heat/energy value of food, 187

canal of Schlemm, opening through which aqueous humor must flow out, or pressure in eye increases, 237

cancer abbreviations, 411–412

Candida, **candidiasis:** yeastlike fungus infection of vagina, 203, 215; of the mouth, 244

canthus, canthi, corner of eye, 237

capillaries, tiny blood vessels connecting arteries and veins, 154

carbuncles, pustular lesions, boils, abscesses, 130

carcinoma: abbreviations referring to, 411–412; broncho geniccarcinomas originate in bronchi, 170; in female reproductive system, 203; of male reproductive system, 213; malignant tumor (GI organ), 183; skin cancer, 130

cardiac arrest, cessation of heart action, 158

cardiac catheterization, catheter passed into heart through vein in arm or leg to detect abnormal flow in coronary arteries, 160

cardiac muscle, heart, 138

cardiectomy, surgical excision of donor heart, 86, 160

cardiomyopathy. See idiopathic cardiomyopathy

cardiovascular system: circulatory—heart and vessels, 122; abbreviations used for, 162–163; anatomy and physiology of, 152–157; pathophysiology of, 158–163

cardioversion, treatment for tachycardia (rapid heart rate) using does of electrical energy or medication, 160

caridovascular diseases, cardiologist, treats diseases of the heart and blood vessels/cardiovascular surgery, 34

caries, cavities, 244

carotid endarterectomy, surgically cleaning the carotid artery, 160, 223

carpal tunnel syndrome, pain, edema, and atrophy, due to pressure on median nerve of wrist, 142

cataract, progressively blurred, double or halo vision, opaque lens (instead of clear), 233, 254

cataract extraction, with or without intraocular lens implant, the lens is removed surgically, 236

catatonic, does not talk, move, or react, 226

CAT, CT: computerized (axial) tomography, 92, 174, 179, 223, 224; illustration of, 172

cathartics/laxatives, purgatives/any substance taken orally to induce bowel movement, 187

catheterization, emptying bladder with a catheter (tube), 196

cauda equina, "horse's tail" at the end of the spinal cord/also group of nerves that supply the rectal area, 225

caudal, tail or base of spine, 76

cautery, machine or methods used to destroy tissue by electricity, freezing, or chemicals, 130

CBD(E), common bile duct/union of hepatic and cystic ducts, 187

cc, with correction (lenses), 237

cecum, first part of large intestine, 179

cell membrane, holds the cell together, 122

cells, basic unit of all living things, 122

cellulitis, inflammation of skin and subcutaneous tissue, 130, 132

central nervous system (CNS). See **nervous system**

central retinal artery occlusion, may be due to embolism or thrombus in sclerotic central artery, cranial arteritis, or fat emboli, 233

central retinal vein occlusion, occurs in elderly arteriosclerotic patients/blindness may develop in hours, 233

cephalic, head, 76

cerebellum, occupies posterior cranial fossa behind brain stem, 218

cerebral palsy, paralysis resulting from developmental defects or trauma, 222

cerebrospinal fluid (CSF), fluid that circulates around cord and brain, 218

cerebrovascular accident (CVA), change in blood supply of brain, 158

cerebrum, largest part of brain, consciousness and voluntary movement, 218

certified medical technologist (CMT), performs all laboratory procedures, 40

certified nursing assistant (CNA), one who helps nursing staff perform routine tasks, 40

cervical biopsy, excision for examination, 204

cervical dysplasia, abnormal cell growth in cervix, 203

chairside dental assistant, assists dentist with fillings, suction, instruments, 41

chalazion, meibomian cyst on eyelid, 234

cheiloplasty, plastic surgery on lip, usually for cleft lip, 186

chemical name, chemical formula, 114

chemical process (digestion), food reacts with enzymes, 182

chemonucleolysis, dissolving herniated nucleus pulposus by injecting an enzyme, 145

Cheyne-Stokes, irregular breathing/ slow and shallow, increasing in rate and depth, then decreasing until breathing stops for 10–20 seconds, 173

chiropractor, Doctor of Chiropractic/treats with manipulation only, 37

chlamydia, 215

cholangiography, X-ray examination of the bile ducts using contrast medium, 184

cholecystectomy, excision of the gallbladder, 186

cholecystitis, inflammation of the gallbladder, 183

cholecytography and choledochography, oral dye is ingested that outlines the gallbladder and bile duct so that X-ray detects stones, 184

choledochoduodenostomy, permanent opening between the common bile duct and duodenum, 186

choledocholithotomy, removal of gallstone through incision in the common bile duct (CBD), 186

cholelithiasis, condition of gallstones, 183

cholesteremia, cholesterolemia, or hypercholesterolemia, high cholesterol levels, 158

cholesterol, chemical component of oils and fats/synthesized in the liver and a normal constituent of bile, 187

chorionic villus sampling (CVS), collecting chorionic cells that surround embryo via a catheter through the vagina to uterus, 206

choroid, dark-brown layer between sclera and retina, 233

chromosome, linkage structure of specific genetic information, 206

chromosome engineering, incorporation of parts of or whole alien chromosomes into given set of chromosomes, 206

chronic brain syndrome (organic brain syndrome), symptoms of senile variety, 222

cicatrix, scar, 132

ciliary body, muscle that changes shape of the lens by contracting and relaxing, 233

circumcision, cutting foreskin of newborn male, 204, 213

cirrhosis, replacement of liver cells by fibrous tissue, 183

claudication, cramplike pains in legs due to insufficient arterial blood supply to muscles, 160

clavicle, collarbone, 138

clear liquids, liquid you can see through, 92

cleft lip/palate, congenital failure of lip and/or palate to fuse, 183

Clinitest (also Testate), convenient, inexpensive method of testing urine, 196

clonic, muscular relaxation and contraction, 142

closed reduction, restoring bone in a cast, 146

coarctation, compression or narrowing of the walls of a vessel, 158

cocci, round or spherical shape bacteria, 68

coccidioidomycosis, "valley fever" caused by fungus that lies dormant in spore form in hot, dusty climates, 170

cochlear implant, procedure to restore some hearing, 240

colitis (ulcerative, spastic), inflammation of colon, 183

collagen disease, any of several diseases of the connective tissue, 142

collateral circulation, "new" expanded small vessels that try to accommodate ischemic area when primary circulation has been locked, 160

colonies, how bacteria grow, 68

colonoscopy, procedure of looking into the colon with flexible fiber-optic scope, 184

color blindness, most cases are congenital (in males) but can be caused by injury, disease, or drugs, 234

colostomy, permanent opening of colon to surface of abdomen with a stoma, 186

colporrhaphy, surgical repair of vagina (A & P repair), 204

colposcopy, procedure of using colposcope for magnified view of cervix, 204

comatose, in a deep stupor, cannot be aroused, 225

combining form, adding "o" to root word, 4

commercial dental laboratory, impressions are sent to this lab instead of made up in dentist's office, 245

commissurotomy, cutting defective heart valve to improve flow of blood, 160

community resources: listed in disease report, 273; locating, 275–276

complications (toxemia), during pregnancy/characterized by hypertension, edema, weight gain/ a serious complication, 206

compound words, words made up of two root words, 4

compression sclerotherapy, injection along with compression for treatment of varicose veins and spider veins, 160

concussion, injury to brain due to blow on head, 222

cones, light-sensitive nerve cells responsible for bright light and color vision, 233

congenital, present at birth/may be hereditary or acquired in the uterus or birth canal, 123

congenital defects, include septal defects, patenductus arteriosus, tetralogy of Fallot, 158

congestion, "stuffy feeling" experienced with colds and other respiratory ailments, 173

congestive heart failure (CHF), inability to pump blood effectively throughout the body, 158

conjunctiva, mucous membrane covering eyeballs and eyelids, 233

conjunctivitis, inflamed conjunctiva/ acute type called "pink eye," 234

connective tissue, connects and supports and forms blood cells, 122

consolidation, solidification of lung tissue, 173

constriction, making something smaller or narrower, 123

contact dermatitis, allergic reaction caused by contact, 131

continent, capable of controlling voiding and defecation, 196

contrecoup, occurring on opposite side, injury in which brain literally bounces back and forth, 225

contusion, bruise, black-and-blue mark, 132

convulsion (seizure), sudden disturbances in mental functions and body movements, some with loss of consciousness, 222, 254

Coombs' test, blood test used to diagnose hemolytic anemias in newborn, 204

cordotomy, cutting of nerve fibers to relieve intractable pain, 223

corium, deeper layer connective tissue containing nerves, nerve endings, blood vessels, sebaceous glands, and sweat glands, 128

corneal transplant, surgical procedure with donor cornea used, 236

corneal ulcer, usually result of injury or inflammation, 234

coronal (frontal), vertical body plane, 76

coronary arteries, supply the heart muscle with blood, arise from base of aorta, 154

coronary artery bypass graft, substituting vein from the leg to bypass the occluded artery in MI patients, 160

coronary occlusion and coronary thrombosis (heart attack): clot in a coronary artery, cutting off circulation to the heart muscle, 158; illustration of, 154

cor pulmonale, heart failure due to pulmonary disease, 170

cortex (kidney), outer layer, 195

coryza, the common cold, caused by viruses, 170

crab lice, 215

cranial cavity (skull), contains brain, 122, 141

cranial nerves: listed, 220; testing of, 224

craniotomy, incision to gain access to the brain when burr holes are inadequate for procedure, 223

cretinism (in children), slow, physically and mentally, 253

Crohn's, inflammatory disease of the colon, 183

crown, made of enamel/portion above the gums, 241

crusts, flaking type of lesions, 128

cryoextraction, fixation of detached retina with cold/scar tissue forms and reattaches the retina, 236

cryopreservation, freezing of tissue for future use, 207

cryoprobe, surgical instrument used with liquid nitrogen, 237

cryptitis, inflammation of "crypts," especially those in anus and penis, 183

cryptorchidism, "hidden testes," undescended, 213

CT, CAT scan: computerized (axial) tomography, 92, 174, 197, 223, 224; illustration of, 172

culture media, bacteria food, 68

Cushing's disease, weak, obese, hypertensive, hyperglycemic, moon facies, 253

CVA (cerebrovascular accident), any interruption of blood supply to brain causing brain damage with neurologic symptoms, 222

cyanosis, condition of blueness due to insufficient oxygen, especially in nailbeds and skin, 173

cyst, type of nodule that is usually somewhat moveable, 128

cystic fibrosis, mucoviscidosis/ disorder of mucous glands leading to pancreatic insufficiency, 170

cystitis, inflammation of bladder, 195

cystocele, hernia of the bladder, 195

cystogram, X-ray of bladder, 196

cystoscopy, using a cystoscope to examine the bladder, 196

cystotome, instrument for cutting anterior lens capsule, 237

cytoplasm, protoplasm of the cell, 122

D

dacryoadenitis, inflammation of the lacrimal (tear) gland, 234

dacryocystitis, inflammation and obstruction of lacrimal sac following nasal trauma, deviated septum, nasal polyps, 234

dacryocystotomy, incision of the lacrimal sac, 236

dacryolith, a "stone" in the lacrimal duct, 234

deafness, hearing loss, 239

debridement, removal of dead tissue around a wound, 130

decibel, unit of measure for sound, 240

deciduous (baby) teeth, "falling away" and total of 20, 241

decubitus: lying down, 76; ulcers on bony prominences due to prolonged lying down, 132

degenerative, result of wear and tear, 124

deglutition, swallowing, 187

delirium, mental confusion or excitement, 226

delusion, false belief, 226

dental anesthesia, topical, local injection, general anesthesia, hypnosis, 244

dental chart, teeth are numbered and notation made regarding condition, 245

Dental Claim Form (illustrated), 243

dental hygienist, does prophylactic dental care, cleaning, teaching patients proper prophylactic care, takes X-rays, 41

dental practice, 244

dental practitioners and specialists, listed, 40–41

dentition, eruption of teeth, 241

depression, lack of hope, symptoms of irritability, exhaustion, overeating or weight loss, difficulty concentrating or making decisions, 226

de Quervain's disease, tenosynovitis caused by narrowing of tendon sheath, 142

dermabrasion, scraping off surface layers to remove scars or wrinkles, 130

dermatology, dermatologist, deals with disease of the skin, 34, 133

dermatome, instrument for cutting thin sections of skin for grafts, 130

dermatosis, any skin condition without inflammation, 132

dermis, deeper layer connective tissue containing nerves, nerve endings, blood vessels, sebaceous glands, and sweat glands, 128

descending colon, large intestine, 179

desensitization, building tolerance to an antigen, 132

detached retina: detachment occurs in myopics, may be the result of injury, 234; illustration of, 235

detail rep, representative of pharmaceutical company who calls upon physicians and introduces new drugs, 114

deviated septum, defect in wall between nostrils that can cause partial or complete obstruction, 170

dextro, to the right, 79

diabetes mellitus: low insulin production affects metabolism, 131, 253; long-term complications of, 255; short-term complications of, 255

diagnostic/laboratory abbreviations, 99–109. *See also* abbreviations

diagnostic microbiology, 277–278

dialysis, filtering blood with artificial kidney, 196

diaphoresis, excessive perspiring, 254

diaphragm, dome-shaped muscle that separates the pleural cavity from the abdominopelvic cavity, 168

diastolic pressure, bottom number in B/P reading, 157

diet orders, abbreviations for, 92

digital examination, insertion of the gloved finger into rectum, 184

digitalized, subjection of patient to drug digitalis to maintain heart contraction force without side effects, 160

digital subtraction angiogram (angiography), uses computer/ unwanted parts of X-ray picture are subtracted to give clear image of vessels, 160

dilatation or dilation, making something wider or opened up, 123

diopters, unit of measure for lenses, 237

diphtheria, acute bacterial disease, 170

disclosing products, exposes areas not being brushed adequately, 245

disease report outline, 273

distal, farthest from center, 76

distress, "excessive" and/or "difficult" stress, 256

distribution, of blood types, 156

diuresis, increased urinary output, due to diuretic drug, 196

diuretic, medication (water pill) that lowers blood pressure by reducing blood volume, 160

diverticulitis, diverticulosis, inflammation or condition of having diverticula, 183

DJD (degenerative joint disease), inflammation of a joint in older people, 142

donor egg program, using eggs donated by relatives or other women undergoing IVF, 207

donor embryo program, using embryos donated by women who underwent IVF, 207

Doppler, ultrasonic probe that checks blood flow in artery under it, 160

drug names: generic, 113–114, 384–394; trade/brand, 112–113, 384–394

drug reactions, rash-type lesions caused by medication and/or photosensitivity, 131

dry eye, tear production decreases with age/also associated with a type of arthritis, 234

DTR (deep tendon reflex), body movement at unconscious level, 225

ducts, fallopian tube where fertilization occurs, 203

duodenum, jejunum, ileum, three small parts of the small intestine, 179

duramater, tough outer covering of brain, 218

dyscrasia (blood), any abnormal condition, 160

dysentery, severe dehydrating diarrhea (Montezuma's revenge), 183

dysphonia, impaired voice, 173

dyspnea, difficulty breathing, 173

dystocia, difficult labor, 204

dysuria, difficult or painful urination, 196

E

ear: abbreviations for, 241; anatomy and physiology of, 238–239; illustration of, 238; pathophysiology of, 239–240

eating disorders, emotional and psychological disorders related to eating behavior, 226

ecchymosis, bruise, black-and-blue mark due to bleeding under skin, 132

echocardiogram, using ultrasound to visualize internal heart structures, 160

echolalia, repetition of anything that is said instead of answering, 226

ectomy: to excise or cut out surgically, 5; four ways of using, 6

ectopic (extrauterine), pregnancy outside of uterus, 204

eczema, redness of skin due to allergic reaction, 131

edentulous, edentia, without teeth, 244

EEG (echoencephalogram), use of ultrasound to show displacement of brain structures, 224

EEG (electroencephalogram), record of electrical activity of the brain, 224

ejaculatory duct, canal formed by union of ductus (vas) deferens and excretory duct of seminal vesicle, 213

electrical stimulation, used to quickly heal fractures or injuries to cartilage or tendons, 146

electrocardiogram (ECG, EKG): picture of electrical impulses of the heart, 160; illustration of, 161

electrodesiccation, destruction and drying out with electricity, 130

electrodynogram, computer measurement of foot movement, 146

electromyography (EMG), recording of muscular contraction for diagnostic purposes or treatment, 146

electronystagmography, method of testing vestibular function by assessing eye motion, 240

ELECTZ, procedure to treat cervical dysplasia by shaving tissue away from cervix, 204

elimination (digestion), of solid wastes in form of feces, 182

emaciation, wasting, extremely thin condition, 254

embolus, embolism, thrombus that has broken loose and is carried in the circulation until it blocks a vessel, 158

embryo, term used from 3rd to 8th week after fertilization, 204

embryology, embryologist, monitors prenatal development between stages of ovum and fetus, 34

emergency medical technician (EMT), emergency specialist, 40

emergency medicine, traumatologist, deals with injury, accidental or physiological, 34

emesis (emetic), to vomit, 187

emmetropia, normal vision, 237

emphysema, distended or rupture alveoli/irreversible condition characterized by severe dyspnea, 170

empyema, pus in pleural cavity (abscess), 170

encephalitis, inflammation of the brain, many types, 222

encephalon, the brain, 225

encopresis, repeated, uncontrolled passage of feces, 183

endarterectomy, "boring out" inner lining of artery to increase size of lumen, 160

endocarditis, inflammation of the endocardium, 158

endocardium, membranes inside of heart chamber, 153

endocrine system: ductless glands, 122; anatomy and physiology of, 251–252; illustration of, 252; pathophysiology of, 253–254

endodontist, treats diseases of pulp, root canal work, 40

endometriosis, cells of inner lining of uterus spreading into pelvis, 203

endoscopic retrograde cholaniopancreatography (ERCP), flexible tube is passed through the small intestine into the bile duct/after dye is injected an X-ray is taken, 184

enema, introduction of fluid into rectum for cleansing and/or diagnostic purposes, 187

enucleation, surgical removal of eye, 236

enuresis, bedwetting, 196

enzymes, more than 650 complex proteins manufactured by living tissue which stimulate chemical changes, 187

eosinophils, WBCs which increase in allergic conditions, 156

epidemiology, frequency, distribution, occurrence, prevalence, 123

epidermis (cuticle), nonvascular outer layer of skin, 128

epididymis (ducts), top of each testis, spermatozoa stored here, 213

epididymitis, inflammation of epididymis, 213

epiglottis, flap that covers entrance to trachea, 168

epilepsy, seizure disorder, may be caused by injury, 222

epinephrine, medication used to open bronchioles during asthma attack or allergic reaction, 173

episiotomy, incision of perineum to facilitate delivery and avoid laceration, 204

epistaxis, nosebleed caused by trauma, hypertension, or hormones, 170

epithelial tissue, protects, absorbs, and secretes, 122

erosion, "eating away"/an early ulcer, 128

eruption, any rash or breaking out, 132

erysipelas, acute febrile disease causes by "strep" infection, 131

erythema, redness, 132

eschar, hard crust over a burn, 132

escharotomy, removal of burn scar tissue, 130

esophageal varices, enlarged, incompetent veins in distal esophagus due to portal hypertension in cirrhosis, 183

esophagitis, inflammation of the esophagus (food tube), 183

esophagogastroduodenoscopy (EGD), using scope to examine these structures, 184

esophagus, tube to stomach, behind the trachea, 179

esotropia, type of strabismus involving one or both eyes turning in, 234

essential hypertension, high blood pressure with no apparent cause, 157, 158

ethmoid cranial bones, upper nasal, between eyes, 141

etiology, cause, 123, 273

eustachian salpingitis, inflammation of eustachian tube, 239

eustachian tubes (auditory tubes): from middle ear to pharynx (throat), 239; tubes from pharynx to middle ear, 168

eustress, "good" stress that increases person's health or performance, 256

eversion, turning outward, or inside out, 79

eviscerate, internal organs come out (through a wound), 187

exanthem, rose-colored eruption, 132

excoriation, severe abrasion, 132

exfoliation, scaling, flaking, 132

exodontia, extraction, 245

exophthalmic goiter, swelling of the thyroid gland in neck, 253

exotropia, type of strabismus involving one or both eyes turning out, 234

expectorants, medications that loosen secretions, 173

extension (extending), straightening, 79

external, outside, 79

external ear, auricle, pinna, and auditory meatus, 239

external fixation, fracture reduction devices, 146

external genitalia, scrotum and penis, 203, 213

extracorporeal shockwave lithotripsy, patient partially submerged in a tube/lithotriptor produces shock waves to pulverize stones, 186, 196

extraction, surgical procedures to remove tooth, 245

exudate, exit or drainage of cellular debris secondary to inflammation, 240

eye bank, for donor corneas, 237

eye drops, for treatment of several conditions, 237

eye muscle surgery, shortening and/or lengthening muscles that regulate eye movement for correction of deviation, 236

eyes: rest in eye sockets/in orbital cavities of cranium, 233; abbrevia-tions for, 238; anatomy and physi-ology of, 232–233; illustration of normal, 232; pathophysiology of, 233–235

F

facial nerves, muscles of face, ears, scalp, 220

facultative, growing with/without oxygen, 68

family practice specialty, family practice specialist, similar to general practice but qualified as a specialty, 35

fascia(ae), connective tissue sheath/holds muscle fibers, 141

FDA, Food and Drug Administra-tion/regulatory agency which approves new drugs, 114

female reproductive system: abbrevia-tions regarding, 207–208; anatomy and physiology of, 202–203; illustration of, 202; pathophysiology of, 203–204

femur, thigh, 138

fenestration, artificial opening is made to bypass the damaged middle ear, allowing sound waves to reach inner ear, 240

fertility, ability to conceive, 204

fertilization: fusion of two opposite-sex gametes to produce zygote, 204; alternative methods of, 206–207

fetus: term used starting 9th week after fertilization, 205; illustration of sonograms of, 206

fibrillation, quivering or trembling type of contraction caused by injury to heart, 158

fibrocystic disease, benign cysts in breasts, 132, 203

fibroids, benign tumors of uterus, 203

fibrosis, abnormal formation of fibrous tissue, 170

fibula, lower leg, 138

fissure: crack in skin surface, 128; deep furrow in the brain, 225; groove in tooth enamel, 245

fistula, abnormal opening between two organs or to surface of skin, 187, 203

flaccid, flabby, poor muscle tone, 225

flail chest, erratic movement of chest due to multiple injuries of ribs or sternum, 170

flat plate of abdomen, X-ray film of abdomen, 184

flatus, flatulence, excessive gas in the GI tract, 187

Fleet's (enema), prepackaged, disposable type of enema, 187

flexion (flexing), bending, 79

flexure, a turning or angle, as the hepatic flexure of the colon near the liver, 187

"floaters" (in vitreous), bits of protein or cells floating in vitreous fluid that cause visual disturbances, 234

"floating kidney," displaced and movable, 195

"flu," term that has come to mean almost anything (used by laypeople), 170

fluorescein angiography, injection of a dye intravenously to detect retinal blood vessels, 160, 236

food poisoning (gastroenteritis), acute nausea and vomiting, cramps, and diarrhea due to a variety of ingested toxins or bacteria, 183

foramen magnum, opening in occipital bone through which cord passes, 225

forceps delivery, low-forceps for routine delivery/mid- and high-forceps for complicated deliveries, 205

foreign bodies in eye, may require surgery, chemicals in eye should be washed out immediately, use safety goggles to prevent injuries, 234

foreign body in ear, insects, beans, and so on, 239

formen (foramina), holes in a bone for large vessels and nerves to pass through, 141

fossa(ae), depressions or hollows, 141

Fowler's position, head of bed raised 1½ feet, knees elevated, 80

fracture reductions, restoring bone to normal position without surgery, 146

fractures: illustrated, 143; listed, 142

fracture (skull), usually comminuted with bony fragments in brain making surgery imperative, 222

frequency and urgency, frequent, urgent trips to bathroom but voiding small amounts (painfully), 196

frontal cranial bones, forehead, 141

fulguration, destruction of tissue with electric sparks, 130

full liquids, all types of liquids, 92

fundoscopy, funduscopy, examination of the inner eye with ophthalmoscope or funduscope, 236

fundus: in back part of eye, 237; body or larger part of a hollow organ, as the fundus of the stomach, 187

fungicide, medication that destroys fungi, 132

furuncles, pustular lesions, boils, abscesses, 130

G

gallbladder, behind liver/stores and concentrates bile, 181

gallbladder series (GBS), X-ray film is taken after patient has been given a dye that will outline a gallbladder, second X-ray films taken after fatty meal, 184

gamete, one of two cells (male and female) needed for sexual reproduction, 206

gamete intrafallopian transfer (GIFT), eggs are retrieved, mixed with sperm in catheter, and injected into fallopian tubes for natural fertilization, 207

gamma globulin, substance containing antibodies, used to provide passive immunity in people exposed to infectious disease, 187

ganglion, "knot" of many cell bodies outside cord and brain, 225

gangrene, necrotic tissue, 132, 254

gastrectomy, usually subtotal removal of stomach, 186

gastric ulcers (peptic, duodenal), inflamed area with destruction of tissue, 183

gastritis, gastroenteritis, inflammation of stomach or entire GI tract, 183

gastroenterology, gastroenterologist, deals with diseases of the digestive system, 35

gastrointestinal series (GI series), UGI or barium swallow/lower GI or barium enema (BE)/opaque substance (barium) is given by mouth or enema and X-ray films are taken, 186

gastrointestinal system (GI): digestive organs, 122; abbreviations used for, 188; anatomy and physiology of, 179–182; illustration showing pathologic conditions, 180; surgical/miscellaneous terms for, 186–188

gastroscopy, examining the stomach with a gastroscope, 186

gavage, feeding by tube, 187

gene, the unit of heredity, 59

general dentist (DDS and DMD), treats all ages but may restrict practice to adults only, 40

generic, drug comparable to trade name substance, 114

generic drug names, 113–114, 384–394

genetic counseling, service providing people with information regarding risk of genetically abnormal progeny, 206

genetic engineering, DNA manipulation with in vitro techniques for deliberate gene changes, 206

genetics: branch of biology that deals with heredity, 59, 206; medical terms regarding, 204–206

genetic therapy, addition of functional gene(s) to cell by insertion to correct a hereditary disease, 206

genitals, organs of reproduction, 59

genitourinary system (GU), reproductive and urinary organs, 122

genu, means "knee," 142

geriatrics, geriatrician, deals with all aspects of aging and disorder thereof, 35

gerodontist, gerodontologist, specializes in dental problems of aged, 40

gestation, period of pregnancy, 205

gestational diabetes, increased maternal insulin produced due to placental hormones, 254

gingivectomy (or gingivoplasty), gum surgery, 245

gingivitis, inflammation of the gums, 244

gland, any organ that secretes something, 254

glaucoma, increase in intraocular pressure due to closing of canal of Schlemm/fluid cannot circulate, and pressure builds up, 234

glomerulonephritis, form of nephritis involving glomeruli, 195

glossal, pertaining to the tongue, 187

glossitis, inflammation of the tongue, 183

glossopharyngeal nerves, secretion of parotid gland, taste, 220

goiter, swollen thyroid caused by lack of iodine in diet, 253

gonioscopy, using a special optical instrument to inspect angle of anterior chamber, 236

gonorrhea, 215

gonorrheal conjunctivitis of newborn, purulent conjunctivitis usually due to GC and passed to newborn in the birth canal, 235

gout, type of acute arthritis, 142

grafts, tissue taken from one place to replace defect elsewhere, 130

granulocytes, category of white blood cells, 156

gravida, pregnant woman, 205

grid test, used to detect blind spots or distortions of vision via vertical/horizontal lines on charts, 236

grooves, shallow linear depressions in bone, 141

guide dogs, for the blind, 237

Guillain-Barré syndrome, acute, rapidly progressive polyneuropathy with muscular weakness and sensory loss, 222

gyrus, gyri, convolutions of the cerebrum, 225

H

hair, appendage of skin, 128

hallucination, auditory or visual/hearing or seeing things not really present, 226

halocath laser, used to widen vascular openings in lower limbs, 160

harvest, taking an organ, 86

hay fever, allergic coryza, pollinosis, 170

head and neck, brain, skull, ear, sinuses, 92

hearing aids, types include bone conduction receiver and air conduction receiver, 240

hearing-ear dogs, dogs trained to respond to sounds and alert the hearing-impaired person, 240

heart: lies in the mediastinum between the lungs, has four chambers, 153; illustrations of, 152–155. *See also* **cardiovascular system**

heart attack: clot in a coronary artery, cutting off circulation to the heart muscle, 158; illustration of, 154

heart block, type of arrhythmia/conduction of impulses from atrium to ventricle disturbed, 158

heart murmur, soft, blowing sound heard on auscultation, indicating valve may be incompetent and does not close properly, 158

hematology, hematologist treats disorders of the blood and blood-forming organs, 35

hematoma, "blood tumor" (clot), 222

hematuria, blood in the urine, 196

hemiplegia, paralysis of only one side of body, 225

hemisphere, either half of the brain, 225

hemoglobin, iron-containing pigment in red blood cells, 160

hemophilia, congenital lack of clotting factor in blood, 158

hemoptysis, expectoration of blood from lungs, 173

hemorrhages (subconjunctival), blood under the membrane as result of injury/may occur spontaneously, 234

hemothorax, blood in thoracic cavity, 170

heparin, anticoagulant in the blood, also given as medication, 160

hepatitis, liver disease/one type is spread by blood, 158, 183

hereditary, transmitted genetically from parent, 123

hernias: protrusion of a part out of its natural place, many types, 183; hiatal, 170; hydrocele (fluid) in scrotum, 213; illustration of inguinal, 185; of meninges (meningocele), 222; rectocele (of rectum), 184

herniated nucleus pulposus (HNP): ruptured intervertebral disk, 142; illustrated, 144

hernioplasty (or herniorrhaphy), surgical repair of hernia, 186

herpes genitalis, blister-type lesions in genital area, 130, 215

herpes ophthalmicus, severe type of herpes zoster affecting fifth cranial nerve (eye), 130

herpes simplex, "cold sores" or fever blisters, 131

herpes zoster, "shingles" lesions follow the course of a nerve, 131, 222

herpes zoster (ophthalmic), involvement of the fifth cranial nerve with herpes virus, 234

hiatal hernia, diaphragmatic hernia/opening in diaphragm allows part of the stomach to move up into chest, 170

hiatus, an opening, especially in diaphragm, 173

hiccough, hiccup, spasm of diaphragm due to many things, 170

hilus, root of lung where vessels, nerves, and bronchi enter, 173

hinge joint, elbows, knees, fingers, 141

hirsutism, excessive body hair, 132

histoplasmosis, fungus disease of lungs, 170

HIV (Human Immunodeficiency Virus), 214

Hodgkin's disease, type of malignant tumor of the lymph nodes and spleen, itching of skin may occur, 131, 158

Holter monitor, portable ECG, 160

homeostasis, state of equilibrium or relative constancy body strives to maintain, 123

homogenous (homogeneous), derived from like source, 59

humerus, upper arm, 138

Huntington's chorea, hereditary disorder due to gene on chromosome 4, 222

hyaline membrane disease, poorly developed alveoli leading to collapse of lungs in premature infants, 171

hydrocele, hernia (of fluid) in scrotum, 213

hydrocephalus, "water in the head": increased accumulation of CSF in ventricles of brain, 222

hydronephrosis, collection of urine in pelvis of kidney due to obstructed outflow, 195

hydrosalpinx, fluid collection in fallopian tubes, 203

hyfrecator, type of machine for destroying tissue, 130

hyperalimentation, TPN (total parenteral nutrition) with a subclavian catheter, 187

hypercapnia, increased CO_2 in blood, 173

hypercholesterolemia, high cholesterol levels, 158

hyperopia, farsightedness/cannot see at close range, 234

hypertension, high blood pressure, 157, 158

hypertropia, type of strabismus involving one eye turning up, 234

hyperventilation, increased rate and/or depth of respiration, 173

hypochondria, preoccupation with body, imaginary illnesses, 226

hypoglossal nerves, tongue, 220

hypoglycemia, abnormally low blood glucose level/reactive and spontaneous, 253

hypophysectomy, excision of pituitary gland, 254

hyposensitization, type of allergy treatment: increasing doses of offending substance to build tolerance, 173

hypotropia, type of strabismus involving one eye turning down, 234

hysterectomy, excision of uterus, 204

hysteria, extremely emotional state, 226

hysterosalpinogram, "picture" of uterus and tubes to determine whether tubes are open, 204

I

iatrogenic, caused by treatment by physician, 124

idiopathic, disease for which no cause can be determined, 124

idiopathic cardiomyopathy, thickening of heart walls and septum that obstructs the flow of blood, 158

ileostomy, permanent opening into ileum, 186

illusion, false interpretation of something seen or heard, 226

immunization abbreviations, 93

immunologic, immune-related diseases, 124

immunosuppressant, suppression (by drugs) of natural immune responses, 86

impacted cerumen, hard, dry cerumen which causes discomfort or infection, 239

impaction (dental), tooth embedded in alveolus so that eruption is prevented, 244

impaction (fecal), hard stool impacted in rectum that usually must be removed manually, 184

impetigo, pustular lesions, 130

implantation, setting tooth into socket after injury/replacing lost tooth with artificial tooth, 244

impressions, molds made by dentist for inlay, crown, and so on, 245

incontinent, inability to control urination and bowels, 196

IND, investigational new drug, 114

induction, starting labor by artificial means, 205

infection, caused by any pathogenic agent, 123

influenza, "la grippe"/group of virus-caused acute febrile pulmonary diseases, 171

inguinal hernias (illustration), 185

injuries, foreign body, lacerations, contusions (black eye), and burns, 234

inner ear, vestibule, semicircular canals, and cochlea, 239

insect bites, local reaction due to bite or sting, 131

insemination, impregnating with sperm from mate or donor, 205

insulin, antidiabetic hormone made from a combination of beef and pork sources, 254

integumentary system: skin, 122; abbreviations for, 133; anatomy and physiology of, 127–128; pathophysiology of the, 128–133

interaction, chemical reaction when two or more drugs are taken simultaneously, 114

intercostal muscles, muscles between ribs, 168

interior (sub) (infra), below, 76

internal, inside, 79

internal medicine, focuses on medical conditions, 35

interphalangeal joints, fingers and toes, 141

intervertebral disks, cartilaginous material between vertebrae, 141

intra-aortic balloon pumping, to push more blood into coronary arteries following severe MI or open-heart surgery, 160

intracytoplasmic sperm injection (ICSI), helps sperm enter eggs by using microneedle to pierce egg's shell, fertilized eggs are placed in Petri dish, embryos are inserted in uterus, 207

intraocular pressure, increased due to closing of canal of Schlemm/fluid cannot circulate, and pressure builds up resulting in glaucoma, 234

intrauterine insemination (IUI), at ovulation sperm is delivered via catheter to uterus, 207

introitus, vaginal cavity, 123

intubate, to insert an airway, 173

intussusception, telescoping of intestine causing obstruction, 184

in vitro, studies under artificially controlled conditions outside the organism, 206

in vitro fertilization (IVF), ovaries are stimulated to produce multiple eggs which are retrieved, mixed with sperm in Petri dish where fertilization occurs, 206

involutional melancholia, mental illness in menopause, 226

IPPB, intermittent positive-pressure breathing, ventilator method used to assist breathing, 173

ipsilateral, on the same side, affecting the same side, 225

iridectomy, excision of part of iris, 236

iris, colored band of choroid surrounding pupil and behind cornea, 233

iritis, inflammation of the iris, 234

irritable bowel syndrome (IBS), spastic bowel causing frequent, loose stools, 184

ischemia, insufficient blood supply to body part, 158

IVF, in vitro fertilization, 205

J

joints, 141

K

Kaposi's, varicelliform eruption, 131

keloid, abnormal scar tissue, 128, 130

keratoconus, cone-shaped cornea causing severe myopia, 234

keratomileusis, cornea removed, frozen, ground to a new shape, thawed, and replaced, 236

keratoplasty, corneal transplant (using donor cornea), 236

keratosis, thickened, horny skin, 130

keratotomy (RK), surgical slits made in cornea to treat myopia, 236

ketosis, accumulation of ketone bodies due to incomplete metabolism of fatty acids, 254

kidneys, two, lie behind the abdominal organs against muscles of the back, 195

knee-chest position, kneeling, chest on table, 80

Korsakoff's syndrome, deficiency of vitamin B complex, usually secondary to alcoholism, 222

Kussmaul breathing, deep, gasping type of breathing, 173

kyphosis, hunchback deformity of spine, 142

L

laboratory: abbreviations/terms used in, 100–108; arthritis tests in, 146; blood chemistry tests (SMA) in, 100, 109, 184, 254; communication within the, 108–109; examination of cerebrospinal fluid, 224; skin tests in, 133. *See also* blood chemistry tests (SMA)

laboratory report (sample), 101–106

labyrinthitis, otitis internal, inner ear disturbance, 239

lacerations, cuts/deep lacerations, 132

lacrimal apparatus, tear ducts and glands, 233

lacrimation, production of tears by lacrimal apparatus, 237

lamina(ae), flattened part of the vertebral arch, 141

laminectomy, excision of the arches of vertebrae to view spinal cord, 224

laminectomy with diskectomy, surgical excision of part or whole of intervertebral disk by incising the lamina, 146

Landsteiner types, based on type of red blood cells: A, B, AB, and O, 156

laparoscope, endoscope inserted through small abdominal incision to view and work on abdominopelvic organs, 204

laparoscopic sterilization, "band-aid surgery"/patency of tube is destroyed, 204

laparotomy, incision into abdomen, usually "exploratory," 186

laryngectomy, excision of larynx, 173

laryngitis, inflammation of larynx, 171

laryngotracheobronchitis, "croup"/named because of croupy cough with air hunger, 171

larynx, voice box/vocal cords, 168

laser, produces highly concentrated beam of light and creates tiny stop of intense heat, 130, 237

laser photocoagulation, laser produces intense heat to treat retinal detachment and other conditions, 236

lateral, side, 76

lavage, to wash out, especially the stomach after ingestion of poison, 187

lavage of sinuses, washing out or irrigating sinuses, 173

laxatives/cathartics, purgatives/any substance taken orally to induce bowel movement, 187

Legg-Calve-Perthes disease, osteochondritis of head of femur, 142

lens, transparent, colorless structure encapsulated and held in place by a ligament, 233

lesion, any kind of a "sore," 132

leukemias, group of diseases of the blood-forming organs and WBCs, 159

leukoplakia, white spots or patches on mucous membranes of cheek and/or tongue, 244

leukorrhea, white vaginal discharge, 203

licensed practical nurse (LPN/LVN), may perform some duties similar to RN in limited hospital settings/graduate of one-year program, 40

ligament, strong fibrous tissue connecting bone to bone, 141

limbic system, "edge or border of a part," refers to that part of the brain controlling emotions, 225

lingual, pertaining to the tongue, 187

lithotomy position, lying flat on back, legs in stirrups, 80

lithotriptor (extracorporeal shockwave lithotripsy), patient partially submerged in a tube/lithotriptor produces shock waves to pulverize stones, 186, 196

liver: largest gland/responsible for hundreds of chemical reactions, 179; transplant of, 186

lobectomy, excision of lobe of lung, 173

lobotomy (amygdalotomy), operation used to be performed for severe mental illness/helps control behavior, 224

lochia, vaginal discharge following delivery, 205

lordosis, convex curvature of spine (swayback), 142

Lou Gehrig's disease, syndrome marked by muscular weakness and atrophy with spasticity and hyperreflexia, 142

low-salt diet, lowers blood pressure by reducing blood volume, 162

lumbar puncture (LP), spinal tap, insertion of needle into subarachnoid space to measure pressure, 224

lumbar sympathectomy, cutting fibers of sympathetic nerves that contract walls of blood vessels of lower leg, 224

lumen, opening within hollow tube or organ, 123, 162

lungs: right, three lobes/left, two lobes, 168; abscess of, 170; illustration of, 169

lupus erythematosus, inflammatory dermatitis that may precede systemic lupus, 131

lupus erythematosus, systemic, collagen disease affecting connective tissues, 142

Lyme disease (LD), symptoms resemble arthritis, caused by spirochete transmitted by a tick, 144, 222

lymphatic vessels, lymph fluid returns to blood via, 156

lymph fluid, comes from blood and filters out into spaces between tissue cells and returns to blood, 156

lymph nodes, numerous in certain parts of body, help filter out harmful substances, 156

lymphocytes, WBCs which produce antibodies, 156

M

macular degeneration, damage to macula, layers of retina separate due to fluid under the retina, 234

macule, spots/not elevated, 128

malar, cheekbone, 141

male reproductive system: anatomy and physiology of, 212–213; illustration of, 212; pathophysiology of, 213

malingering, making believe, pretending, 226

malleolus, hammerlike protuberance on either side of ankle, 141

malocclusion, poor alignment of teeth, may require braces, 244

mammilliplasty, plastic surgery of the nipple, 130

mammogram, mammography, X-ray of breasts to detect early cancer, 204

mammoplasty, surgery to reconstruct breasts after radical mastectomy, 130

mandible cranial bone, lower jaw, 141

manometer, apparatus to measure pressure of spinal fluid, 225

Mantoux, TB skin test, 173

Marie-Strümpell disease, chronic, progressive inflammation of the vertebrae with spontaneous fusion causing deformity, 142

Marshall Marchetti, surgical repair of cystocele (stress incontinence), 204

mastitis, breast inflammation, 130

mastoidectomy, excision of mastoid cells, 240

mastoiditis, inflammation of mastoid process, 239

maxilla cranial bone, upper jaw, 141

meatus, passage or opening, 123

mechanical process (digestion), food is broken up and mixed with digestive juices, 182

meconium, first bowel movement passed by newborn, 205

medial, middle, 76

mediastinum, heart lies here, 122

medical conditions/diseases suffixes, 20–21

medical dictionary, 274

medical examiner, performs investigative examinations of bodies to determine cause of death, 35

medical instruments/machines suffixes, 26–28

medical transcriptionist, technician who transcribes medical data, 40

medical words: directional and positional, 77; organ transplant, 86–87; symbols for, 408. *See also* abbreviations; word parts

medications: generic names, 113–114, 384–394; over-the-counter (OTC), 114; trade or brand names, 112–113, 384–394; use of, 384–394

medulla (kidney), inner portion, 195

megalomania, delusions of being someone important, 226

meibomian cyst (chalazion), cyst on eyelid, 234

melanoma, skin cancer, 130

menarche, onset of menses, 206

Ménière's disease, characterized by tinnitus, dizziness, feeling of pressure in ear, 239

meninges, membranes which cover the spinal cord and brain, 218

meningitis, inflammation of meninges due to infection, 222

meningocele (myelomeningocele), hernia of meninges (and cord) to surface of back, 222

meniscectomy, excision of part or whole of meniscus of the knee, 146

meniscus, lateral and medial knee cartilage, 141

menopause, change of life, cessation of menses, 206

menstruation, flow from uterus when conception does not take place/approximately every 28 days, 206

mental status, intellect, orientation as to time and place, disordered thought, 224

metabolic, hypoactive or hyperactive endocrine gland disorders, 123

metabolism (digestion), sum of all physical and chemical changes taking place within the body and cells, 122, 182

metastasizes, cancer which spreads to underlying tissues, 130

micturate, urinate, void, 196

middle ear, from tympanic membrane/lined with mucous membrane, three ears, 239

MI (myocardial infarct, heart attack): clot in a coronary artery, cutting off circulation to the heart muscle, 158; illustration of, 154

miotic (myotic), drug used to contract pupil, 237

miscarriage, spontaneous interruption of pregnancy before fetus is viable, 203

mitral, between left atrium and left ventricle, 153

monilia, moniliasis, yeastlike fungus infection of vaginal area, 203

monocytes, WBCs which perform phagocytosis of invaders, 156

mouth: oral cavity, 179; anatomy and physiology of, 241–242; pathophysiology of, 244

MRI, magnetic resonance imaging, 92

MTBE, chemical name of stone-dissolving medication, 186

mucolytic, type of medication to "dissolve" mucus, 173

multipara, woman who has borne more than one term infant, 205

multiple sclerosis (MS), brain and cord contain areas of degenerated myelin, 222

muscle tissue: contracts/three types, 122, 138; myocardium (heart muscle), 153

muscular dystrophies (MD), motor dysfunction and weakness/ inherited diseases with progressive degeneration of muscle fibers, 144

musculoskeletal system: muscles, bones, and connective tissues, 122, 137–147; illustrations of, 137–139

mutation, any heritable alteration in the genetic material of a living cell or virus, 206

myasthenia gravis, severe fatigability and weakness of muscles, 144

mydriatic, drug that dilates pupil, 237

myelin, white fatty substance that surrounds certain nerve fibers, 225

myelogram, diagnostic X-ray exam of the spinal cord after dye has been introduced into the spinal cavity, 146, 224

myelomeningocele, congenital defect of the spine allowing spinal cord and meninges to protrude on surface of back, 145

myocarditis, inflammation of heart muscle, 159

myocardium, the heart muscle, 153

myopia, nearsightedness, usually corrected with lens, 234

myositis (or myitis), inflammation of muscles, 145

myringitis, inflammation of eardrum due to infection or trauma, 239

myringotomy (tympanotomy), incision into eardrum when eardrum is in danger of rupturing spontaneously, 240

myxedema, obesity, sluggishness, dry puffy skin due to mucous accumulations under skin, 253

N

nails, appendage of skin, 128

narcissistic, grandiose feeling and preoccupation with entitlement, arrogance, and self-importance, 226

nasal cavity, nose/nares/nasal septum divides cavity, 168

nasogastric tube, soft, flexible tube introduced through nose into stomach, 187

naturopath, treats with natural forces or substances, 37

nausea and vomiting, N and V/common symptoms in GI disorders, 184

neonatal period, first 4 weeks of life, 205

neonatology, neonatologist, treats high-risk infants in first six weeks of life, 35, 204–206

neonatorum conjunctivitis, purulent conjunctivitis usually due to GC and passed to newborn in the birth canal, 235

neoplasms: malignancies/abnormal tissue formation, 123, 128; malignant growth in oral cavity, 243

nephrolithiasis (calculus, renal), kidney stones, cause blockage with severe pain, 195

nephrons (kidney), kidney cells and capillaries, 195

nephroptosis, prolapse or downward displacement of kidney, 195

nephrorrhaphy, surgical repair of kidney, 196

nerve block, injection of anesthetic into nerve to produce loss of sensation, 224

nerve tissue, conducts impulses, 122

nervous breakdown, layperson's term for mental illness, 226

nervous system: includes brain, spinal cord, and special senses, 122; abbreviations regarding, 227; anatomy and physiology of, 218–221; illustration of, 219; pathophysiology of the, 221–225

neurasthenia, ill-defined weakness/ weak, tired feeling that rest does not alleviate, 226

neurilemma (sheath of Schwann), membrane enveloping peripheral nerves, 225

neurodermatitis, usually severe itching and excoriation with unknown cause, 132

neurofibromatosis (or von Recklinghausen's disease), hereditary peripheral nerve disorder, 222

neurons, respond to stimuli and specialize in transmitting impulses, 221

neuropathy, any disease of nerves, often observed in diabetes, 255

neuropathy (neuritis), disease of peripheral and cranial nerves, 222

neurosis, having a feeling of extreme anxiety, 226

neutrophils, WBCs which defend the body by means of phagocytosis, 156

nevus(i), mole/discolored, flat or fleshy growth, 130

nocturia, nycturia, getting up during the night to void, 196

nodule, larger raised lesion, 128

nonstriated muscle, smooth, involuntary, 138

normal B/P, pressure up to about 140/90 reading, 157

nosocomial, caused by being in hospital or treatment facility, 124

NPO ("nothing by mouth"), in preparation for tests and before/after surgery, 187

nuclear medicine, makes diagnostic and therapeutic use of radionuclides, 35

nucleus, contains chromosomes, 122

nummular, having shape of coin, 132

nurse midwife, RN with additional training for delivery in uncomplicated births, 40

nurse practitioner (NP), RN with additional training/does examinations and some treatment, 40

nursing unit clerk, assistant to nurses on a nursing unit, 40

nutrients, food/proteins, fats, carbohydrates, plus vitamins and essential minerals, 182

nystagmus, rapid, side-to-side movement of eyeball, 235

O

obesity, overweight/20–30% above normal, 184

OB index, number of pregnancies, term deliveries, abortions, stillborn, 205

oblique, at an angle, 76

obsessive-compulsive, neutralizing or suppressing thoughts, impulses, or actions by engaging in repetitive behaviors, 227

obstetrics-gynecology, concerned with female reproductive tract disorders, prenatal, delivery, postpartum care, 35, 204–206

occipital cranial bones, back of head, 141

occupational therapist (OTR), similar to RPT but accent on fine motor skills, daily living activities, and job skills, 40

oculomotor nerve, movement of eyes, 220

odontalgia, dentalgia, toothache, 244

olecranon, process on the ulnar bone (elbow), 141

olfactory nerve, sense of smell, 220

oliguria, scanty output of urine, 196

oncology, oncologist, uses radiation, surgery, and chemotherapy in treatment of tumors/cancers, 35

oophorectomy, excision of ovary, 204

open heart surgery, coronary artery bypass and other surgical procedures in which heart is exposed, 162

ophthalmology, ophthalmologist, deals with eye diseases, eye surgery and does eye examinations/prescribes glasses, 35, 237

ophthalmometer (ophthalmoscope), instrument for looking into the eye, 237

optician, (not a medical doctor) eye product specialist, 237

optic nerve, transmits images from retina to the brain, 220, 233

optometrist, Doctor of Optometry/treats refractive errors and fits glasses, 37, 237

oral medications (hypoglycemic), medications used by some non-insulin-dependent diabetics, 255

oral mucosa, mucous membranes of mouth including palate, cheek surfaces, tongue, 245

oral surgeon, extractions, especially complicated ones/maxillofacial trauma cases, congenital defects such as cleft palate, 40

orchiectomy, excision of a testicle (castration), 213

orchiopexy, operative transfer of undescended testis into scrotum and suturing it there, 213

orchitis, inflammation of testes, 213

organic brain syndrome (chronic brain syndrome), symptoms of senile variety, 222

organs, made up of more than one kind of tissue, 122

ORIF, open reduction with internal fixation, 146

orifice, entrance of any body cavity, 123

orthodontist, treats malocclusion with braces, retainers, 40

orthopedics, orthopedist, orthopedic surgeon, or orthopod, treats disorders of musculoskeletal system, joint diseases, 35

orthopnea, able to breathe only in sitting position, 173

os, mouth/opening, 123

Osgood-Schlatter disease, osteochondrosis of end of tibia (knee), 145

osteoarthritis, inflammation of a joint in older people, 142

osteochondrosis (and osteochondritis), degenerative changes and chronic inflammation of bone and cartilage, 145

osteogenesis imperfecta, congenital, cause unknown, brittle bones, and fractures, 145

OTC, over-the-counter drugs, 114

otic, pertaining to ear, 240

otitis externa, bacterial, fungal ear canal infection, 239

otitis media, middle ear inflammation, 239

otolaryngologist, medical doctor specialist of ears and larynx, 240

otology, otologist, deals with ear surgery, hearing problems, hearing aids, 35, 240

otoplasty, surgical repair or plastic surgery on the ear, 240

otorhinolaryngology, otorhinolaryngologist, treats ear, nose, and throat disorders and performs surgery, 35

otosclerosis, ankylosis of the stapes causing deafness, 239

otoscope, otoscopy, instrument and procedure for looking into ear, 240

ovaries, female sex glands located in pelvis, 203

P

pacemaker, battery-powered device implanted under skin to regulate heart rate, 162

palate, roof of the mouth, hard and soft portions, 245

pancreas: behind stomach, controls use of sugar and starch, insulin, 179, 251; blood chemistry tests for, 254

pancreatitis, inflammation of the pancreas, 184

papilledema, swelling of the optic nerve (choked disk), 235

papule, small, raised spots, 128

paradental personnel, 41

paralysis, inability to use muscles due to nerve damage, 225

paramedic, ambulance attendant, 40

paramedical personnel, 40

paranasal sinuses, air spaces in cranium connected to nasal cavity, 169, 171

paranoid, having feelings of persecution, 227

parasympathetic, cell bodies originate in craniosacral sections/brings body functions back to normal after stressful situation has ended, 221

parathyroids, behind thyroid, regulates calcium and phosphorus content of blood and bones, 251

parenchyma, essential parts of organ concerned with function, 122, 173

paresis, incomplete or partial paralysis, 225

paresthesia, abnormal sensation, such as numbness and tingling without apparent cause, 225

parietal cranial bones, top of head, 141

Parkinson's disease, usually occurs after age 50/manifested by expressionless face, slow movement, muscular tremors, 223

paronychia, inflammation around a nail, 132

parotid, results when salivary glands near the ear become inflamed, 187

patent, adjective meaning open or not plugged, 123

pathogenic organisms (pathogen): bacteria which cause disease, 59, 69; listed under Latinized names, 277–278

pathologist, diagnoses morbid changes in tissues from biopsy or postmortem, 35, 108

pathology, study of nature and cause of disease, 35, 108, 123

pathophysiology: study of nature and cause of disease, 123, 128–133; of endocrine system, 253–254; of eyes, 233–235; of female reproductive system, 203–204; of the integumentary system, 128–133; of mouth, 244; of the nervous system, 221–225; of the respiratory system, 170–174; of urinary system, 195–197

patients: community resources for, 273, 275–276; illustrated quadrants of, 79; laboratory report (sample) on, 101–106; support groups for, 276

PDR, Physicians' Desk Reference, 112–114

pediatrics, pediatrician, deals with disease prevention, diagnosis, and treatment of children, 35

pediculosis capitis, head lice, 131

pediculosis corporis, body lice, 131

pediculosis pubis, pubic lice or crabs, 131

pedodontist, specializes in treating children, 41

pelvic exam, using speculum to dilate vagina for inspection of cervix and Pap smear, 204

pelvimeter, pelvimetry, instrument to estimate pelvic diameter for delivery, 205

percutaneous excimer laser angioplasty (PELA), uses high-energy "cool" laser to open blocked arteries, 162

percutaneous nephrolithotomy, incision into kidney for removal of kidney stone, 196

percutaneous transhepatic cholangiography (PTC), thin needle is passed through abdomen into the duct network of the liver to insert dye to enhance X-ray, 186

percutaneous transluminal coronary angioplasty (PTCA), alternative to bypass surgery in selected cases/balloon-type catheter exerts pressure on area of plaque opening the blocked area of vessel, 162

perforation, hole in something, 123

perfusion, injecting fluid to thoroughly permeate (blood), 162

perfusion, perfusionist, heart/lung machine, and operator, 86

pericarditis, inflammation of double membranes surrounding the heart, 159

periodontist, treats gums diseases such as gingivitis/performs surgery and deep cleaning, gingivectomy, 41

peripheral, outer edges, 76

peripheral nervous system (PNS), involuntary functions, 218, 220

peripheral vision, vision out to the side, 237

peritoneal cavity, contains stomach, intestines, liver, gallbladder, pancreas, spleen, reproduction organs, and urinary bladder, 122

peritoneum, membrane lining the abdominal cavity, 188

peritonitis, inflammation of the peritoneal cavity, 184

permanent teeth, starting at age 6–7 and total of 32, complete at age 12–13 except for wisdom teeth, 241

pertussis, acute febrile disease (whooping cough) caused by bacterial infection, 171

phacoemulsification, treating cataract by disintegrating it with ultrasound for extraction, 236

pharmacist, Doctor of Pharmacy/licensed to prepare and dispense drugs, 37

pharmacology: PDR and, 112–114; terms related to, 114

pharyngitis, "sore throat"/inflammation of the pharynx, 171

pharynx, throat, 168, 179

pheochromocytoma, tumor of the adremal medulla, producing hypertension, weight loss, personality changes, 254

phlebotomy, incision of vein when venipuncture is unsuccessful, 162

phobia, exaggerated fear, 227

physiatry, physiatrist, deals with physical medicine and rehabilitation, 35

physical therapist (RPT), performs treatments by physical means such as heat, cold, and exercise/accent on gross motor skills, 40

physical therapy abbreviations, 409

physician orders abbreviations, 91–94

physicians: education of, 33–34; related professions listed, 37–38; specialists/specialties of, 34–36

physician's assistant (PA), usually has served internship, may have medical corpsman experience/does examinations, simple suturing, 40

piamater, internal membrane layer of brain, 218

pineal gland, base of brain, produces melatonin, affects body's day/night cycles, 251

pituitary gland, master gland/deep in cranial cavity, 251

PKU, phenylketonuria, a congenital inability to metabolize phenylalanine leading to mental retardation, 184

placebo, inert substance substituted for a drug, 114

placenta, the afterbirth, 205

plaque: sticky mass of microorganisms that grows on crown of tooth and erodes the gums and bone, 244; used to described silvery scales of psoriasis, 128

plasma, liquid part of the blood, minus the cells, 156

platelets, also called thrombocytes (clotting particles), 156

pleura, double mucous membrane that covers the lungs and lines the thoracic cavity, 169

pleural cavity, contains lungs, trachea, esophagus, thymus, 122

pleurisy, fluid discharged by inflamed pleural membranes, 171

plexus, network of nerves or blood vessels, 221, 225

plural endings, 46–47. *See also* word parts

pneumoconiosis, any of the pulmonary disorders caused by irritating dusts, 171

pneumocystis, type of pneumonia developed due to suppression of immune system, 86

pneumocystis carinii, opportunistic pneumonia common in AIDS patients and other immunosuppressed patients, 171

pneumoencephalogram (PEG), picture of brain after air has been injected into subarachnoid space by lumbar puncture, 224

pneumogastric, vagus nerves, controls voice and swallowing, 220

pneumonias, lung inflammation/many causes and types, 171

pneumothorax, introduction into thoracic cavity as therapeutic measure as the result of injury, 173

podiatrist, Doctor of Podiatric Medicine/specialist in care of feet, 38

poliomyelitis, viral infection affecting all areas of the brain, brain stem, and cord, 223

polyposis, condition of having polyps in colon, 184

population affected, factors of age, sex, and race, 273

portacaval shunt, portal vein stitched to inferior vena cava to bypass the obstructed cirrhotic liver, 186

portal circulation, circulation from intestines, stomach, pancreas, and spleen to liver, 155

posterior (dorsal), toward the back, 76

postpartum, six-week period following childbirth, 205

posttraumatic stress disorder (PTSD), recurrent replay of some traumatic event that intrudes via thoughts, images, or dreams, 227

postural drainage, "postures" assumed by the patient to facilitate loosening and expectoration of secretions to improve ventilation, 173

Pott's disease, osteitis of the vertebrae, usually of tuberculous origin, 145

Pott's fracture, fracture of the lower end of the fibula and medialmalleolus of the tibia with dislocation of foot outwards and backwards, 145

PPH, primary pulmonary hypertension/candidate for heart-lung transplant, 86

prefixes: directional and positional, 80–81; listing of, 23–24, 49–51, 54–56; numerical, 83; word part at beginning a word, 3. *See also* word parts

prenatal, before birth, 205

presbycusis, form of nerve deafness in older people, 239

presbyopia, affliction of older-age people/lens loses elasticity, 235

prescription abbreviations, 95

presentation, position infant is in for delivery, 205

pressure-equalizing (PE) tubes, inserted following a myringotomy to promote drainage from and air flow to eustachian tube, 240

preventive dentistry, prophylactic care, 244

primipara, woman who is bearing her first child, 205

proctology, proctologist, treats diseases of the rectum, sigmoid colon, 35

proctoscopy, examining the rectum, sigmoid, with scope, 186

procurement coordinator, person responsible for obtaining donor organ/getting permission, arranging transportation, 86

productive cough, cough that produces sputum, 173

progeny, offspring from a given mating, 206

prognosis, predicted outcome, 273

prolapse of uterus, uterus dropping down into vagina, 203

prominences, processes, projections, 141

prone, pronation, face down, or palm down, 79

prostatectomy, excision of prostate, 213

prostate gland, surrounds urethra/secretes alkaline fluid forming part of semen, 213

prosthodontist, works on dentures, bridgework, artificial appliances, 41

proximal, nearest to center, 76

pruritus, itching, 133

psoriasis, chronic, hereditary dermatosis associated with arthritis, 133

psychiatric medical terms, 226–227

psychiatry, psychiatrist, diagnoses and treats mental disorders, 35

psychological tests, 227

psychologist, Doctor of Philosophy/group and individual counseling and testing, 38

psychoneuroimmunology, psychoneuroimmunologist, explores the relationship between immune system and psychological factors, 35

psychosis, mental illness in which person is out of touch with reality, 227

pterygium surgery, growth of conjunctiva over inner portion of eye, 236

ptyalism, excessive saliva production, 184

public health, administrative medicine, concerned with epidemiology and communicable disease, 36

public health nurse (PHN), has BS degree/works for health departments, schools, or health agencies, 40

pulmonary circulation, starts in right side of heart and returns to left atrium by pulmonary veins, 155

pulmonary function: various tests used to evaluate ventilation, 173, 174; abbreviations used for, 409–410

pulmonary semilunar, between right ventricle and pulmonary artery, 153

pupil, "hole" in the iris/iris regulates size of, 233

pustule, lesion contained pus, 128

pyelitis, inflammation of renal pelvis, 195

pyloric stenosis, congenital condition/outlet of stomach is narrow and will not allow food to pass into duodenum/causing projectile vomiting, 184

pyorrhea, gum disease with pus pocket formation around tooth, 244

pyuria, pus in the urine, 196

Q

quadrants, right and left upper abdomen, 79

R

rachitis, inflammation of the spine, 145

radiologic technologist (RT), takes X-ray films, prepares patient for X-ray films, 40

radiology, radiologist also roentgenology, roentgenologist, uses radiant energy, X-rays, radium, and cobalt in diagnosis/ treatment, 36

radius, forearm, 138

rales, rhonchi, sounds in the chest indicating pathology, 173

rarefaction, term used to describe decreased density in X-ray films, 173

reconstructive knee surgery, arthroscopic surgery to replace torn ligaments, 146

records technician (MRT), collects, files, organizes, and retrieves medical data, 40

rectocele, hernia of rectum, 184

rectum, large intestine, 179

recumbent, lying down, 76

red blood cells (RBCs), contain hemoglobin and carry oxygen to the cells and carbon dioxide away from cells, 156

reflex, involuntary response to stimulus, 225

refractive errors, vision disorders that are correctable with lenses, 237

registered nurse (RN), graduate nurse/may work in hospitals, clinics, or offices/often has BSN, 40

registered physical therapist (RPT), performs treatments by physical means such as heat, cold, and exercise/accent on gross motor skills, 40

renal failure, due to trauma or any condition that impairs flow of blood to kidneys, 195

renal pelvis, wide, upper end of the ureter, 195

renal transplant, transplanting donor kidney to recipient, 196

replantation, reattaching a severed body part, 146

residual air, air remaining in lungs after expiration, 173

respiration, breathing, consists of inspiration and expiration, 168

respirators (ventilators), mechanical assistance in breathing, 174

respiratory system: lungs and airways, 122; abbreviations used for, 174; anatomy and physiology of, 168–170; pathophysiology of the, 170–174

respiratory therapist or pulmonary therapist (ARRT), treats patients with breathing difficulties/uses machines to facilitate breathing/teaches breathing exercises/conducts postural drainage and nebulizer treatments, 40

restorative dentistry, fillings, bonding, inlays, crowns, bridgework, caps, dentures, cosmetic measures, 244

reticulocyte, immature red blood cell, in bone marrow, 156

retina: innermost layer of the eye, receives images formed by lens, 233; detached, 234, 235

retinitis, chronic progressive degeneration of retina, 235

retinoblastoma, malignant glioma of retina, 235

retinopathies, any disorder of retina, 235

retrieve, taking an organ, 86

retrograde pyelogram, introduction of dye through urethra for X-ray examination of renal pelvis, 197

Reye's syndrome, acute encephalopathy following viral infection, 223

rheumatic heart disease, form of myocarditis with mitral valve insufficiency/occurs as a sequela to rheumatic fever, 159

rheumatism, general term for soreness and stiffness of joint, tendons, muscles, bones, 145

rheumatoid arthritis, severe inflammation of joint, 142

Rh factor, acts like a foreign substance to anyone negative for it, mother's blood may produce antibodies against baby's blood unless RhoGAM is given to prevent Rh antibodies from forming, 157

rhinitis, rhinorrhea, inflammation of nose/"runny nose" or "common cold" due to virus or allergy, 171

rhinoplasty, plastic surgery on nose, 174

rhizotomy, cutting roots of spinal nerves to relieve incurable pain, 224

rhytidectomy, face lift, 133

rickets, juvenile osteomalacia, 145

rods, light-sensitive nerve cells that work in dim light and provide black-and-white images, 233

Romberg test, checking balance by having person touch tip of nose with index finger with eyes closed, 224

root (tooth), portion embedded in socket of jawbones, 241

root words: compound words from, 4; listing of, 8, 11–12, 63–65. See *also* word parts

rotation (version), turning, 79

rotoblator, burrowing instrument used for endarterectomy, 162

routes of administration abbreviations, 95

routine immunizations abbreviations, 93

RSV or RS virus, respiratory syncytial virus type of myxovirus that causes formation of giant cells or syncytia, 171

rubber dam, used by some dentists to cover everything but the tooth being worked on, 245

rubella, three-day or German measles, 131

rubeola, regular or hard measles, 131

Rx, prescription symbol meaning recipe or take, 114

S

sagittal, vertical body plane, 76

salivary glands, three pairs/parotid, sublingual, and submandibular, 179

salpingectomy, excision of fallopian tube, 204

salpingitis, inflammation of fallopian tube, 203

sarcoma (osteogenic), malignant bone tumor, 145

scabies, small parasite called a mite, 131

scales, flaking type of lesions, 128

scans: using a special device (CT or CAT) to produce a picture of any organ, 92, 186, 224; brain, 223; lung, 174; renal, 197

scapula, shoulder blade, 138

scar, mark left by healing of wound, 128

schizophrenia, major mental illness usually affecting young people, delusions, hallucinations, incoherent speech, 227

sciatica, severe pain in leg along course of sciatic nerve, 223

sclera, outer covering of eye, 233

scoliosis, lateral curve of the spine, 145

seminal duct, excretory duct of the seminal vesicle, 213

septum, wall that divides the right and left sides of the heart, 153

serum, plasma minus the fibrinogen that promotes clotting, 156

sex glands (gonads), ovaries secrete estrogens and progesterone, testes secrete testosterone, 251

sexually transmitted diseases (STDs), 214–216

shock, inadequate amount of circulating blood, 159

shunts, types of bypass, via catheter, for drainage of CSF, 224

sialolith, stone in salivary duct, 184

sigmoid colon, large intestine, 179

sign language, use of hands to communicate, 240

signs and symptoms, subjective and objective/part of diagnosis, 273

Simmonds' disease, atrophy of the pituitary, causes exhaustion, emaciation, cachexia, 254

Sims' position, lying on left side, right leg slightly forward, knees flexed, 80

sinistro, to the left, 79

sinoatrial node (SA node), pacemaker for right atrium, 153

sinuses: air spaces in cranium which lighten the skull, 141; lavage (washing out of), 173; paranasal, 169, 171

sinusitis: inflammation of paranasal sinuses, 171; illustration of CAT scan for, 172

sinus rhythm, normal cardiac rhythm initiated by SA node, 162

Sjögren's syndrome, autoimmune disorder, progressive type of collagen disease that occurs post menopause, 145

skin, integument or external covering, 128

SLE (lupus erythematosus, systemic), collagen disease affecting connective tissues, 142

slit lamp examination, microscope that illuminates and magnifies structures within the eye, 236

Snellen eye chart, with letters, or "illiterate E," chart for vision screening, 237

sonograms, a record of ultrasonic echoes as they locate tissues of varying densities, 205; illustration, 205

spastic, having forceful uncontrollable contractions, 225

spermicide, sperm-killing agent, 206

sphenoid cranial bones, behind eyes, 141

sphygmomanometer, B/P cuff (mercury and aneroid types), 157

spina bifida, congenital defect of the spine, 145, 223

spinal cavity, contains spinal cord, 122

spinal column (illustrated), 140

spinal cord: lies inside the spinal column, 218; illustrations of, 144, 220; testing of, 225

spinal cord injuries, three types: compression, transection, or contusion, 223

spinal nerves, thirty-one pairs attached to spinal cord, 220

spinal tap, lumbar puncture, insertion of needle into subarachnoid space to measure pressure, 224

spirometer, spirometry, instrument and its use in pulmonary function tests, 174

spleen, largest lymphatic organ of the body, 156

spondylitis (ankylosing spondylitis), chronic, progressive inflammation of the vertebrae with spontaneous fusion causing deformity, 142

spondylosyndesis, spinal fusion via surgical formation of ankylosis, 146

sports medicine, concerned with injuries peculiar to sports activities, 36

sputum, secretions from bronchi, not saliva, 174

stapedectomy, excision of stapes to restore hearing, 240

steatoma, a sebaceous cyst or fatty tumor, 130

stent, metallic support mounted on balloon catheter and passed into artery, 162

sterility, inability to conceive, 205

sternotomy, incision for heart and heart-lung transplant, 86, 162

sternum, breastbone, 138

stillborn, fetus dead at birth, 205

stimulus, anything that brings about a response, 225

stoma, artificial opening established by colostomy, ileostomy, and tracheostomy, 123, 188

stomach, has cardiac sphincter at entrance, pyloric sphincter at exit, 179

stomach stapling, staples across stomach to allow only small amount of food to be eaten, 186

stomatitis, canker sores, sores in mouth, 184

stool specimen, sent to laboratory for occult blood (guaiac) or for parasites, 186

strabismus, misaligned (or squinted) eyes/any deviation from normal, 235

street drugs, illegal drugs sold "on the street" to users and addicts, 114

streptococcal sore throat, "strep throat"/communicable, may be asymptomatic, 171

stress: forces that disrupt equilibrium or produce strain in amounts that the system cannot handle, 227; illustration of adrenal gland and, 256

stress ECG, electrocardiogram taken while patient is on treadmill, 162 stressor, pressure, force, or strain on system, 256

stress response, how a body responds to stressors, 256

striated muscle, striped, voluntary, skeletal, 138

stroke, cerebrovascular accident (CVA), 159

stroma, type of connective tissue supporting organs, 122

stye (hordeolum), inflammation of sebaceous gland of eyelid, 235

subcutaneous, "under the skin"/contains adipose and connective tissue, vessels, and nerves, 128

suction, device to keep mouth area dry of saliva during procedures, 245

suffixes: group of letters at end of word that alters word's meaning, 4; "ectomy," 5, 6; listed, 58–59; for medical conditions/diseases, 20–21; for medical instruments/machines, 26–28; "ol ogy," 33–36; for surgical procedures, 15–16

sulcus, in dentistry, gum area between teeth, 245

sulcus, sulci, deep furrow in the brain, 225

superfluous hair, excessive hair on face of women, 133

superior, above, 76

supine, supination, face up, or palm up, 79

support groups, 276

surgery, surgeon, performs general surgery, 36

surgical procedures suffixes: ectomy, 5, 6; listed, 15–16

sutures, articulations in the cranial bones, 141

Swan-Ganz catheter, pulmonary-artery balloon catheter/used to measure pressures within the heart, 162

symbols (medical), 408

sympathetic, cell bodies originate in thoracolumbar sections T-1 to L-2, 221

syncope, fainting, loss of consciousness, 225

synovectomy, excision of synovial membrane, 146

synovial fluid, clear joint fluid that acts as lubricant, 141

syphilis, chronic venereal disease with cutaneous lesions, 132, 215

systemic circulation, from the left atrium, blood flows to left ventri-cle and is pumped out through aortic valve to aorta and to entire body, 155

systems, groups of organs working together, 122

systolic pressure, top number in B/P reading, 157

T

tachycardia, rapid heart rate, 162

tachypnea, rapid breathing, 174

talipes, any of a number of deformities of the foot, 145

target organ, any organ affected by stress, 256

teeth: incisors/cuspids or canines/bicuspids or premolars/molars, 179, 241–242; anatomy and physiology of, 241–242; illustration of, 242; surfaces of, 241–242

temporal cranial bones, temples, 141

temporomandibular joint (TMJ), connecting point of lower jawbone and temporal bone, 141

10/10 vision, not perfect vision, means a child can see at 10 feet, screening term, 237

tendinitis (tendonitis), inflammation of a tendon, 145

tendon, fibrous tissue attaching muscle to bone, 141

testes (testis), male sex glands located in scrotum, 213

"test-tube baby" (in vitro fertilization), ovaries are stimulated to produce multiple eggs which are retrieved, mixed with sperm in Petri dish where fertilization occurs, 206

tetanus (lockjaw), caused by toxin produced by anaerobic organism in puncture-type wound, 223

tetany, severe muscle and nerve weakness causing spasm, twitching, convulsions, 254

theca, covering or sheath of tendon, 141

theleplasty, plastic surgery of the nipple, 130

thoracentesis (or thoracocentesis), "tapping" of chest to remove fluid, 174

thoracic outlet syndrome, brachial neuritis with or without vasomotor disturbance in upper extremities, 145

thoracoplasty, multiple rib resection to collapse diseased area of lung, 174

thorax, lungs, heart, 92

thrombophlebitis, inflammation in a vein with clot formation, 159

thrombus, blood clot in a vessel, 159

thymus, pleural cavity, decreases in size in adult, 251

thyroid function studies, blood chemistry tests for thyroid, 254

thyroid gland, aside of in front of larynx, alters metabolic rate and secretes thyroxine, 251

tibia, lower leg, 138

tinea, ringworm, 131

tinea barbae, beard ringworm, 131

tinea capitis, scalp ringworm, 131

tinea corporis, body ringworm, 131

tinea cruris, groin ringworm/ "jock itch," 131

tinea pedis, foot ringworm/athlete's foot, 131

tinea unguium, nail ringworm, 131

Tine test, TB test, 174

tinnitus, "ringing" and other sounds in the ear, 240

tissues, groups of cells that are alike, 122

TMJ (temporomandibular joint disorder), bones of temple and jaw malaligned, 244

toileting abbreviations, 91

tolerance, capacity for ingesting an increasing amount without effect, 114

tongue, muscular organ/covered with mucous membrane/taste buds are present on surface of papillae, 179

tonic, muscular tension, 145

tonometry (tonometer), instrument for measuring pressure within eyeball to diagnose glaucoma before it destroys vision, 236

tonsillitis, highly communicable, inflammation of tonsils with "crypts" of pus formation, 171

tonsils, part of the lymphatic system, 169

total hip replacement, hip joint replaced using prosthetic devices for head of femur and the ace tabulum, 146

Tourette's syndrome, genetic disorder characterized by uncontrolled blinking, facial twitching/tics, and/or obscenity spoken, 223

toxemia, during pregnancy/ characterized by hypertension, edema, weight gain/a serious complication, 206

trabeculectomy, excision of fibrous bands, 236

trachea, windpipe, 168

tracheostomy, new permanent opening into trachea, 174

tracheotomy, incision into trachea when airway is obstructed, 174

trachoma, chronic infection of conjunctiva and cornea, 235

traction, process of drawing or pulling, 146

transient ischemic attack (TIA), brief period of inadequate blood supply to brain, sometimes called "small strokes," 159, 223

transplant: donor heart, 162; heart-lung, 174; liver, 186; renal, 196

transverse, horizontal body plane, 76

transverse colon, large intestine, 179

trauma, ear, occurs as result of a blow to the head or inserted objects, 239

traumatic (trauma), accidental injuries/any physical or emotional injury, 34, 123

treatment, general kinds of treatment available, 273

Trendelenburg position, lying on back, face up, body straight on bed tilted at 45 degrees with head low, 80

trephination, drilling hole in skull of evacuate clots or inject air for diagnostic procedure, 224

trichomonas, trichomoniasis, parasite-caused vaginitis, 203, 215

tricuspid, between right atrium and right ventricle, 153

trigeminal nerve, facial movements, 220

trimester, three-month period in pregnancy, 206

triple coronary artery bypass graft (illustration), 159

trochlear nerve, muscle of eyes, 220

TSS (toxic shock syndrome), produced by "blood poisoning" due to staphylococcus toxin, 203

tubal ligation, "tying" fallopian tubes/sterilization, 204

tubal occlusion, with silicone/ reversible, 204

tuberculosis (TB), infectious bacterial disease that produces "ubercles" in the lung, 171

tuberosities, projections, 141

tumors, malignancies/abnormal tissue formation, 123, 128, 223

tuning fork, forklike steel instrument used in testing hearing, 240

turbinates, cone-shaped nasal bones, 141

20/20 vision, not perfect vision, means person can see at 20 feet, not nearsighted, 237

tympanic membrane (eardrum or myringa), separates middle ear from external ear, 239

tympanoplasty, plastic surgery on eardrum using skin graft to refashion a tympanic membrane, 240

tympanotomy (myringotomy), incision into eardrum when eardrum is in danger of rupturing spontaneously, 240

type and crossmatch (x-match), done to determine compatibility before a transfusion is given, 156

U

ulcers: tissue destruction/deep lesion extending into subcutaneous tissue, 128; corneal, 234; gastric, 183

ulna, forearm, 138

ultrasonography, using ultrasound method to obtain a picture of any organ, 93, 186, 197

ultrasound test, uses sound waves to explore structures in eye, 236

upright, standing, 76

uremia (azotemia), toxic condition/nitrogenous wastes not being excreted, 195

ureterostomy, new opening for drainage of ureter, 197

ureters, two narrow tubes lined with mucous membrane, 195

urethra, in female, one narrow short tube from bladder to exterior/in male, narrow long tube, 195, 213

urethritis, inflammation of urethra/often spread through sexual contact, 195

urinary bladder, lined with mucous membrane, urine collects there, 195

urinary meatus, opening of the urethra to exterior, 195

urinary retention, inability to void, 197

urinary system: abbreviations pertaining to, 197–198; anatomy and physiology of, 194–195; illustration of normal, 194; pathophysiology of, 195–197

URI (upper respiratory infection), general term for colds or what people call the "flu," 171

urology, urologist, treats urinary tract diseases/male reproductive organs, 36

ursodiol, stone-dissolving drug, 187

urticaria, hives, 133

USP, United States Pharmacopeia, 114

uterus, top part called the tundus/ neck opens into the vagina, 203

uveitis, inflammation of iris and blood vessels, 235

uvula, muscle tissue that hangs down from the soft palate/guards the opening from nasal cavity, preventing food from entering, 170

V

vagina, birth canal, 203

vaginal speculum (pelvic exam), using speculum to dilate vagina for inspection of cervix and Pap smear, 204

vagotomy: cutting vagus nerve as treatment for peptic ulcer, 224; cutting vagus nerve/used to treat ulcers or to prevent pain in terminal pregnancy, 187

"valley fever" (coccidioidomycosis), caused by fungus that lies dormant in spore form in hot, dusty climates, 170

valves, keep blood from backflowing, 153

valvulotomy, valvuloplasty, surgical procedures to repair or replace heart valves, 162

varicella, chickenpox, 132

varicocele, varicose veins near testes, 213

varicose veins, dilated veins caused by defective valves/also called varices, 159

vascular, occlusion or rupture of vessels, 124

vas deferens (ducts), ductus deferens, excretory duct of the testis, 213

vasectomy, male sterilization procedure, 213

vasoconstriction, narrowing of vessels, 123

vasodilator, agent that causes dilatation, 162

vasopressor, agent that causes constriction, 162

vasovasostomy, vasectomy reversal, 213

veins, always carry blood toward the heart, 154

vena cava, largest heart vein, 154

venereal warts, 215

venipuncture, puncturing a vein for any purpose, 162

ventilators (respirators), mechanical assistance in breathing, 174

ventricle (brain), cavity in the brain, 225

ventriculography, injection of air directly into ventricles when PEG cannot be done, 224

vernix caseosa, cheesy white substance on skin of newborn, 206

verruca, wart, 131

verruca(ae), wart or epithelial tumor, 130

vertebral column, starting at neck, 138

vertigo, sensation of whirling motion, dizziness, 240

vesicle, lesion containing fluid, 128

vesico, combining word part meaning "bladder," 197

viable, capable of survival/standard for premature infants, 206

viruses, 278

visual field testing, test for peripheral vision, 236

vital capacity, amount of air that can be forcibly expelled from lungs after deep inspiration (pulmonary function test), 174

vitiligo, loss of pigment, 133

vitrectomy, aspiration of vitreous fluid and replacement with saline solution or vitreous to clear opaque vitreous, 236

vitreous humor, jellylike transparent substance inside eyeball, 233

void, to empty (bladder), 197

W

wheal, elevation or "bleb" produced by injection or skin test, 128

"whiplash," imprecise term for injury to cervical vertebrae and adjacent soft tissues, 223

white blood cells (WBCs), five types, help destroy foreign material and bacteria, 156

Wilms' tumor, nephroblastoma, malignant tumor in children, 195

word parts: introduction to, 3–4; plural endings, 46–47; prefixes, 3, 23–24, 49–51, 54–56, 80–81, 83; suffixes, 4, 6, 15–16, 20–21, 26–28, 33–36, 58–59. *See also* medical words; root words

X

xenograft, organ from an animal for transplant, 86

xerostomia, dry mouth, common in many disease conditions, 184, 244

X-ray examination, routine, of chest/AP and lat, 174

X-ray, laboratory abbreviations, 92

Y

Yag laser, to make small opening in membrane during extracapsular cataract surgery, 237

Z

zygote intrafallopian transfer (ZIFT), eggs are retrieved, fertilized by sperm in Petri dish, and embryos are placed in fallopian tubes, 207

zygotes, cell resulting from union of male/female gametes, 206

NOTES

NOTES